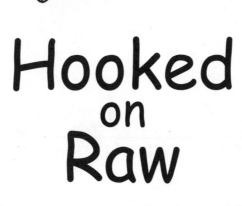

Hooked
on
Raw

Rejuvenate Your Body and Soul
with Nature's Living Foods

by *Rhio*

Illustrations by Gary Bell

Photographs by Steve Ladner

Graphic Design by Pauline Wolstencroft

Food Styling by Rhio

Book Publishing Company
Summertown, TN

Fourth Edition

Copyright © 2000 by
Beso Entertainment/Alternative Media, Inc.

Published in the United States by
Book Publishing Company
PO Box 99
Summertown, TN 38483
888-260-8458
www.bookpubco.com

Printed in the U.S.

ISBN: 987-1-57067-250-7

DISCLAIMER

This book presents information gleaned from personal experiences, along with research and nutritional information regarding the use of plant foods in harmony with Nature's laws for healing and rejuvenation. The information contained herein is not intended as a diagnosis, cure, or treatment for any disease or ailment or to be used as a prescription by the reader. The author and publisher are not offering or dispensing medical advice. Use the information in this book only if you are willing to accept the sole responsibility for choosing and deciding your own diet and lifestyle. Since every individual's health condition and circumstances are unique, the author and publisher advise that you seek the services of a qualified healthcare professional before using any information offered in this book.

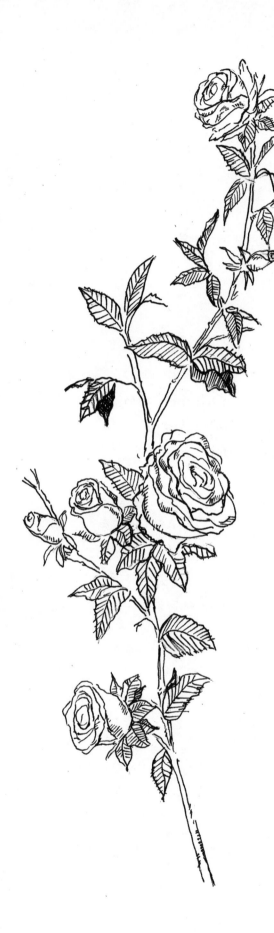

I gratefully dedicate this book to all those who came before me; to those who discovered the incredible value of the raw food diet and were kind enough to write about it so that I, in my time, could discover it also. I thank them and honor them for their tenacity and perseverance in the face of monumental opposition to these ideas.

Other Creations by Rhio

DVD: What's Not Cookin' In Rhio's Kitchen - Vol. I
Music CD: Time to Start Believin' Again
Latin Music CD: Sigue Adelante

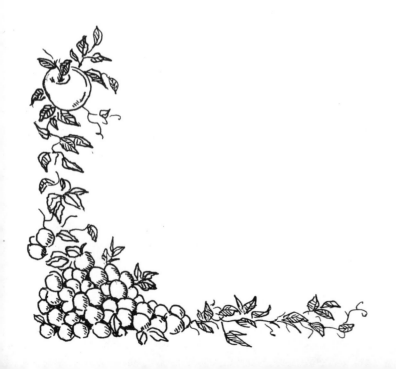

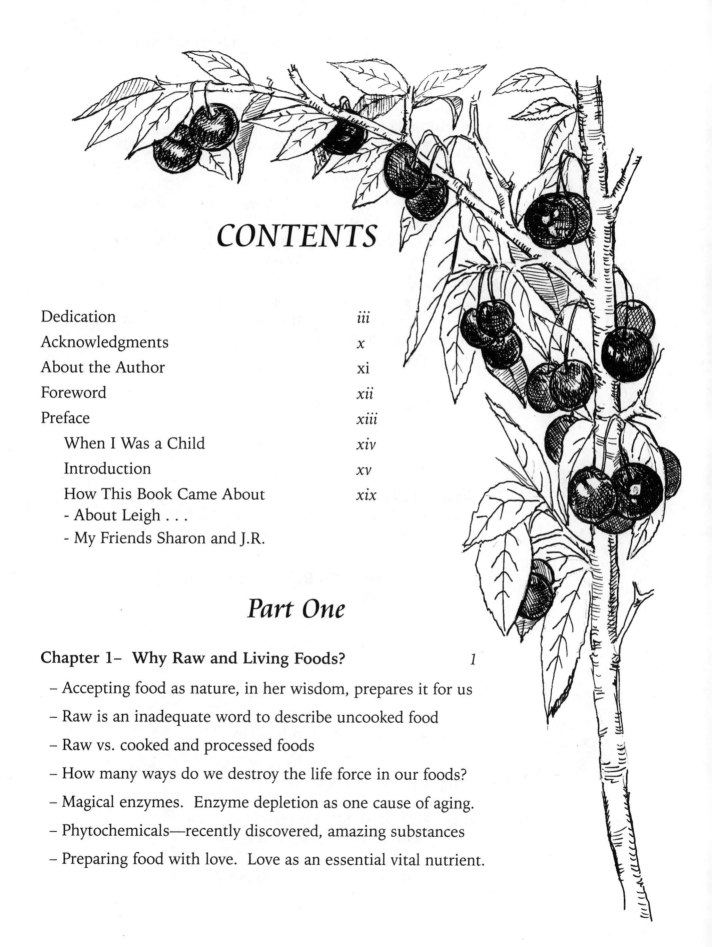

CONTENTS

Part One

  – Accepting food as nature, in her wisdom, prepares it for us

  – Raw is an inadequate word to describe uncooked food

  – Raw vs. cooked and processed foods

  – How many ways do we destroy the life force in our foods?

  – Magical enzymes. Enzyme depletion as one cause of aging.

  – Phytochemicals—recently discovered, amazing substances

  – Preparing food with love. Love as an essential vital nutrient.

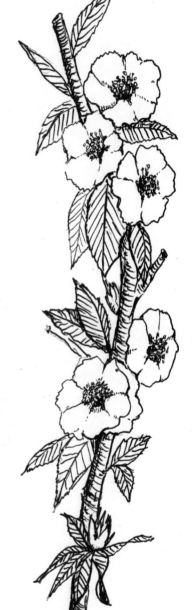

Part Two

Part Three
The Recipes

ACKNOWLEDGMENTS

First, I want to thank Leigh Crizoe for his obstinacy, his occasional not-so-gentle challenging of certain ideas, his finicky palate and his almost impossible to please standards, because these things spurred me on to greater culinary successes, and helped to make the ideas expressed in this book clearer. I am also grateful to Leigh for his ever present support and understanding, his asking every once in a while "Is the book finished yet?" and his nurturing patience when I replied "almost, almost," as yet more pages were added. I appreciated his input even when I didn't use the suggestions, but he did come up with some pretty good recipes.

The most heartfelt thanks to Shaune V., for his loyalty to my dreams and for his enthusiasm for this book.

Next I am very grateful to Arthur Goldberg, my editor, because he made the text so much better and clearer than it was originally, without destroying or overriding my characteristic "childlike" (in his words) style of writing. I gained an awesome respect for the work that editors do through working with him, and it was also a lot of fun being challenged by someone who had no knowledge of the raw/live foods lifestyle when we started. He was very gracious even when I rejected some of his "highfalutin" revisions and insisted on saying the same thing in "just plain talk." Five months into the project, Arthur called me and said that he wanted me to know that, intellectually, he had come to accept as valid the reasoning behind the raw food lifestyle. By the end of the project, Arthur was sprouting, experimenting with recipes and adding more raw and living foods into his diet. This was a great compliment to my powers of persuasion, I thought, until Arthur told me, "You know, Rhio, no one is going to read and reread your book as much as I have done while editing it." Oh, well, I've been cut down to size!

Warmest gratitude and much, much appreciation goes to Gary Bell for his beautiful illustrations which greatly enhance the recipes and other sections; to Steve Ladner for his striking photographs and to Pauline Wolstencroft for her artful graphic design.

Sherry Crespin was wonderful for testing a majority of the recipes, for giving me her valuable input and for generally improving the clarity of the instructions. I regret losing her when she moved to Geneva. I also thank Felicia Watkis and Sybil Walker for their suggestions.

A special thanks to Leola Brooks and Lalita Salas of the Ann Wigmore Institute in Puerto Rico. Thank you for teaching me, gently challenging me and supporting me, even though our ideas did not always coincide. And thank you both for carrying on the work of Dr. Ann Wigmore by providing such a wonderful oasis where people can go to rest, recuperate and rejuvenate.

David Wolfe (author of *The Sunfood Diet Success System*) gave me some valuable advice when he suggested I let as many people as possible read the manuscript in order to obtain their comments before, rather than after publication, when it would be too late to change anything. Thank you David.

Thanks to Dr. Martin Teitle, of the Council for Responsible Genetics in Massachusetts, for reviewing my chapter on genetic engineering for accuracy.

Joan Zaccharias helped immeasurably with the book's punctuation and other editorial suggestions.

Finally, thanks to all those who had enough faith (and patience) to advance order this book, thereby providing the funds that allowed me to pay for editing, illustrations, photographs, typesetting and ultimately printing.

ABOUT THE AUTHOR

Rhio is a singer and author, as well as an investigative reporter in the area of health and environmental issues. Rhio is of Hungarian-Cuban descent, raised in the U.S., but completely fluent in Spanish.

CNN and American Journal aired stories on raw foods featuring Rhio. She is considered an expert in the area of raw and living foods and lectures on both the raw/live food lifestyle and the genetic engineering of seeds/plants.

As a singer, Rhio has appeared on numerous TV shows. 2010 saw the completion of her third CD album entitled *Time to Start Believin' Again*, which tackles environmental issues and includes some humorous raw food songs. For more information on Rhio's music projects, visit: www.rhiosmusic.com

Rhio hosts an internet radio show called *Hooked on Raw* which can be heard worldwide at: www.NYTalkRadio.net and on her website.

Rhio's Raw Energy website: www.rawfoodinfo.com also provides extensive information on the raw/live food lifestyle, as well as organic agriculture, environmental, human rights, civil rights, globalization and economic justice issues.

On the horizon: Rhio's video series on raw food preparation entitled *What's Not Cookin' in Rhio's Kitchen - Volumes 2 & 3* are set for release in Fall 2010.

Rhio and her partner Leigh, are also fledgling permaculture, biodynamic, eco-farmers in Upstate New York with a focus on growing edible wild foods, heirloom vegetables, leafy greens and lettuces, fruit, berries and nuts.

FOREWORD

As a writer in the field of health, I am always glad to welcome a comprehensive book on "Raw and Living Foods." Rhio's book delivers a most timely and much needed message. It shows us how we can move towards a raw/live food lifestyle, and how to incorporate more of these foods into our diet. Rhio has created hundreds of delicious recipes to excite any palate. They include everything from easy-to-prepare main courses to the most exotic desserts.

Hooked on Raw is a can't-go-wrong approach to getting in tune with your body and with nature. The book gives you a blueprint for helping yourself and others. Today, most of us have friends who have just come home from the hospital, where they have been fed only foodless foods, sugar shakes and gelatin. Rhio has an endless supply of power food recipes which can be an important part of taking charge of your own health. When you start to incorporate more of these foods into your diet you'll be giving your body **Nature's own tools** to heal and rebuild.

We are living in an age in which the public has been conditioned to expect instant solutions to complex problems. People are repeatedly exposed to slick TV ads that hypnotize them into purchasing so-called magic pills, which generally suppress symptoms, but do not solve the real problems. In many cases, the side effects of these drugs cause more harm than good. The drug companies have been allowed to come right into our homes to push prescription drugs that are only available from your doctor. Many of these advertisements don't even tell you what the drug is for, or what it really does. People are instructed to ask their doctors about these glorified drugs. The ads may rattle off a list of side effects that can take up a substantial part of the commercial. The spokespeople, however, through their demeanor and vocal inflections, as well as the scenery and background sounds of the commercial, give you the impression that they are selling something as pleasant as ice cream!

As the graying of America creates serious new challenges for an already ailing health care system, *Hooked on Raw* offers new insight into taking charge of your body, mind and spirit to maintain optimum health in a world of synthetic foods and overwhelming pollution.

We receive constant reminders that Western medicine does not have all the answers, and many billions of dollars have been spent to find cures for problems like cancer and heart disease. People are now ready to go back to basics, and with a little effort and planning, let Nature do what it does best—KEEP US HEALTHY.

Harvey Diamond

PREFACE

This book will become a necessity for every family in this country if the American diet, and the practices of the conventional medical community, continue on their present course. The powers that be are so afraid that the relationship between our food supply and illness will be exposed, that unconstitutional laws have been passed to stop concerned citizens from speaking out. Food Disparagement Laws, aka "Veggie Libel Laws," are now on the books in 13 states. A mega-star, Oprah Winfrey, was sued for over $20 million for voicing her concerns, on television, about eating meat. She was acquitted of all charges. The cost of fighting a case of this magnitude however, would break the back of others who lack Oprah's financial backing, and thus effectively shut them up. And this is exactly what these "Food Disparagement Laws," backed by industry, are designed to do.

HMOs are in the news daily, with horror stories of people who were denied proper care. The rates of health insurance are at an all-time high and getting higher by the minute. Big corporations are downsizing to eliminate medical benefit programs promised to their employees. Untold numbers of people are already out in the street, with no medical insurance at all.

This book is a guide for taking charge of your own health and well-being. I know I will practice the ideas outlined in this book in my own life, rather than face the alternatives. I was the willing guinea pig for the majority of recipes given here, which were developed by Rhio over a four-year period. And I was a hard guy to please. A lot of food was dumped into the compost before the best of the best recipes were put into this wonderful book, written with Rhio's love for humanity and concern that people should live to a ripe old age with their God-given ability to be healthy, vibrant and productive, and without having to "fight" disease.

Rhio speaks in plain language and guides you to an opportunity to make the choice to experience life to the fullest.

Leigh Crizoe

WHEN I WAS A CHILD . . .

When I was a child my father brought two very large turtles (tortoises) from Mexico to our home in Los Angeles. My sister and I played with those turtles for months. They became our friends. One day they disappeared and we never saw them again. I don't remember what daddy told us, but soon we had a lot of "chicken" to eat. Sometime later it dawned on me that the "chicken" was our friends, the turtles. That may have been the moment when the concept of vegetarianism was born in my heart. It just lay there until I grew up and then, first chance I got, I converted.

INTRODUCTION

Hi, my name is Rhio and I want to introduce you to a way of eating and a lifestyle to which I have become hopelessly addicted. Because of all the negative "addictions" existing in our society today, we have come to believe that every addiction is destructive. However, the older dictionary meaning of addiction is "a habitual inclination." The bad connotation comes about only because the older, broader definition is no longer in use.[1]

An addiction then, in the older sense, is not necessarily an undesirable thing; it all depends on **what** one is addicted to. Allowing yourself to become addicted (habitually inclined) to eating in a healthy way is a good thing; just as it's a good thing to be habitually loving, or friendly or patient or kind.

Yes, I am hopelessly HOOKED ON RAW, because of all the wonderful benefits I derive from it. What do I mean by Raw? I'm talking about eating food in its prime, primary and natural state, as nature provides it for us; **uncooked**, and **unheated**.

It all started with . . .

The first job I ever had, as a teen, was in a health food store. It wasn't a job that I was specifically looking for that summer; but after putting in many applications, it was just the one that came through first. Once they hired me, I was put to work at the juice bar making all kinds of fresh juices, shakes and blended drinks. It was my first introduction to "natural foods," and it fascinated me. I don't think I even took home any money that summer; I just left it all there because I bought so many books.

As I began to educate myself, I went through many phases. First I became a lacto-ovo vegetarian (one who eats dairy, but no meat). Then I let the dairy go, becoming mostly vegan. Next, I checked out macrobiotics and other ways of eating. Though I was introduced to the concept of eating raw foods early, it took me a while to come back to it. When I finally embraced it, I knew that for me, it was the way to go.

Every time I ate this way, I had loads of energy and felt great. The idea that the Creator has provided us with the very best food and that there wasn't anything we "had to do" to it to make it "better" also made a lot of sense to me. In addition, the books and studies I read on the subject proved very convincing. I will share some of this with you later.

---

[1] The dictionary definition of the word "addiction" has changed with the times. Now it's defined as "the state of being enslaved to a habit or practice or to something that is psychologically or physically habit forming . . . to such an extent that its cessation causes severe trauma." (Random House Compact Unabridged Dictionary, 1996.)

It has been my experience that most people who come to this way of eating do so because they have some illness that the allopathic[2] doctors have given up on. They have been told they have to learn to live with the illness, or, if things are critical, to go home and get their affairs in order. Before I became a raw food enthusiast, I had a very traumatic experience and, as a result of overstressed nerves and emotional overeating, gained 88 extra pounds. On my 5 foot frame, this was devastating. It could have turned into a serious health problem, had I not regained control. I lost all the extra weight by raw-juice fasting and exercise. Through this experience I became much more aware of the *power* of raw foods; it just made good sense for me to continue to eat this way to stay well.

I wanted to learn all I could about eating raw and live food, so I went to several institutes offering programs that teach people how to adopt the lifestyle. One of them was the Optimum Health Institute of San Diego, a comfortable and affordable facility, whose driving force and founder was Raychel Solomon. I signed up here for two weeks and stayed for six. I then returned a couple of weeks later with my mom in tow.

I also went several times to the Ann Wigmore Institute in Aguada, Puerto Rico. In a beautiful tropical setting fanned by ocean breezes, I was transported to an atmosphere of utter simplicity, conducive to leaving worry, fear and doubt behind. This institute encouraged me to find the healing power within, while reconnecting with nature and with my own body. The staff here inspired me to develop my intuition so that I increasingly recognize what my unique body needs really are. The Ann Wigmore Institute provides an excellent program with a caring and loving staff.

I then visited the Centro Naturista Daniel Areola, a clinic in El Grullo, Mexico, where components of the raw food program are provided.[3] Mexico does not have the restrictions we have here in the United States, so in Mexico these programs not only teach you how to care for yourself to keep healthy and well, but they also provide services not readily obtained in the US.

I stayed, as well, at the Hippocrates Health Institute in West Palm Beach, Florida. Hippocrates was founded by Dr. Ann Wigmore in Boston. Many years later, it was acquired by Brian Clement and moved to Florida. Ann Wigmore remained in Boston and started a new institute named after herself.

Hippocrates offers one of the most advanced diagnostic programs available, including live blood analysis to monitor the changes in your own blood picture. They do an analysis when you first come in, then again before you leave. On a video

---

[2]The allopathic system of medical care is the one that is entrenched in the US. This system emphasizes healing through drugs, surgery, chemotherapy and radiation. (The Random House Dictionary definition of "allopathy" states "The method of treating disease by the use of agents that produce effects different from those of the disease treated (opposed to homeopathy).")

[3]The director of Centro Naturista had received instruction at the Optimum Health Institute of San Diego, and he implemented parts of their program in his clinic.

screen, you can actually see how your blood cleans up during your three-week program.

In the United States, all the institutes are set up as schools where you can learn the entire living-foods lifestyle. In addition to food issues and preparation, these programs offer comprehensive instruction covering the mental, emotional and spiritual aspects of health maintenance and recuperation.

At all these places, I saw many wonderful things happen. All around me, people with so-called "incurable diseases" were getting well!

Due to my extraordinary experiences at the various institutes, I became inspired to disseminate information about this lifestyle. Back in New York City, I set up a Raw-Energy Hotline on one of my phone lines. On the hotline, I provide listings as to who is lecturing and where, who is teaching live-food preparation, what events are coming up, etc. Through the hotline, I have talked to hundreds of people from all over the world and heard their inspiring testimonials of recovery. In 2006 I retired the hotline and now provide information through an internet radio show *Hooked on Raw*. Tune in at www.NYTalkRadio.net or at my website.

By now, it may be obvious to you that I am "Hooked on Raw." I am convinced that this way of eating and living has provided huge benefits for me. It is a built-in insurance policy, but instead of paying premiums, I just spend that money on buying the best quality food I can find. As a singer and entertainer it is very important for me to look, sing and be at my best. This diet[4] allows me to do so easily. I have boundless energy and I seldom get hoarse anymore, even when singing under extremely adverse conditions (such as in a club with the air conditioner blowing directly on me while I'm hot and perspiring and, at the same time, experiencing all the cigarette smoke that has drifted to me—ugh!). I am able to handle stress, pressure and disappointments much better than before and I feel happy and joyful most of the time. I don't need a lot of sleep (5-6 hours per night), yet I wake up refreshed and ready to go. And I don't get colds or the flu, aches, pains, or headaches.

One thing you will discover if you go on a High-Raw or All-Raw Diet is the true effect foods have on your body. When you eat raw or almost all raw and living foods for a period of time, and then eat something cooked, you will be able to feel **clearly** the effect this cooked food has on your body and mind. It is unmistakable. You will be able to ascertain for yourself what type of energy each kind of food gives you. **In my personal experience, cooked foods bring me down, weigh me down and slow me down.**

In doing research for this book I asked a lot of questions of food suppliers because I wanted to get to the bottom of what really is raw and unheated food. Although some hesitated, when I presented to them my interest in providing accurate information to the growing number of consumers interested in this lifestyle, most finally did cooperate.

---

[4]The original Greek meaning of the word "diet" was "way of life."

I had a lot of surprises along the way. I didn't know that some figs, dates and prunes are steamed; or that "raw" oat groats are damaged by heat in processing, rendering them unsproutable. I didn't know that the only way to be certain you are purchasing really raw honey is to make sure the label says "**unheated.**" The words "uncooked" or "raw" do not ensure that you are getting what you want, which is **no heat applied**, period (or at least no heat applied higher than body temperature). If the label doesn't say "unheated," you could call the company and ask them about the processing of their honey. I didn't know that the milling process, used to make the "raw" sesame tahini sold on store shelves, generates heat to the tune of 150 to 160 degrees F. I didn't know that some spice blends have been toasted or roasted—which is why, in case you want to make your own, I've included the section "Spice Blends from Scratch." I didn't know the dried coconut on the shelf was pasteurized. I didn't know many things, but I have learned to ask the right questions and you can too, and **the more we ask for what we want, the more it will become available to us.**

It was a little disheartening to discover that so many things we have assumed were unheated really **were heated**, and they can still be labeled as "raw," a complete contradiction in terms. It was disheartening to learn about the extensive hybridization of foods that has rendered them less—much, much less—nourishing than what nature originally provided for us. I tell you this not to discourage you, but rather to empower you to be a better and more informed consumer. In my Source Index, where possible, I have included suppliers who sell these items in their unheated, primary and prime condition. Organically grown foods have become more available to us because we've been asking for them. Heirloom and open-pollinated varieties of produce will become more available to us as soon as we start asking for them, too. **We, the consuming public, have an astounding amount of collective power available with our purchasing dollars. The use of these dollars can be OUR VOTE for better health for ourselves and our loved ones. More than a vote, this kind of citizen action, would ensure the renewal and preservation of our home, our Mother, our beloved—Earth.**

HOW THIS BOOK CAME ABOUT

ABOUT LEIGH

Let me tell you about Leigh because he is such an integral part of the creation of this book. Leigh is my sweetheart, honey, friend, business partner, and confidant, my almost everything.

When I first met Leigh, I knew he was a special man. Since he was not a vegetarian, I wondered how things would work out with him on a day-to-day basis. I had quite a dilemma weighing all his many wonderful qualities and my growing feelings for him against his consumption of meat. Since I had come from a meat-eating background myself, I decided to take the risk. Maybe he could change, I thought, but I didn't ask him to. Maybe it would work out even if he didn't change (doubtful!).

For the first six months we were together, I prepared the food and would prepare two different meals each evening; one vegetarian and one meat or fish-based. This was a very difficult thing for me to do, given my strong commitment and convictions, but I toughed it out. Of course I would always give him some of my food, which he liked. Sometimes he suggested I only make a vegetarian meal and many times he even made the food himself.

One day, about six months later, after we'd enjoyed a very tasty vegetarian meal, Leigh said to me "You know what? From now on let's just make one meal . . . vegetarian." **Hallelujah, I Was So Happy!**

Of course, I wasn't sitting around all those months twiddling my thumbs. While saying almost nothing, I had quietly brought all kinds of delicious vegetables, fruits, nuts and seeds into the house. (I went through my very modest savings pretty fast, too!) I introduced Leigh to fresh pineapple, and he loved it. Previously he had only tasted canned pineapple. Although he liked bell peppers, they would repeat on him. I just said, "Keep eating them, soon they won't repeat," and they didn't.

Every time Leigh opened the refrigerator, there was a virtual cornucopia of luscious, fresh produce awaiting him. Four months into the experiment, he got a bill, a quite substantial bill, from a health food store that had given me credit. But, by that time, he was already hooked. He later told me that he thought I was Wonder Woman for bringing all that wonderful food into the house on the modest budget we had set.

During that first six-month period, two problems surfaced with Leigh's health. The first, which occurred a few weeks into our living together experiment, was a very painful urinary bladder infection, for which he was ready to run to Kaiser (Leigh and his whole family belonged to this HMO). I said to him, "What are they going to give you—drugs? Are you willing to try something different?" Cautiously, he said, "Well, what is it?" So I said, "Why not drink a quart of fresh juice each day for a few days to see if it has any effect?" He replied, "But this is really painful!" I said, "Do you think you could give it five days?" So he started on a quart of carrot, celery, cucumber and parsley juices mixed together each day. By the third day he already knew he was not going to Kaiser. In less than a week the infection was gone.

The second crisis had us traveling over a bumpy little road before it was worked out. We found out Leigh had high blood pressure. So, since I knew garlic would lower it (based on the knowledge that it had worked for others), I made up a "gorilla brew" of raw garlic juice and then I told him to drink it. He did not want to cooperate, but since I was standing there taunting him (YES, sometimes I was terrible!), he finished it up. The garlic juice went down, took a look around, did a U-turn and then came right back up. OH WELL, I guess I overdid it! We went to the health food store and got "Kyolic" (aged garlic capsules) instead, and they worked very well. After a while, his blood pressure was normal.

Because of these experiences, Leigh became a true believer in the value of healthy eating. A couple of years later we unwittingly created a mini-scandal in Leigh's family when he decided he was going to resign from the HMO. The rest of the family most emphatically thought he was doing the wrong thing. But by not having insurance, we became more responsible for our own wellness and more motivated to look around for folk or home remedies when we had health problems; and for us at least, this has worked very well. **I'm not advising anybody else to do this, but this was and is our personal choice.**

Leigh's conversion to vegetarianism was nothing, let me tell you, compared to his making the switch-over to raw and living foods. This he definitely rebelled against. My efforts in trying to make things tasty and palatable for him is what helped inspire this book.

Further incentive came from indirectly experiencing the struggles of two dear friends, J.R. Funk and Sharon.

MY FRIEND SHARON

I met Sharon a few years back, while attending a Louise Hay weekend seminar on love and forgiveness. We became instant friends. Sharon had cancer and was looking for some solutions to her problem. At the time we met, Sharon was adhering to a raw food diet that she learned at a retreat in upstate New York, and was doing very well. After consuming raw foods for about a year, she had reduced her cancerous tumor from the size of a grapefruit to the size of a pea. During that time Sharon had been so strict with herself that she wouldn't even put dressing on her salad. Feeling that nature would return her to health even if she was a little less austere in her approach, I suggested that she make delicious dressings out of herbs and seed cheeses, all acceptable on the live food program. Sharon did not take my suggestions, however, opting to follow in every detail the program given to her. And it was wonderfully effective, as evidenced by the reduction of her tumor.

The problem with overly restrictive diets though, is that people cannot usually continue them for very long. So it was with Sharon. One day she decided to eat without restriction. This was like opening a dam. From that point on she had no control and went back completely to the SAD (Standard American Diet), including chocolate cake, spareribs—you name it. Because she had denied herself flavorful food for a year, it seemed to me that she felt greatly deprived and this undermined her resolve to get back into control.

When the cancer began to grow again, Sharon chose to go the conventional medical route. First she lost her beautiful long hair. Then she was in such pain that her husband tried to alleviate her suffering by providing her with marijuana. Needless to say, we all know the end to this story. A beautiful young woman in the prime of her life is no longer with us.

I miss my friend Sharon, and though we only knew each other for a short year and a half, her needless death had a profound impact on me. I truly believe Sharon would have continued her recovery by eating delicious raw food rather than by following the austere version of the diet that she was taught. Her experience, though sad, was my second motivation for writing this book. I want to dispel the erroneous belief that a raw food diet must be restrictive, devoid of flavor and boring.

Sharon did not die only as a result of a faulty diet. Food is only one component, though a very important one, creating our health. Other factors to be considered include the mental, emotional and spiritual aspects of living. I believe that at some point, because of other things going on, Sharon gave up on life. Once she gave up, death became a possibility.

J.R. FUNK

When I moved from Southern California to New York City, one of the first people I met was J.R. Funk. In a rented room at a rehearsal studio, Leigh and I were auditioning drummers for a musical group we were putting together. After each drummer would leave, a man kept sticking his head in the door and smiling at us with a silly grin. We thought he was kind of strange, but we were newcomers to New York ways. At the end of a long day, we still had found no drummer who performed to our satisfaction.

Again, this person stuck his head in the door, smiled, and for the first time said, "I'm a drummer." By that time we were tired and disgusted, and we thought: "What the hell, let's listen to one more." J.R. turned out to be an excellent drummer, and as a bonus, sang wonderfully too. He just happened to be hanging around the studio that day . . . probably waiting for us.

That was the beginning of a five-year association, during which time we went through a lot of highs and lows together, as musicians are apt to do. During those years we didn't work much, but the three of us shared a lot of dreams. It was through the bond of those commonly shared dreams and aspirations that we became very close friends.

J.R. had an act that brought the house down every time. First the lights in the club would be dimmed. Then J.R. appeared to set his drums on fire and play them while he threw the lighted mallets around. In the finale, he would eat the fire. It was a showstopper! Very flashy! The fire would burn on the lighter fluid that he used to douse his mallets.

We never gave a second thought to the toxic constituents of the lighter fluid, until one day we heard that J.R. had developed a tumor in his throat. I then realized that J.R., over a long period of time, had been swallowing residues of poisonous lighter fluid.

Around that time, I was staying at the Optimum Health Institute in San Diego, learning their program. I called J.R. from California and asked him—no, I begged him—to come down to San Diego and go on their raw/live food program. I told him I would help him through it. I wish I could have convinced him, but he refused.

A few months later, I visited J.R. at the Veteran's Hospital in New Jersey. He was living on gelatin, and on canned, so-called nutritional malts that contained nothing but refined sugars mixed with some synthetic vitamins and additives. I offered to bring in some real food, but the hospital discouraged it.

One of the saddest things is having to stand back and watch people you love die. Would J.R. have recovered if he had gone through the detoxification program? Based on the experiences of other people that I've witnessed, I believe so. People make their own choices for their own reasons, and we must respect that. Still, it's never easy.

If the raw/live food lifestyle was more generally known and accepted, then people wouldn't be so reluctant to give Nature's ways a try. My experiences have motivated me to bring this information to a wider audience.

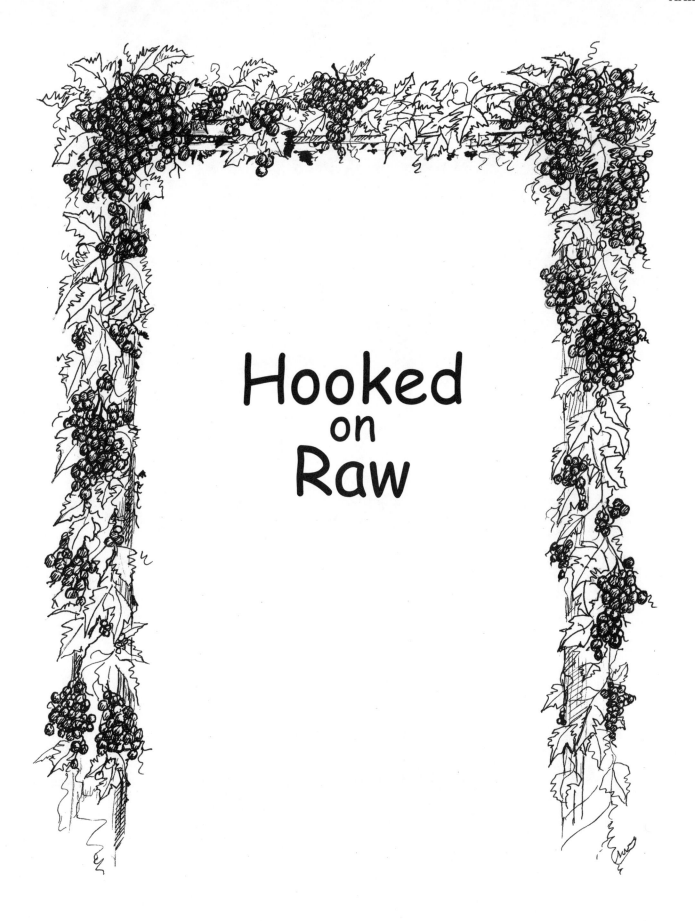

Hooked
on
Raw

CHAPTER ONE:
Why Raw and Living Foods?

ACCEPTING FOOD, AS NATURE IN HER WISDOM PREPARES IT FOR US

I am a child of Nature, and I am a child of God; therefore I accept what Nature/God has put here before me. Yes, there is much discovery I must still do on my own, but as I observe the natural animals[1] in their natural environments, undisrupted by man (and they are getting increasingly difficult to find), I see that they eat things as nature produced them. They have no stoves, broilers, ovens or microwaves; they do not cook. Usually, they eat the whole food. They do not peel, pare, fragment or discard tops and seeds. The natural animals eat a variety of food. Depending on the species, they eat fruit, roots, leaves, grass, weeds, seeds and berries, and they've been known to eat the vegetables out of people's gardens. Even the carnivores eat their catch raw and in its entirety; e.g., they do not eat just the muscle meat but also the contents of the stomach, the organs and even the bones.

As I observe further, I see that these animals do not suffer from the diseases of civilization. They have no cancer, heart disease, osteoporosis, arthritis, diabetes or any of the other 27,000 diseases of civilized mankind.[2]

Eating raw is nature's first law; every species on the planet does it, except man and his domesticated animals. How is it that we, perhaps the most intelligent of the species, cannot make the simple connection to this basic truth? Could it be that by living in unnatural environments, we have increasingly isolated ourselves from our mother, the earth . . . and from the soil? And yet, what person has not felt something—infinite, timeless, enduring—a distant, internal longing, when exposed to the beau-

---

[1]Here I refer to the (so-called) "wild animals" which existed long before the encroachment of civilization and long before the effects of the industrial age compromised their health. Even though there is no total escape from the consequences of our modern age, there are still places where these animals exist in excellent health, surpassing that of any civilized human.

[2]For purposes of simplicity, I use the terms man or mankind to refer to both genders. This is not intended as a slight to women.

ties of nature, such as we experience in isolated beaches or in pristine mountains and forests?

Nature does call to us in our soul, but living as we do, in cities of concrete, and in houses of steel construction, immersed in plastic, without the resonance of natural materials surrounding us, we become increasingly alienated from these connections. Living the modern life has created a deficiency in our exposure to nature, but the deficiency does not become obvious to us until we actually spend some time in natural surroundings. Then we are able to feel the nurturing which takes place between us and the trees and plants, the air and the vibrations of the natural world—and the loss of this nurturing in our daily lives.

HOW DO WE GET BACK IN TOUCH SO WE CAN FEEL THE TRUTH AND WISDOM IN OUR SOUL?

Spend time outdoors in natural environments. Put your hands into the good, rich earth of an organic farm. Touch the trees, and breathe deeply of the fresh air, which contains the negatively charged ions the plants provide for us. We are perfectly synchronized with plants: They need the carbon dioxide we expel and we need the oxygen they expel. Spend time picking apples off the trees, or berries off the bushes. It gives you a first-hand appreciation of what nature is doing for us, and you will come to realize, as expressed so eloquently by Chief Seattle of the Divamish Indians:

> "The earth does not belong to man; man belongs to the earth. This we know. All things are connected, like the blood which unites one family. All things are connected.
>
> Whatever befalls the earth befalls the sons of the earth. Man did not weave the web of life; he is merely a strand in it. Whatever he does to the web, he does to himself."

By spending time in natural environments you will increasingly glimpse heaven, not as an abstract, nebulous place way above or far away somewhere, but as a concrete way to feel about things right here and now. Heaven is here on earth. The earth knows it and we know it . . . we've just forgotten.

Nothing we can do will improve upon the perfection of the food, as nature, through the wonder of the solar system, has prepared it for us. Some authorities have stated that cooked food is easier for the body to digest and assimilate. I suggest this is **not** the case. If it were so, then we would be the healthy ones and the natural animals would suffer from 27,000 diseases.

RAW IS AN INADEQUATE WORD TO DESCRIBE UNCOOKED FOODS

Raw is an inadequate word to describe uncooked foods. It connotes something somehow unfinished, undesirable and needing something to be done to it to make it right or OK. A ripe, succulent peach or luscious cherry needs nothing from us to complete its perfection, yet the very language we use to describe it, "raw," while technically accurate, is inadequate. This is why some proponents of this lifestyle use terms like "Sun-Fired Foods." This word was coined by Aris La Tham, a gourmet live-food chef who teaches both in the United States and internationally. Other terms used are "LifeFood," "Live-Foods," "Living-Foods," "Sunfoods," or my favorite, "Raw-Energy Foods." The proponents of this lifestyle are trying to get away from using the term "raw" with all of its negative cargo attached.

My dictionary has these definitions for "raw," most of them negative in some way.

Uncooked

Indecent

Bawdy

Harsh

Inexperienced

Bare

Sore

Bleak

and the synonyms are:

Unprepared

Unfinished

Unripe

Crude

Rude

Rough

Unseasoned

Fresh (here's a good one for a change)

Green

Undisciplined

Unskilled

Unpracticed

Untried

Exposed

Since our language helps shape the way we feel about something, people who have never heard of this "new" (actually ancient)[3] cuisine may look at you askance when you say you eat everything raw. In addition to the negative feelings they associate with "raw" things, they may ask: "But what about beans and potatoes?" "What about rice?" "What about etc., etc., etc.?" They just have no idea what a world of wonderful eating is out here . . . in the RAW.[4]

RAW VS. COOKED & PROCESSED FOODS

WHAT ARE SOME OF THE KNOWN DIFFERENCES?

Cooked foods cannot create true health because they are missing some very vital elements needed by the body for its optimal functioning; things like enzymes, oxygen, hormones, phytochemicals, bio-electrical energy and life-force. When foods are heated above 105° F they **begin** to lose all of these. By 118° F, most food is dead. Yes, the vitamins, minerals, carbohydrates, fats and proteins are still there, but in a greatly altered state—not at all what nature provided.

Each cell of the body is like a tiny battery, and raw and living foods supply the bio-electricity which charges these batteries. The bio-electrical energy of raw food can be clearly seen in Kirlian photographs of the food. This photographic process shows electrical discharges that naturally emanate from all living things as luminescent, aura-like flares surrounding the subject. The glow is bright and radiant in raw foods, yet almost totally absent in Kirlian photographs of comparable cooked foods.

To me "life-force" means "the energy that is able to create life." The sprouting ability of raw foods demonstrates the presence of the life-force within them. All grains, legumes, beans and seeds sprout. Nuts in the shell sprout. Potatoes sprout and create new potato plants. (Do not eat potato sprouts as they are poisonous.) If you stick the top part of a pineapple into water, it will sprout roots. Apple seeds create apple trees. Avocado pits and mango pits sprout.

Now, take cooked versions of all the above, put them into soil and see if a plant will grow. Cooked food rots, rather than sprouts, and a new plant does not come forth. Through observation, you can easily demonstrate for yourself what you are losing by eating cooked foods. A food that is cooked cannot create life and cannot maintain the life-force energy in our bodies.

Cooking food disrupts its molecular structure and kills all the enzymes too. Enzymes are the indispensable biological catalysts (infused with "energy charges") which

---

[3]The Essenes were a religious sect before and during the time of Christ, who reportedly advocated the use of raw foods. Reference: *The Essene Gospel of Peace.*

[4]You may wonder why, despite these negative connotations, I continue to use the term "raw" in this book? The answer is that words such as "SunFired" or "LifeFood" would require explanation; but "raw" is raw, and no one misunderstands the term.

enable the body to utilize vitamins and minerals. (Think of enzymes as the workmen and vitamins and minerals as the bricks and mortar. Without the workmen, the bricks and mortar don't get put into place.) Enzymes are extremely heat-sensitive and thus do not survive in cooked foods. The vitamins and phytochemicals also are injured, greatly diminished, and left in an altered molecular state. The minerals are made less soluble. The fats have turned from life enhancing *cis* fatty acids to *trans* fatty acids, which create damaging free radicals in the body. Trans fatty acids also interfere with respiration of the cells. The proteins (including vegetable proteins), become denatured; they then coagulate (like the white of an egg) and are very difficult to digest. Some researchers report that unmetabolized protein particles in the bloodstream are a possible cause of allergies.

When you eat cooked (enzymeless) foods, you put a heavy burden on your body, which then has to produce the enzymes missing in the food. One of the reasons you feel lethargic or sleepy after a cooked meal is because the body is diverting its energy to replacing the enzymes that were not supplied. By comparison, a raw food meal leaves you feeling light and full of energy. You can judge this for yourself. Uncooked foods digest in 1/3 to 1/2 the time of cooked foods. The stress of creating and replacing enzymes, meal after meal, day after day, year after year, greatly contributes to accelerated aging.

Ingesting cooked food also causes the body to produce a surge of white blood cells (leukocytosis). These cells normally defend against disease, infection and injury to the body, but their production is a routine effect of ingesting cooked foods (as if the body considers such food a threat or danger). Because leukocytes carry a variety of enzymes, there is another possible explanation for the increase in white blood cells. The leukocytes may be delivering the missing enzymes so that digestion can proceed unhindered. **Leukocytosis does not occur when raw, unheated foods are eaten.** According to Viktoras Kulvinskas,[5] "in any pathological condition, including the intoxification of the digestive system with cooked food or other toxic materials, these white cells increase from 5 or 6 thousand per cubic millimeter to 7, 8, or 9 thousand per cu.m.m." Leukocytosis also occurs when additives, pesticides and chemically based supplements are ingested. And, of course, producing these cells creates an additional stress upon the body.

Raw foods are full of oxygen, especially green leafy vegetables which contain an abundance of chlorophyll. The chemical structure of chlorophyll is almost identical to the hemoglobin in our red blood cells. The only difference is that the hemoglobin molecule has iron in its nucleus and the chlorophyll molecule has magnesium. Chlorophyll detoxifies the bloodstream and every other part of the body better than anything else you could eat. When you eat raw green chlorophyll foods, you oxygenate the blood. The bloodstream, through its capillary system, then delivers this oxygen to every cell in your body. And when you eat greens in blended form, such as in Dr. Ann's Energy Soups (*see* page 198), this process is even more efficient.

---

[5]*Survival Into The 21st Century*, Viktoras Kulvinskas. Iowa: 21st Century Publications, 1975.

Sprouted seeds contain vital elements which nourish our glands, nerves and brain. The hormones needed by the body are created out of the natural fat and other essential principles found in seeds. Think about how few seeds are found in the average diet. The plant breeders are hybridizing most of the seeds out of our foods. Now we can get seedless watermelons, seedless grapes, seedless citrus, and the list goes on. Even if we did find a seed, most of us don't understand the value of eating it and thus, it would be discarded.

When you eat cooked starch, the body absorbs more than it needs. Getting rid of the excess starch then becomes another burden to the body. Those who favor cooked foods often make the point that since the body cannot absorb raw starch, this is a sign the food should be cooked. Another way to look at it, however, is that the body absorbs just enough of the raw starch for its needs and then passes out the rest. (When pig farmers feed their pigs raw potatoes, the pigs stay slender. Since farmers sell their pigs by the pound, they have learned to feed them cooked potatoes, which fattens them up.)

Cellulose—the woody, fibrous part of food—was previously believed to be unnecessary to the body. Because the body did not absorb it, it wasn't deemed important. Now we know that this fiber is what keeps things moving through our body so that we don't become constipated. Nature is vindicated again! I believe, in addition, that **raw** fiber has the ability to act as a broom which sweeps the intestinal tract and keeps it clean. Cooked fiber has lost the ability to do this for us. Enemas and colonics serve their purpose, but they are a poor substitute for what nature, by putting (raw) fiber into foods, has provided.

Raw and live foods nourish and improve the body's inner environment. Raw and live foods enable the body to dislodge and expel accumulated wastes. A member of my family had a tiny sliver of metal lodged in his hand as a result of an accident. For two years he tried to get it out by squeezing, pushing, and probing with sterilized needles, etc., but it wouldn't budge. He went to the Optimum Health Institute (to learn about live foods) for a week and, when he returned home, decided he would continue on raw foods. Four weeks later, a bubble formed on his hand and inside the bubble was the sliver of metal. The bubble then burst and the sliver came out. This is an example of what raw and live foods do. If something is not supposed to be in your body, it will be expelled.

Eating cooked food prevents the immune system from working on what is really important in keeping us superbly healthy and young in body, mind and soul. We exhaust and dissipate the body's strength by using the immune system to combat the unnatural cooked foods, chemically based supplements, pesticides, herbicides, fungicides, hormones (in meats, poultry, fish and dairy) and numerous other toxins we ingest, breathe in or absorb through our skin. When we really need the immune system to support us (as when a disease or infection develops or an injury occurs), it then lacks the strength to defend us properly.

Eating healthy means giving your body *power* foods it can easily assimilate and use for regeneration and rejuvenation. Life comes from life. So the more foods you eat which are organic and straight from nature's **raw** garden, the better you are going to feel.

HOW MANY WAYS DO WE DESTROY THE LIFE-FORCE IN OUR FOODS?

Fry
Grill
Bake
Barbecue
Boil
Pressure Cook
Roast
Simmer
Toast
Stir Fry
Deep Fry
Bain Marie
Flambeau
Scorch
Sear
Broil
Fricassee
Pasteurize
Caramelize
Steam
Parch
Crock Pot (all day cooking)
Braise
Parboil
Scramble
Stew
Smoke
Scald
Sauté
Poach
Char
Brown
Blanch

AND THE LATEST ENTRIES:

Microwave

Irradiate

Flashbake

There's no doubt we've been VERRRRY creative in our cooking! One of the goals of this book is to point out alternative ways of preparing foods so as to **preserve** the life-force in them. I hope more talented chefs than I will use the book as a starting point, and then go on to create world-class live food recipes which become standards that people universally enjoy. We can be just as creative in our **UN**cooking; we just have to keep our priorities straight because our goal is to:

**Keep The Life-Force Intact So Food Will Nourish
Our Body and Soul Optimally, As Nature Intended**

MAGICAL ENZYMES

**"Enzymes are the bridge between the physical
and the spiritual worlds."**

This quote, attributed to Rudolf Steiner,[6] is thought-provoking and evocative. Could there be some truth in it? Enzymes carry a unique energy; they seem to have their own intelligence which leads them to act in highly specific ways in response to different bodily needs. Some researchers have stated that enzymes emit a particular type of radiation unmeasurable by conventional means. Yet others have attributed to enzymes "biotic energy" or the "spark of life." Enzymes have also been described as "matter impregnated with energy values" and "protein carriers infused with energy charges." These are not terms usually used by scientists. What are they really saying? It seems that at a certain point in their research, scientists are faced with an unknown factor. The "spark" of the enzyme appears to be more than what can be found in physical matter or measured in physical terms. When the protein portion of the enzyme is separated from the "spark," it becomes inert. The protein is merely a carrier of "the spark." The true nature of enzymes cannot be explained either by biology or chemistry at this time. And, modern science is not yet geared to testing for, much less accepting, the possibility of spiritual realities.

Nearly all life processes depend on the functioning of enzymes. Enzymes can be likened to (but are much more than) biological catalysts that make everything work. Vitamins and minerals (known as co-enzymes) and hormones cannot function in the absence of enzymes. This is why cooking food is so destructive. Enzymes are completely destroyed by heating them above 118° F. Some enzymes are destroyed at even lower temperatures.

People usually understand the destruction of which fire is capable. A forest fire destroys natural habitats, extinguishes life and creates devastation in its wake.[7] If you set fire to something (almost anything you can think of, with some exceptions), it usually does not improve it or make it better.[8] But when we apply fire to food, all of a sudden we don't seem to realize that we are destroying something. Now we think we are improving it.

---

[6]Best known for his writings on Anthroposophy or Spiritual Science.

[7]Nature, of course, regenerates itself after a forest fire and some specialized plants even arise to help the process. These plants practically never appear, except under these conditions.

[8]Even when fire benefits us by providing warmth, the benefit is usually gained at the expense of something being destroyed or polluting the atmosphere.

Evaluating the nutritional value of food by calculating its vitamin, mineral, protein, carbohydrate and fat content is useless unless you also tabulate its enzyme content because, without the enzymes, all these other factors will not be properly assimilated by the body.

There are three categories of enzymes utilized by the body— food enzymes, digestive enzymes and metabolic enzymes. **Food enzymes** are supposed to be in the food you eat, but, in our modern diet, they are mostly missing (deactivated by heat, never to revive). **Digestive enzymes** are produced by the body to assist in digestion. **Metabolic enzymes** are produced by the body to repair cells, tissues and organs and to generally keep the body in an optimal functioning condition. Any action the body/mind takes involves enzymes. They are the housekeepers and enablers, making sure everything that needs to be done gets done. **Eating cooked food deprives you of one complete category of enzymes, and puts a great strain on your body's supply of the others.**

In order for the body to digest food lacking in enzymes it must call upon itself to produce those enzymes that are missing. In this way the salivary glands, stomach, intestines, pancreas and other organs, as well as the cells, work overtime to supply the obligatory enzymes. Without them the food will not digest properly. The pancreas was not designed to handle cooked and processed foods, lacking in enzymes. As stated by Howard R. Loomis, Jr., D.C. in his book, *Enzymes: The Key to Health, Volume 1,* "When any tissue of the body cannot secrete enough substance it is responsible for providing, it hypertrophies (enlarges)—that is, it swells and gets larger trying to provide more tissue to make more secretion." **The pancreas of a cooked food eater is enlarged, denoting its overworked condition.**[9] This condition has been observed many times in autopsies performed on both humans and laboratory animals whose diets had been composed of heat-treated and processed foods. Wild animals, on the other hand, eating the raw food available in their natural habitats, do not have enlarged pancreases. Many interesting enzyme studies have been reported by Dr. Edward Howell, one of the pioneers of food enzyme research in this country. When metabolic enzymes are diverted from their designated work, the body is robbed of its valuable reserves. This squandering of valuable enzymes may be one of the primary causes of accelerated aging.

Another indication that lack or loss of enzymes (enzyme exhaustion) leads to or is associated with aging comes from comparison studies which show that the salivary enzymes of young adults (average age of 25) are 30 times stronger than the salivary enzymes of older adults (average age of 81). This waning of enzyme activity in older adults leads to digestive and nutrient assimilation problems. In his books,[10] Dr. Howell cites many studies detailing the decline of enzyme availability with age, to support his belief that life slowly ebbs away with the depletion of enzymes. Studies also show that in acute disease conditions, there is first an acceleration of enzyme activity; but when that same disease condition becomes chronic, the enzymes are then reduced

---

[9]An enlarged pancreas can also be an indication of a pathological condition.

[10]*See* Bibliography.

to below normal levels. According to Dr. William Campbell Douglass "The main reason for aging . . . is the failure of enzymatic systems that are responsible for your body's uptake and utilization of oxygen." And we all know the importance of oxygen!

Billions of enzymes are working in our bodies, and it is estimated that there may be thousands of different kinds, each performing specific functions. While too numerous to cover here, I'll just mention a few of these functions:

- Enzymes are involved in all metabolic processes.

- Enzymes assist the immune system in neutralizing toxins.

- Enzymes break food down into simple components which can then be taken up by the bloodstream and assimilated into the cells. The components of food enzymes and digestive enzymes are essentially the same, except for the differing pH medium in which they work. When food is eaten with its enzymes intact, fewer digestive enzymes are secreted by our bodies.

- Enzymes, paired with co-enzymes, repair and rebuild the body and the brain.

Simply put, enzymes are needed to bring the nourishment into the cells and take the wastes out of the cells.

Supplemental plant enzymes can be very beneficial. According to DicQie Fuller, Ph.D., D.Sc., in her book *The Healing Power of Enzymes*, protease enzyme supplements taken on an empty stomach help hydrolyze and remove proteinaceous debris from the blood and from extracellular fluid. Dr. Fuller also states, "Clinical observations . . . have noted that upon high intake of oral protease, heavy metal concentrations have been significantly decreased in the blood."

Dr. Howell came to believe that every degenerative disease may have its origin based on enzyme deficiencies. He stated **"To say that the body can easily digest and assimilate cooked foods, may someday prove to be the most grievous oversight yet committed by science."**

Dr. Howell writes that we are born with a healthy enzymatic bank account based on what he calls our "enzyme potential." This is the ability of the body to have enzymes available at all times for metabolic functions, as well as to produce them as needed. Enzymes also need to be present in optimal amounts in our cells and tissues. According to Dr. Howell, by eating cooked and processed foods, our "enzyme account" becomes depleted over time. When that account gets too low, disease, old age and finally death will be the result. Dr. Howell also believed that the "enzyme bank account" was finite, and once depleted, could not be built up again. I hope that the good doctor was not correct on this point. Enzymes are produced by the body and recycled many times (except for those lost in the urine and feces) before being discarded. The daily ingestion of enzyme-rich food to add to the body's own supplies and perhaps food enzyme supplements for those that continue to eat some cooked foods can, to a great extent, alleviate the strain on the body's own production. With judicious care, why can't the body be kept in condition to produce all the enzymes it needs, no matter what the age? The riddle is, how do we continuously maintain the body in such a prime condition? I believe some of the answers can be found in Chapter 5, "Is Aging Inevitable?"

WHY ARE ENZYMES MOSTLY MISSING IN THE MODERN DIET?

In order for food products to have an extended shelf life, their enzymes MUST BE DEAC-TIVATED. Extended shelf life is a quality of food that does not have the least bene-fit to the health of the consumer. Purveyors of this food, however, do get an economic benefit; they avoid losing any part of their investment to spoilage, because dead, life-less food will last almost indefinitely. In addition, we are conditioned to eat cooked food and have become addicted to it. When we think of food, we picture cooked food, and cooking is regarded as the normal way to prepare food. But there is nothing at all normal about eating cooked food in light of the losses suffered by our health as a result. Live food, with its enzyme activity, has the ability to rot. Bringing the "spark of life" to our cells depends on this. For true health, we must eat food that has the ability to rot, only we must eat it while it is still fresh and live.

A machine will keep working indefinitely until one of its parts breaks down; then, if that part is replaced it keeps on working until something else breaks down or wears out. If that part is replaced, it works once again. The human body is infinite-ly more unique and spectacular than the most advanced machine of our creation. The human body is constantly being repaired or replaced biologically. In fact, no person is ever more than seven years old. That's how long it takes for every single part of the body to be replaced. (Of course, some parts are replaced many times in seven years.) In seven years of right living, you can have a completely new body that is stronger, younger and more vital than the one you have right now. If we were to provide our bodies with all the materials needed for perpetual repair and replacement of our parts, we would be immortal. In fact, we are potentially immortal. I suggest that the tools of choice, the means to attain these ends (youth, health), were put here for us by Mother Nature and have been here since the beginning of life as we know it. Some-times the truth is just so simple—too simple—that we tend to overlook it. We seek instead a more complicated explanation or solution. We look for artificial ways, technological methods, and medical interventions to extend life. But what of life's qual-ity? If we have extended life only to spend our remaining years in nursing homes under medication, then what kind of **life** is that?

There are two types of truth. One type of truth is malleable, ever changing, in the field of possibility and potential. Then there are immutable truths, the kind that never change, no matter what era we are living in, no matter what the latest scientif-ic discovery, no matter what. One of the immutable truths, as I perceive it, is that we were meant to live in a state of abundant health. Disease does not come to us out of the blue, and God (or the higher power) does not send it. Life, in its essence, is perfection. We take this perfection and degrade it to our own purposes. We create disease for many different reasons,[11] perhaps to learn some lessons that need to be learned, perhaps to come to an awakening, or to spur us to embark on a personal trans-formation. Disease may have certain benefits for us in our spiritual education, but **dis-ease is man-made**, not nature-made.

---

[11] I have not covered them all here.

Organic, raw fruits and vegetables, sprouted nuts and seeds, fresh, unpolluted air and clean water, a place to call home, an optimistic outlook, peace of mind, a loving attitude towards ourselves and others and creative endeavors — these are the basis of a good life, a healthy life, and most of all, a rewarding life. As David Wolfe, author of the *Sunfood Diet Success System*, states with his infectious exuberance, "When you consciously resolve to have **the best day ever**, it leads, day by day, to the best life ever. A life where you squeeze the 'raw' juice out of every single moment."

PHYTOCHEMICALS: *What are they?*

Phytochemicals are substances, which have recently been discovered by the thousands, in various plant foods. They are found locked in the vivid color pigments of fruits and vegetables. Researchers seem to be confused about these substances, sometimes calling them phytochemicals, and other times phytonutrients. When they are found to contain estrogenic properties, they are also referred to as phytoestrogens.

As far as the experts know at this time, they are not nutrients (like vitamins, minerals or amino acids) because the body does not assimilate them into its cell structure and does not use them for fuel.

SOME BENEFICIAL FUNCTIONS OF PHYTOCHEMICALS:

1)   The amazing thing about phytochemicals is that they seem to assist or aid the body organs in their work; in other words, they somehow help the organs to function better. They also stimulate the immune system.

2)   They serve as protective factors for the various body systems and processes. The function of phytochemicals in a plant is to protect the plant from pollutants, radiation, insect predators, disease and other potential damage. These protective factors are transferred to our bodies when we eat and then assimilate raw plant foods (and to a lesser degree, cooked plant foods), and then protect us in the same way that they protected the plant.

3)   They serve as antioxidants which assist the nutrient antioxidants (Vitamin A, C, E, Selenium, etc.) in detoxifying our body. They prevent or mitigate cell damage caused by free radicals.

4)   They assist in the formation of enzymes which process and remove carcinogenic substances from our cells. Broccoli and other vegetables of the cabbage family contain sulforaphane, a well-studied antitumor compound.

5)   Some phytochemicals assist in the transfer of nutrients through the blood vessel walls into the cells.

6)   They block or interfere with processes that lead to disease conditions in the body by inactivating or inhibiting the enzymes associated with these disease conditions. For example, isoflavones found in legumes deactivate cancergene enzymes.

7)   They block carcinogenic substances from entering the cells and they inhibit growth of malignant cells.

8)   Some phytochemicals calm and quiet the nervous system, and also reduce blood pressure through the regulation of hormones. One of these, 3-n-butyl phthalid, is found in celery.

9)   They reduce cholesterol levels by blocking its absorption in the intestines. Saponins, found in soybeans and fenugreek seeds, have this capability.

Phytochemicals have a favorable effect on many other body functions, and numerous other benefits are being revealed daily. To me the discovery of phytochemicals denotes one more reason (as if I needed one) to stick with Mother Nature.

Phytochemicals are being studied intensively—but not for the purpose of telling people to eat foods which contain them, as nature provides, but to foster the expansion of a budding industry that isolates phytochemicals in the manufacture of supplements. As I mention in my supplement chapter,[12] nature does not create isolates—she puts things together as complexes, where everything works together synergistically.

Industry is also very interested in creating **"designer super foods,"** with the aid of biotechnology. On the surface, the creation of prescriptive foods which may have the potential to fight or prevent disease would appear to be a positive development. The real reason that these companies are turning to gene manipulation, however, is to patent the new products that are thereby "created." Phytochemicals, as they now exist in nature, cannot be patented, but when "new," gene-spliced versions are developed, these can be patented. Formulated into "nutraceuticals," the most common term used for this new category, and claiming to lower blood pressure or cholesterol, reduce inflammations or relieve any number of symptoms, they can then be sold for high prices. Some other names used for this new category that manufacturers are trying to establish are pharm foods, medical foods, functional foods and phytofoods. As U.S. Food and Drug Administration regulations now stand, any substance that can relieve or cure a disease condition has to be classified as a drug, even though it may be a naturally occurring substance found in a food. This is ridiculous, of course, but it is also the reason that nutraceuticals, this new category which falls somewhere "between a food and a drug," is being created.

A nutraceutical professes to deliver the health benefits of a food substance in a pharmaceutical dose much larger than the daily allowance recommended by our FDA. But what about receiving the health benefits of phytochemicals in the proportions and ratios that are delivered by nature in her vegetables and tree-ripened fruits? If we are just beginning to discover the benefits of these compounds, how can we know better than nature what dosage is optimal?

By consuming raw plant foods, as served up by nature, you can have the benefits of these marvelous body protectors. **Raw/live food was, is and will always be your best medicine**... as long as it's not genetically engineered.

---

[12]*See* Chapter 10, "Supplements—Yes, No, or Maybe?"

PREPARING FOOD WITH LOVE

The importance of preparing food with love cannot be overstressed. When food is prepared lovingly, an intangible vital nutrient is added to the food. As far as I know, there is no name for this nutrient, so, for the purposes of this book, I'll call it Vitamin L-complex. (Of course, researchers would dispute the existence of this nutrient, as it has not been located in the physical realm.) I submit that the food tastes better and is more nourishing when Vitamin L-complex is imparted to it.

"Oh, no, now she's really lost it!" I can hear you say. But, bear with me and I will try to explain. Author and lecturer Dr. Deepak Chopra, in his audio tape series, *Magical Mind, Magical Body,* talks about an experiment that was done with newborn premature babies at the University of Miami. In the experiment, the newborn babies were divided into two groups. Both groups were fed identical diets, but the experimental group was touched and stroked for 10 minutes, three times a day (they referred to this stroking as "tactile kinesthetic stimulation"), while the control group was just fed, but neither touched nor stroked. At the end of the experiment they found that the group which was touched had gained 49 percent more weight per day than the control group. As a result, this group of babies could be released from the hospital much sooner, saving the hospital $3,000 per baby in costs.

Stroking stimulates the secretion of growth hormone (such as occurs when dogs and cats lick their young). I question whether this effect results from just the physical stroking alone. It may be more likely that stroking, in conjunction with the loving feelings that are generated by the very act of stroking, stimulates growth hormone. In the case of the newborn babies above, I don't see how a caring nurse in a hospital could mechanically stroke a baby without communicating some tender, loving feelings.

As Chopra says, "Heaven forbid they should call this stroking 'love,'" but that's just what it was and you can plainly see the result. It's intangible, but it nourishes. Is it not possible then to affect the foods as we prepare them by touching with our hands and our loving thoughts? And as a result, would not this food be more nourishing to those who ate it?

Another example of how we impart intangibles into things is a humorous incident that occurred to Edgar Cayce, as reported by his son, Hugh Lynn Cayce. Edgar Cayce,[13] in some of his readings, had given detailed instructions for building an appliance which was supposed to help people, especially insomniacs, sleep better. After a number of these readings, a close friend of the Cayces, Marsden Godfrey, decided to manufacture the appliances to send to people, as called for in some of the readings. One client, who received an appliance, sent a letter to Cayce stating, "Mr. Cayce, I was

---

[13] Edgar Cayce was a psychic during the early part of the 20th century who was able (by going into a trance state), to diagnose people's illnesses and offer remedies for their healing. If people followed his suggestions faithfully, a large percentage of them regained their health. The readings, over the course of years, numbered into the thousands. An organization known as The Association for Research and Enlightenment sprang up as a result of Edgar Cayce's work. It is located, to this day, in Virginia Beach, Virginia. The readings are available for perusal.

sleeping part of the night before I got this appliance that you recommended and now I can't sleep at all. I have gotten so nervous. What should I do?" Cayce didn't know what to do either, but he told her to send the appliance back. When it arrived, it was decided that they would set up another reading to find out how to proceed.

Cayce, in the trance state, suggested that they use a strong magnet to remove the anger which had been programmed into it. It seems that Godfrey, on the day he was building the appliance, had a violent argument with his wife and the "inanimate" object had picked up the vibration. After being cleared by the magnet, the appliance worked as it was supposed to, as later reported by the client.

"Of course, we could never explain to the woman what was wrong with her appliance because the explanation was harder to accept than the original malfunction," mused Hugh Lynn.

What I got out of this incident is that feelings—especially strong feelings—can impart intangible qualities into things.

Many cultures on earth adhere to a tradition of blessing food before eating it. This is usually in the form of being grateful to nature, to God or to the universe for providing sustenance. This consciously charges the food with loving energy, which makes it more harmonious and nutritious to consume.

My third example is that of Grandmother's Chicken Soup. I believe it may work for the ailing grandchild or family member, because when Grandmother is making this soup, she is making it with the love and regard she has for her family. So the Vitamin L-complex is imparted to the food and is picked up by the person who eats it. Love is ever the healer, and we do absorb it any way it comes.

How much love and caring do you think goes into the food prepared in fast food establishments? Or into factory-processed food?

So please, get into a good mood, put on some healing music and impart Vitamin L-complex into the food as you lovingly prepare it. And this will be the most nourishing ingredient of all.

CHAPTER TWO:
Soil Fertility, Wild Foods, Organic Foods

SOIL FERTILITY: FEAST OR FAMINE?

Life on earth, as we know it, depends on just a few inches of topsoil.

While it's important to eat food raw and unprocessed, as provided to us straight from our mother, the good earth, food can only be as healthy as the soil upon which it is grown. In fact, the health of a people is dependent on the fertility of their soil.

Do you know who the very first organic farmer was? Can you guess? The first organic farmer was Mother Nature herself. We can learn everything we need to know about soil fertility by observing how she nurtures and fertilizes her earth. In this chapter, I will briefly go through a few of the fascinating and diverse mechanisms Mother Nature uses to assure soil fertility. It would take a whole book or even several books to cover them all, and I do not believe we even know a fraction of her secrets.

RENEWAL

Mother Nature recycles. In natural environments, such as forests, Nature recycles everything. Leaves, flowers and fruits fall off the trees and create a plush carpet underneath the canopy. This carpet is called a mulch. Mother Nature was the first mulcher. The leaves and organic matter on the bottom of the mulch continuously break down and enrich the earth in a never ending cycle of soil renewal. **In Nature's system, nobody comes in to sweep up the leaves and cart them off to a landfill where they sit for years without decomposing, adding to our already deplorable waste disposal problems. Conditions in a landfill, (where everything is thrown together indiscriminately) are not conducive to the breakdown of organic matter.** If Nature had her way, all organic matter would be returned to the good earth from whence it came. And through this ancient process, the ongoing renewal of our soils would be assured and their fertility preserved.

When a branch falls or a tree dies in a forest, it eventually gets recycled into earth. All the animals living in the forest leave their little gifts of manure which are pulled into the soil. When the animals die, their bodies also are recycled. The end result of all this breakdown of organic matter is what is called "compost" or "humus"—the basic material of healthy soil. With it we have Mother Nature's Garden of Plenty—a feast for the body and soul. **Without it we have man-made deserts, famine, scarcity, blights, massive insect infestations and people suffering from poor health.**

Mulch has the added advantage of keeping moisture from evaporating out of the soil. In a farm or garden situation, you wouldn't need to water as much if you utilized a mulch. Plants growing on a mulched soil are more comfortable because there are fewer fluctuations between moisture and drought. Wherever there are plants, Nature always mulches. **On a conventional farm, the soil between the plants is kept clean of debris because the farm managers think it prevents predator insects from coming; and so the soil becomes parched and baked. With little organic matter to anchor it down and no mulch on top, the soil on these farms simply blows away when it becomes dry enough. Or it washes away when the rains come. This is how we lose tens of millions of tons of topsoil every year. Is this stupid or what!?**

By way of comparison, when there is plenty of organic matter in and on the soil it eventually becomes humus through the action of microorganisms. This humus then acts like a sponge which absorbs and holds moisture. As a natural consequence, the soil does not erode but stays in place, and in fact, slowly builds up. Over time, six inches of topsoil becomes seven and then eight, etc.

FERTILIZER

Mother Nature has arranged for the finest fertilizer to be created right at the location where it is needed. She has provided the earth with tiny little "tractors," and they don't cost big bucks like the tractors made by humans. These tiny little "tractors" are called earthworms.

Earthworms have gotten a bad rap. To be called a worm in our society is not a compliment! In spite of this image problem, earthworms are one of the finest little creatures that ever existed. They do a great service for the soil, and by extension, for human beings and other animals. Earthworms aerate the soil as they burrow through it, to depths of 15 feet or more, breaking up and preventing hardpans. (A hardpan is earth that is hard as a rock and impervious to water.) The burrows also serve as canals for efficient water drainage.

Farm tractors, on the other hand, because of their weight, compact the soil and prevent aeration. In addition, plowing, by turning over the soil, disrupts the natural environment of the soil organisms and decimates their numbers. Farmers plow to break up hard clumps, aerate and prepare for planting. In Nature's garden, the earthworms perform this function admirably. Just push aside the leafy carpet in a forest and stick your finger in and you will see how loose and friable (crumblike) the soil is.

Earthworms eat all kinds of organic matter and then expel "earthworm castings," the finest fertilizer in the world. The castings keep the soil pH nearly neutral—neither too acid nor too alkaline. Over time in this humic medium, rocks break down and release their minerals, which are then available in a form easily absorbed by plants. And, of course, when the earthworms die, their bodies also contribute to the fertility of the soil.

The chemical fertilizers and pesticides that are applied on a conventional farm eventually kill off the earthworms and other life forms in the soil. As this life dies off, the soil becomes more and more barren.

Charles Darwin, in his book *The Formation of Vegetable Mould through the Action of Worms*, estimated that in a field well populated with earthworms, one inch of topsoil is created every five years. Henry Hopp, a scientist formerly with the USDA, estimated that **over five tons** of earthworm castings can be produced each year per acre of good agricultural soil. Other estimates have placed the production of castings as high as **30 tons** per acre per year! What could account for the discrepancy in these estimates is the numbers of earthworms populating the different soils. Where there are larger earhworm populations, more castings are produced.

A soil rich in earthworms and earthworm castings prevents soil erosion.

SOIL LIFE

The life within fertile soil is more prolific in number than all the life that exists on its surface. One gram of fertile soil may contain 29 million bacteria. Rich, organic soil teems with life and is replete with worms, insects, yeasts, bacteria, fungi, tiny algae, protozoa and other microorganisms. Each type of organism plays its own significant role in creating or maintaining the soil's fertility. In a humus-rich soil, for example, there are symbiotic associations formed between various fungi and the roots of plants or trees. These fungi are called mycorrhiza. In this process the fungi form extensive threads (hyphae) that surround or engulf the roots and in essence feed the plant water, minerals and other soluble organic matter. Such associations between organisms are not well understood by biologists at this time. What is known, however, is that these relationships are not parasitic; rather, the plant and the fungi seem to function together as a partnership for the purpose of drawing in sustenance from the soil.

NITROGEN

Nitrogen is a necessary component of plant growth. There is an abundance of free nitrogen in the air. But how does the free nitrogen from the air get into the soil? Nature has various mechanisms, the least known of which has to do with thunder and electrical storms. As lightning comes streaking through the air during an electrical storm, it catalyzes a chemical reaction that converts nitrogen from the air into nitric and nitrous acid and deposits them into the soil with the rain. Approximately 250,000 tons of nitric acid are formed in this way in EACH 24 HOURS!

Certain soil bacteria, which attach to the root nodules of leguminous plants, also attract free nitrogen into the soil. This process is called nitrogen-fixing. Evidence suggests that this natural process ceases in the presence of synthetically produced nitrogen. Nitrogen is also abundant in compost and humus. **Chemical fertilizers are com-**

posed primarily of three ingredients, abbreviated as NPK. The N stands for nitrogen, while the other two-thirds of the trio are phosphorus (P) and potassium (K). With these three ingredients, and a barrage of pesticides, conventional farmers think they can grow healthy crops. The result of using these synthetics is weakened plants, susceptible to disease and insect infestations. In addition, these plants are deficient in trace minerals, as they are not supplied in the NPK fertilizer.

Have you heard of nitrate and phosphate pollution of underground water sources and rivers? This is the result of fertilization of soil by chemicals, which later seep out and contaminate our water. These nitrogen-based fertilizers also release nitrous oxide into the atmosphere, which contributes to global warming. When nitrogen, phosphorus, and potassium are locked up within humus, they can never contaminate the earth. This is because they are only "unlocked" by plants as they are needed.

All the nutrients a plant needs to grow healthy are held in the humus until the plant releases, chelates and absorbs them for its use. In a conventional farm situation, the chemical fertilizers that are spread out on the land overfeed the plants. A plant needs water to transpire but while taking in the water, the plant cannot selectively exclude the soluble synthetic fertilizers; so the plant tissues become saturated with an overload of NPK. This creates an unhealthy plant, short on trace minerals and unable to properly metabolize nutrients.

According to Joe Nichols (founder of Natural Food Associates in Atlanta,TX), when corn was heavily fertilized with synthetic nitrogen, it was unable to convert carotene into vitamin A. The resultant corn was also deficient in vitamins E and D. Other research demonstrated that levels of iron, zinc, copper and manganese in corn were also reduced by heavy chemical fertilization.

BIODIVERSITY

Mother Nature revels in biodiversity. If we tune into her ways, she seems to be saying to us: "Why have one of something when you can have thousands instead?" In Nature's garden there is a great mix of plants, each one attracting its own circle of insects and animals. A natural order is created in which this mixture of plants, insects and animals seems to keep everything in check. No vast disease or insect infestations occur to wipe out everything in their path.

Man favors monoculture in his farming practices. He allocates huge tracts of land to only one crop and then wonders why diseases and insects create such devastation.

WEEDS

Mother Nature has provided a great multitude of weeds. It seems that she has created them for our benefit (to eat) as well as to correct soil imbalances. (Perhaps they are correctors of body imbalances, also.) Weeds are valued in natural systems because they add to soil health and fertility.

Some weeds help to bring minerals up from the subsoil, which are buried at great depths. As companions to domesticated crops, weeds help clear the way for crops' roots to get down to food that they would be deprived of ordinarily. A certain percentage of weeds growing in a crop field also helps assure some of the crop's survival, in case of drought.

When soil is deficient in minerals or elements, certain weeds will come to grow on it, and in some way not yet understood, correct the deficiency. For example, Ehrenfried Pfeiffer, a plant research biochemist, was able to prove that calcium-rich daisies could grow on calcium-deficient soils, as long as the soil was abundant in silicon and microorganisms. He also showed that, when the daisies died, they added calcium back into the soil. He was never able to ascertain, however, how the daisies got the calcium out of the deficient soil in the first place.

I believe (and I'm not alone here) that it has to do with transmutation. Mother Nature, in ways that are still mysterious to us, is able to **change** one element into another.

SELF-PRESERVATION

In order to preserve her systems intact, Nature fights back when humans interfere. One of her ways of maintaining healthy flora is to get rid of the weak or substandard specimens. Since many of the crops raised by conventional farmers are substandard and deficient (at least by Nature's standards), she tries to eliminate them. Bug infestations and diseases are ways to get rid of this inferior vegetation. They only have a significant effect when something in the plant is out of balance. A balanced and healthy plant is resistant to bugs and disease, just as a healthy person is resistant.

It should be obvious to those farmers who spray poisons upon their land and crops that these methods do not give them the results they seek. The bugs just come back stronger the next year. Then the poisons have to be reformulated to make them strong enough (more lethal) to deal with the ever more resistant species of bugs, and this cycle just repeats itself. It is because Nature is fighting back.

There are hundreds of mechanisms, perhaps thousands, by which Mother Nature feeds, balances, nourishes, creates and sustains soil fertility. Other factors which impact soil fertility and plant health include electro-magnetism, bird songs, insect sounds, cosmic and telluric[1] forces, the phases of the moon, planetary influences and water quality.

Are you beginning to see how Mother Nature works her miracles? If our agricultural practices were reversed and we were wise enough to cooperate **with** Nature,

---

[1]Influences emanating or proceeding from the earth

instead of trying to subdue and dominate her, we would truly have a world of abundance and plenty—Feast, not famine.

THE VALUE OF WILD, UNCULTIVATED FOODS

PRESERVING THE HERITAGE OF NON-HYBRIDIZED SEEDS

It is eminently important to preserve the heritage of unhybridized seeds (aka heirloom or open-pollinated seeds) because they are the root source or root stock (germplasm) of all of our domesticated, commercially grown fruits, vegetables, nuts, seeds and grains, and, in fact . . . of all our food. All our food originally came from non-hybridized wild stock, a large percentage of it discovered in the (now diminishing) rainforests.

Non-hybridized seed has the ability to reproduce itself from generation to generation, true to its original form. This means that the seed, when planted, will produce a plant and a fruit that is just like its parent. You can count on it; it will not let you down. When you use non-hybridized seed (and save a small part of your crop for seed), it becomes unnecessary to purchase seed year after year as the farmers do today.

Hybridized seed, on the other hand, which constitutes the bulk of seed used today to raise our crops, does **not** have the ability to reproduce itself true to form. What is the significance of this? For one thing, it has been speculated that if a world-wide crop disease epidemic were to occur, all the usable seed stock (of hybridized corn, for example) could be wiped out. Then, just when we need to go back to the original seeds, there might not be any left to go back to. Why? For several reasons. One is that all the places where most of the original seed stock was found in the first place—like the rainforests—are being destroyed at an alarming rate. Another reason is that there are very few organizations in the world dedicated to preserving original seed stock.

Wheat, rice and corn account for half the world's human diet. A serious disease infestation afflicting any one of these could create famine of unimaginable proportions. This is not as far-fetched as it may sound. We've already had disease epidemics, such as "the Southern Corn Leaf Blight, [which] devastated 15 percent of America's 1970 corn crop . . . costing farmers about $1 billion in losses. Some southern states lost more than 50 percent of their corn crop."[2] This occurred because a mutation in the hybridized seed made the corn susceptible to the blight. The devastation would have been much more serious except that the weather in the corn-growing states remained cool that summer. Had the weather been more hot and humid, the losses would have been even more ruinous. In addition, because this seed was exported to other parts of the world, the potential for this disease to have spread was mind boggling.

Modern agriculture is a chronicle of crop disasters, many caused by reliance on a few hybridized crop varieties that were genetically weak and unable to survive dis-

---

[2]*Altered Harvest*, Jack Doyle. New York: Viking Penguin, 1985.

ease infestations. In 1953, 65 percent of America's durum wheat was destroyed by wheat stem-rust; in 1954, 75 percent was lost. The National Academy of Sciences states in its 1972 report, "The wheat rust epidemics of modern times are clearly genetically based, in that as resistant varieties become available, fungus mutates to a form which attacks the new variety, and an epidemic ensues." In California, in the early 1900s, fire blight almost wiped out the Bartlett pear trees, and, as reported in *Altered Harvest*, "Nearly half of the tomato crop in the Atlantic Coast states fell prey to late blight in 1946, the same year that Victoria blight swept through 86 percent of the nation's oat crop. In the latter epidemic, at least thirty oat varieties, all with a common parent, accounted for the genetic sameness that led to almost a total crop failure."[3]

Because of the uniformity of current seed stock (seed companies have been focusing their attention on hybrids), many of the original unhybridized seeds have been lost. Our government maintains a seed preservation facility at Fort Collins, Colorado, known as the National Seed Storage Laboratory; but because of budget problems, mismanagement, negligence and incredible indifference, a lot of original seeds stored there have not been grown out in years. Many have not even been cataloged.

To remain viable, seeds need to be grown out in a field every few years to produce new seeds, which are again stored for preservation. Then, in a few more years, it needs to be done again. If the seeds are not grown out periodically, then there is no guarantee they will grow, if and when they are needed in the future. When these seeds are allowed to deteriorate, they, in effect, become extinct. Seeds are a living treasure, more precious than gold to ourselves and to future generations.

A better way to preserve seeds, it seems to me, is to let them thrive in their own environment, which is not in a vault, but out in the wild, growing freely year after year, in a natural preserve. (After all, that is where we found their ancestors in the first place.) Perhaps a national park or a few parks in different climates could be set aside for this purpose. Then, original plant varieties in danger of being lost can be replanted (naturalized) where they grow best.

The situation existing in government seed banks worldwide is not much better than here in the United States. There are some private organizations trying to recover and save original seeds so they won't be lost forever, but these organizations are still too few and far between at present.

Biological diversity is about having hundreds of thousands of varieties and species of plants and animals inhabiting the planet. Whereas modern people seem to be satisfied with less than 100 varieties of apples, with only about 15 of them available commercially, nature, over the centuries, has produced maybe 10,000 apple varieties. Nature loves diversity. Man wants to alter one gene[4] (out of thousands) in a plant and then get a patent because he thinks he has created something new!

What is the prime focus of a plant breeder's work? Why do they breed hybrids in the first place? More often than not, it is because industry wants to maximize yield

---

[3]Ibid

[4]*See* Chapter 9, "Frankenfoods: Biotechnology and Genetically Engineered Foods."

and profits.[5] How do they do this? Well, they hybridize to get traits into the plant which will make the crop uniform in size, so it can be easily harvested by machine. They hybridize for toughness, because it was found that these machines were crushing the fruits. They also hybridize for durability in shipping, for keeping qualities, for maximizing yield, etc.

Well, what's wrong with that? Nothing, **if it's not done at the expense of our health.** Many times, however, the very traits that the breeders want to retain are acquired by sacrificing other traits that would make the plant more nutritious, more flavorful or intrinsically resistant to disease. For example, it has been shown over and over again that the gene responsible for maximizing yield in wheat is connected to the gene that lowers the protein content. So, for the purposes of attaining higher yields per acre, the public is consuming a nutritionally impoverished form of wheat.

Hybridization is also done so that the plant can withstand greater applications of chemicals and pesticides without dying. It is no coincidence that many multinational petrochemical companies have gotten into the seed business. They manipulate the seeds so the plants need more chemicals and pesticides and then they also sell these products to the farmers. The use of altered seeds, combined with an artificially contrived need for more chemical fertilizers and pesticides, creates a self-perpetuating vicious cycle that is almost impossible to break out of for today's farmers.

Any profit gained at the expense of destroying the planet or its inhabitants is immoral. For the purpose of earning such undeserved profits, multinational agribusiness corporations, through their relentless destruction of natural environments (including native cultures), are extinguishing the earth's biological diversity—**nature's fail-safe mechanism against extinction.**

ALL HYBRIDIZATION IS NOT NECESSARILY NEGATIVE

Nature practices cross-fertilization, which results in the creation of hybrids. This is how the original agriculturists learned to do it: by observing nature. While most of the hybridization being done in modern times is not positive for our health, that does not mean that intelligent and wise use of the method cannot be achieved. Some hybridized plants have been coaxed to come full circle and are again able to reproduce themselves. This indicates that they have reacquired many of the characteristics and qualities inherent in wild plants.

Many wild plants are very small (though potent), and you would need to gather a lot of them to be able to make a meal. Hybridization, in these instances, has increased the size so there will be more to the meal. The carrot is a hybrid plant, created by humans. Some people reject the carrot because of this. I think development of the carrot is probably an instance where we have done something right.

---

[5]I do not refer, of course, to plant breeders who have worked for the betterment of humanity, such as Luther Burbank, George Washington Carver, and hundreds of thousands of unacknowledged native farmers all over the world, down through the centuries.

Dr. Norman Walker, who lived to be 115 years old, recommended carrot juice, and was able to help people recuperate their health by use of the carrot (as well as other plants).

All hybridization is not necessarily negative. The sagacious use of it can benefit humankind; it's a matter of intent.

WHAT YOU CAN DO TO EAT MORE WILD FOODS AND WHY IT IS NECESSARY TO EAT AT LEAST SOME

Wild plants are tough; they can take care of themselves. Cultivated plants, on the other hand, would not even survive without our assistance. Can extensively hybridized plants provide us with the nutrition that nature, through her original wild plants, intended? Since plants impart their strengths (and weaknesses) to us, how can we possibly gain any strength from those plants that don't even have the energy to reproduce?

Research has indicated that plants from hybridized seed have trouble picking up certain nutrients from the soil. Plants from hybridized seed may not be as abundant in phytochemicals as non-hybridized plants. In addition, the protein content is reduced and the quality of protein is inferior (as shown in the case of hybridized wheat. Ref: *Altered Harvest, see* Bibliography). Modern plant breeders have been tampering with our seeds for decades, but we are just now discovering the real consequences. If these findings are confirmed by further research, it means that, in the interest of big business controlling all the seed stock of the world, our health is again being compromised. This is because hybridized plants are not able to nourish us as optimally as the original plants provided by the creator.

The advent of the genetic modification of seeds (one example; the introduction of fish genes into a tomato by Calgene Co., so the tomato will not freeze in the field) **is causing serious interference with the homeostasis of nature**. With such unconscionable technology, soon the only way to get produce that is not tampered with will be to grow your own from open-pollinated seed. And how many of us will be able to do that?

This is a serious problem. I hope we wake up soon and do something about it. Individually we can help organizations that preserve original seed by supporting their work and by buying these heirloom seeds for our home gardens. (*See* "Heirloom Seeds" and "Seeds of Change" in the Source Index.) We can also learn more about the growing dangers by reading books such as *Shattering—Food, Politics and The Loss of Genetic Diversity* by Cary Fowler and Pat Mooney, and *Seeds of Change; The Living Treasure* by Kenny Ausubel, and then lending our voices to the growing protest.

Maintaining a home garden and planting only heirloom, open-pollinated seed is one way to get better nutrition from the plants you eat. Of course, I encourage you to grow organically to avoid exposing yourself, your family or your environment to pesticides, herbicides, fungicides and chemical fertilizers. By exposure, I mean physically coming into contact with these poisons (as you apply them), as well as by ingesting the fruit of a poisoned harvest. It is a fallacy to think that these poisons can be washed off. If that were the case, the farmer would have to spray after each rainfall. In addition, I believe that the plant picks up some of these poisons from the soil and so the poisons then become part of the body of the plant and its fruit.

Another way to obtain superior nutrition is by learning to forage for wild plants. Wild plants are much higher in nutrients than commercially grown plants. Nature has conditioned them to be strong; otherwise they would not have survived. And since they have the strength to survive, they will impart that strength to you. Lambs-quarters, for example, a wild relative of the spinach family, is much denser in vitamins, minerals and other nutrients than its domestic cousin.

In all instances, it is the same. Plants that grow wild are always stronger and hardier and have higher nutrient values. If you have a wild plant and a cultivated plant growing side by side and a drought occurs, which plant do you think is more likely to survive? Or which plant will more likely regenerate after the drought has ended? The wild one, of course! If you live in a big city, start noticing some of the tenacious wild plants that are surviving, growing out of cracks in the sidewalk and other unlikely places. (I wouldn't recommend eating wild plants growing from cracks in the sidewalk. Seek them out in a cleaner environment, such as in a park, forest or meadow, well away from the flow of traffic.)

Even if you only incorporate a small percentage of wild plants into your diet, the gain to your health would be substantial. This is because a small amount of wild foods equals in nutrient value much larger portions of their cultivated counterparts; and there may be other, as yet undiscovered factors in wild foods, not present in cultivated foods.

Finding these wild, original foods can be done very easily by foraging, but **FIRST**, you must take some classes with an expert forager so you know what you are doing. There are poisonous plants out there too, and to the untrained eye, a few of these poisonous plants look very much like the edible ones. In New York City we have a treasure . . . "Wildman" Steve Brill. "Wildman" takes people for walks through public parks almost every weekend throughout the year and teaches them which plants are food for the taking. In New York City and the surrounding area parks, wild foods are abundant; and thank goodness, New York does not have money in the budget to apply pesticides in its parks.

One summer a few years back, I spent every weekend with the "Wildman" on his sojourns through the different parks and it was an education I will never forget. We found mulberries galore: white, pink, and purple; yet people are largely unaware this fruit is edible and soooooo delicious![6] We also found an abundance of other types of berries, wild cherries, blueberries, apples and green herbs of all kinds. One of my favorites, which I go to pick every year in Inwood Park, is goutweed. It is a leafy-green, herb vegetable with an indescribable flavor and aroma. If you can locate some, try my *Go–Go Goutweed* recipe (*see* page 247).

---

[6]The mulberry trees are here because in some former time there was an effort to create a silk industry in New York and, when it failed, the trees remained.

Most localities have people who are trained in wild plant identification and who are willing to teach others. To find them, check with your local botanical gardens, organic gardening clubs or horticultural organizations.

ORGANIC FOODS

WHAT EXACTLY DOES "ORGANIC" MEAN?

Organically grown produce (verified by organic certification programs) consists of agricultural products grown without pesticides, herbicides, fungicides or chemical fertilizers. In an optimum organic growing situation, this produce would be fertilized with compost, seaweed, cover crops (green manure),[7] clean fish waste, composted manure, rock dust and other natural soil fertilization methods. In organic agriculture, the farmer always works **with** nature instead of against her.

WHY YOU SHOULD MAKE THE EFFORT TO BUY ORGANIC

While tests have been conducted on the toxicity of individual pesticides, etc., and tolerances set by the government (e.g., so many parts per million of a substance allowed), we don't know what the synergistic effects are of combining the myriad of pesticides, herbicides and chemicals which are used in conventional farming. Tests have never been conducted to ascertain these effects, and so we are the unfortunate guinea pigs for this experiment.

I would like to see 0 parts per million as the maximum amount of every toxic substance that is allowed in our food![8] **There is just no need for them**. As cited in *Living Foods for Optimum Health*, "Before DDT, American farmers lost about a third of their crops each year to insects, weeds, and disease. Today, with **twenty-one thousand** pesticide products to choose from and an annual pesticide bill exceeding $4 billion, farmers still lose the same—a one third share."[9] So why not just take the loss, maintain the integrity of the land and stop gambling with the public health?

ORGANIC FOODS TASTE BETTER AND ARE HIGHER IN NUTRIENTS

I've often wondered why so many people just don't seem to like vegetables and I've always come to the same conclusion. Conventionally grown vegetables and fruits often just don't have much flavor. I have eaten tomatoes that taste like soggy cardboard, stone fruits (such as peaches, apricots and nectarines) that taste like flavorless mush and watermelon with definite chemical undertones. Oranges and other citrus fruits

---

[7]Any crop that is grown and then turned into the soil for the purpose of soil improvement.

[8]Of course, I am not referring here to any naturally occurring toxins in the food itself.

[9]*Living Foods for Optimum Health*, Clement & DiGeronimo, Prima Publishing, 1996.

are much too acidic and pineapples can resemble vinegar. Lettuce and other vegetables are usually blah.

By contrast, organic produce is highly flavorful. Tomatoes are sweet and juicy; stone fruits have indescribably succulent, honey-tinged flavors; watermelon is sweet with no chemical undertones; oranges and other citrus are sweet and mellow; pineapples are beyond description and the vegetables are anything but blah.

Any particular fruit or vegetable will have a wide range of nutrient values, but in general, organically grown produce has been found to have a higher nutrient content than conventional produce. In a 1993 study, published in *The Journal of Applied Nutrition*,[10] it was also found that beneficial trace minerals were present in organic fruits and vegetables at approximately twice the level of coventionally grown produce. Organically grown foods are also substantially lower in heavy metals (such as mercury, lead and cadmium), as well as in aluminum.

Conventional produce may look big and beautiful, but the real values are determined when the food is reduced down to its ash weight (what remains after the food is burned). Studies have consistently shown that organically grown foods have a higher ash weight. This may indicate that conventional produce is waterlogged.

HOW YOU CAN REDUCE YOUR COST IN BUYING ORGANIC

Buying organic food is a wonderful way to give yourself the very best health support available, while at the same time supporting our planet, Mother Earth. Our buying dollars **do** make a difference. It is because more people are asking for organic foods that they are becoming more available. "But it's SO expensive!" you say. I know the prices for organic produce can be high in a regular health food store. So look around for ways to lower your cost, such as joining or starting a food co-op, going to farmer's markets, or participating in a CSA group. CSA stands for Community Supported Agriculture, an arrangement where a group of people share the costs of supporting organic farms, in exchange for a share of the produce. (In some communities you even have a say as to what will be grown.) This is a powerful way to support your health AND the small family farmer[11] at the same time.

If you have a backyard, you might consider growing some of your own vegetables, herbs and weeds. As an avid gardener myself, I know how satisfying this can be.

The formation of services that deliver fresh, organic produce right to your door weekly, and for very reasonable prices, is a great new development that is becoming popular in New York, California and other areas of the country. In New York, a

---

[10]Ref: "Organic Foods vs. Supermarket Foods: Element Levels." *Journal of Applied Nutrition*, 1993.

[11]Over the past 15 years, by some estimates, more than 350,000 farmers have been forced out of business. This loss has accelerated and "Currently, we're losing about 100,000 family farms a year." (Ref: *Mad Cowboy* by Howard Lyman). Our government does not help the small family farmer who, in former times, was the very backbone of our communities. The government has set up its supports and subsidies, for the most part, to accomodate and benefit the huge Multinational Agricultural Corporations.

box of fruit and vegetables, enough for two people for a week, costs $37 delivered, as of this writing. In Brooklyn, NY, contact "Urban Organic." (*See* Source Index.) Check around, for this is an idea whose time has come. I hope services such as these will soon be springing up in your community.

When we support community-based agriculture we are taking **direct action** to ensure the resurgence and survival of the small family farms. This is a part of our heritage which most of us value.

One thing to watch out for in the future: The federal government is getting into organic food certification through the USDA's National Organics Program. The problem is that when the government gets involved, the definition of what is "organic" may be loosened up. A cursory look at the new proposed standards will quickly reveal that the USDA, FDA and EPA are trying to reinvent the definition of "organic." Could it be that these government agencies, ostensibly set up to protect the public interest, are bought and paid for by industry?

According to an article entitled "Organics Under Siege" in *The Food & Water Journal* (Winter 1997 issue), "Over half of the substances that are approved by the USDA and set to be on the National List are prohibited for use by the Organic Crop Improvement Association." It may be that a new word will have to be coined in place of "organic" to identify food grown without questionable chemicals or processes. The words "organically grown," as defined by the federal government, may not give the protections that we, as a conscious consuming public, really want.

A VISIT WITH AN ORGANIC FARMER

At the Santa Monica Farmer's Market in Southern California which takes place every Wednesday and Saturday, I met an organic farmer by the name of Truman Kennedy and his wife, Betty. I had been buying his fresh (in season) and dried fruits and nuts every week and they were superb. His nectarines, peaches, plums and prunes had a unique flavor of their own which was luscious. His nuts were incomparable.

One day I struck up a conversation with him and it resulted in an invitation to visit his organic farm. I was intrigued because some of the things he had been saying were meshing with the ideas I already had about preparing and touching food with love. He told me he never hires negative people to pick or handle his produce because he believes they will leave a negative vibration on the food. Bingo! I had to go up to Fresno to learn more.

On a beautiful, late summer's day, Leigh and I went to visit with Truman on his farm. There we were delighted to see acres and acres of diverse heirloom fruit trees and gorgeous grapes. Walking through the groves of plums, peaches, nectarines, walnuts and almonds, we could feel Truman's justifiable pride in his creation of a farm truly in harmony with nature.

Truman's father and grandfather were both farmers; in fact he comes from 10 generations of farmers. Though Truman had spent his earlier years as a schoolteacher, he did eventually find his way to the land. In tracing his genealogical tree (one of his favorite endeavors), he discovered that his great, great grandfather began raising tree fruit back in the 1700s, and judging by the extent of the land he owned, was successful at it.

Perhaps Truman's love of the land is genetic. Truman half-jokingly said that he originally became an organic farmer because he was too cheap to buy the chemicals and too lazy to apply them. Much later, after taking a class on sustainable agriculture, he was surprised to learn he actually was an organic farmer by default. But he then embraced the concept and became a proponent.

Truman says he plants one or two rows of each kind of tree fruit, mixing the different varieties. He says each variety attracts its own insects and, because he hasn't planted the trees in large tracts, everything keeps everything else in check. Culls[12] keep the dust down and thousands of pits create a kind of pavement after a few years. This benefits the plants by keeping the aphids and mites from "flaring" (getting out of control). Culls also attract quail and pheasant who come to visit in the fall. These birds add aesthetic value to the farm because they are very beautiful to watch and listen to. And, if you need the soil to be more acidic for growing blueberries, putting culls on the ground naturally builds up acid in the soil. (Conventional farmers use aluminum sulfate to increase soil acidity.)

Truman plants cover crops[13] of clovers, poppies and wildflowers to attract bees to pollinate plants in the spring, and then disks about twice a year to keep the land more level, to increase safety for the farm workers, and to provide "green manure." After pruning and then shredding the pruned branches, he plows the wood fiber back into the soil. He reports that additional benefits of using the mulch are soil enrichment and retention of moisture. The mulch also "helps keep the bugs living in the 'weed/soil zone' instead of the 'fruit zone' on the trees." Truman said that in the past, crop losses were mostly due to bad weather and not so much to bugs. Crops from good, healthy, **heirloom** stock are naturally resistant to bug and pest infestations.

Truman says his conventional farming neighbors always complain about the high cost of chemicals and pesticides and of **not** making a profit at the end of the season, while at the same time, they kid him about getting into the world of "modern" farming. Truman, who has kept a low profile, says he just laughs to himself, knowing he's doing the right thing. Carving out a special niche for himself and his family by farming with heirloom varieties of tree fruits and grapes has brought him peace, fulfillment and financial independence. This gentle giant of a man is able to live as he wishes, pursuing the things that make him happy and traveling to his favorite places in the world during the off growing season.

Our visit and conversation reinforced my belief that people can get back to the land (if they wish to) by farming organically, and can make a good living at it. Truman says you don't need more than 50 well-managed acres (in orchards) per family

---

[12]Culls are the substandard, not fully developed fruit which fall off the trees or are discarded when picked.

[13]Cover crops are grasses, legumes, wildflowers, etc. which are planted between trees or at the end of a crop growing season. They are then plowed or tilled under to improve soil tilth and fertility.

to be productive and profitable. (Dry farming[14] would require more acreage.) If you were to grow vegetables, much, much less acreage would be required. The public is demanding organically grown produce; so potential future farmers can take heart from the fact that one can live a good life . . . back on the farm. Truman, and hundreds of small organic farmers like him, are laying the groundwork for this new paradigm.

---

[14]In dry farming you let nature do all the watering by means of rainfall.

CHAPTER THREE:
Some Significant Studies

POTTENGER'S CATS

In the 1930s, a physician named Francis M. Pottenger, Jr. undertook a series of studies,[1] which lasted 10 years and involved over 900 cats, to ascertain the effects of a raw food versus a cooked food diet on a cat's physiology. All the cats were fed either milk or meat or both. Some were fed raw meat and raw milk, some were fed cooked meat and raw milk, and others cooked meat and cooked milk. All the cats received cod liver oil. Pottenger kept meticulous records which met the most rigorous scientific standards of the day. The studies,[2] while initially well received, have unfortunately been much criticized in the ensuing years, yet no one has attempted to replicate them in order to disprove the results.

These results were both profound and enlightening. The most startling finding was that the cats fed almost exclusively cooked meat (with one-third of their diet consisting of raw milk) did not survive beyond the third generation. They could not reproduce. There seems to be a parallel in our human family today. As reported by John Robbins in *Diet for a New America* (Stillpoint Publishing, 1987), "Tests done at several major universities have found nearly 25 percent of today's college students are sterile."[3] This finding is substantiated by the increased prevalence of fertility clinics, which are trying to fulfill the needs of couples who cannot produce offspring on their own.

---

[1] *Pottenger's Cats* by Dr. Francis M. Pottenger, Jr., available from the Price-Pottenger Foundation (*see* Source Index).

[2] Some of the results were published in *The American Journal of Orthodontics and Oral Surgery* (Vol. 32, No. 8, August 1946).

[3] Robbins attributes this to the increased presence of PCBs in our environment.

GENERAL OBSERVATIONS FOR CATS FED A DIET OF 2/3 COOKED MEAT, 1/3 RAW MILK:

While the findings are too extensive to describe here in their entirety, it was observed that the skeletal development and size of different kittens in litters fed this diet was widely divergent, with malformations of the face, jaws and teeth occurring frequently. The skulls were smaller than normal, the teeth narrow and crowded. Tissue elasticity and muscle tone were poor. The long bones tended to have greater length, and the internal network of the bones was coarse, showing evidence of calcium loss and general demineralization. In the third generation the deterioration of some bones progressed to the point that they became as soft as rubber, very fragile, and subject to fracture. Unmistakable infections of the bones often appeared to be the cause of death of the animal.

The following were common occurrences in this group:

- Heart problems
- Farsightedness and nearsightedness
- Thyroid gland abnormalities
- Infections of the kidneys, liver, testes, ovaries and bladder
- Inflammation of the nervous system, with paralysis and meningitis
- Arthritis and inflammation of the joints
- Abnormal respiratory tissues, bronchitis and inflammation of the lung
- Frequent parasites, skin lesions and allergies which worsened with each generation. By the third generation almost 100 percent of the cats had allergies.
- The female cats were hyper-irritable with a propensity toward biting and scratching. The males, conversely, were docile and their interest in sex was either lax or they engaged in sexual deviations. They also had a low sperm count.
- 25 percent of the pregnant females aborted in the first generation, increasing to 70 percent in the second generation. Deliveries were difficult, with many dying either in labor or within three months afterward. If a mother cat was kept on cooked food for more than two years, she usually died during delivery. The average weight of the kittens at birth was 100 grams, 19 grams less than the group fed raw food. Kitten mortality was high.

GENERAL OBSERVATIONS FOR CATS FED A DIET OF 2/3 RAW MEAT, 1/3 RAW MILK:

- These cats did not have any of the problems experienced by the cooked meat group.
- Kittens in a litter were uniform in size, with broad faces and dental arches.
- There were no malformations of the face, jaws and teeth.
- Tissue and muscle tone were excellent.
- Fur was of good quality, with very little shedding.

- Inflammation and disease of the gums were almost non-existent.
- This group was resistant to infections, fleas and other parasites.
- There were no signs of allergies.
- The cats were friendly and gregarious with predictable behavior patterns.
- Miscarriages were rare, with birth weight averaging 119 grams.
- These cats reproduced generation after generation with ease.
- Mothers nursed their young without difficulty.

REGENERATING CATS

The study also included cats who had already experienced the physiological effects of eating cooked foods and were then put on a completely raw food diet. It was observed that, with each succeeding generation, the physiology of these regenerating cats would progressively improve; but it took four generations for them to return to a normal state of health.

AGRICULTURAL STUDY

A further extension of the study took place when the researchers used manures of several groups of cats to fertilize different plots of land planted with beans. The plants that were grown on soil fertilized with manure from cats fed cooked meat were tall and spindly, with pale color and flabby thin leaves. One-quarter of the beans were shriveled and yellow in color. The remainder exhibited a peculiar oblong shape and were not as plump as the beans grown on soil using manure from cats fed raw meat.

The bean plants grown on soil fertilized with manure from cats fed raw meat were sturdier, with good leaf color and heavy, firm texture. The beans were uniform in size and plumpness, and their root systems contained strands that were at least twice as numerous, tougher and longer than those fertilized with manure from the cooked food group.

WHAT DO CATS HAVE TO DO WITH PEOPLE?

While cats are natural carnivores and humans are physiologically more suited to vegetarianism (herbivores and fruitarians), cats and humans do share many genetic traits "and so often respond similarly to similar types of medicinal or nutritional input. Consequently, there is much of significance for humans in {these experiments} . . . The results carry heavy implications for human well-being, but have largely been ignored by the medical profession (for whom nutrition has generally seemed irrelevant)."[4]

---

[4]*Instinctive Nutrition*, Severen L. Schaeffer. Berkeley, CA: Celestial Arts, 1987.

DR. WESTON PRICE

In the 1930s and 40s, Dr. Weston Price undertook an extensive study of human physical degeneration, which took him all over the world. As a dentist, Dr. Price sought to ascertain the true genesis of dental decay. Rather than studying the disease conditions he constantly encountered in his practice, he decided to study populations that were free of decay. In 1945, Dr. Price published some of his findings in a monumental work entitled *Nutrition and Physical Degeneration* (*see* "Price-Pottenger Foundation" in the Source Index).

At hundreds of locations on five continents, Dr. Price visited communities of indigenous peoples, made records of their dental conditions, took measurements of their dental and facial arches, made note of other conditions present and documented his observations with amazing photographs. Many of the native peoples studied were following their traditional whole foods diet, whatever it may have been for the area. Dr. Price also sought out others of the same racial group who had been exposed to refined and processed "modern" foods. The diet of these people had changed either because they worked and lived in a port town where these foods were brought in or because they worked for a company or lived on a government reservation where these were the only foods made available.

An astonishingly consistent pattern emerged in Dr. Price's studies. He found that in every instance where indigenous people adhered to their native diet of whole foods, they had little or no dental decay and had perfectly formed facial and dental arches. Their physiques were excellent and they were healthy and happy. In areas where these people had switched to the diet of modern commerce[5] (white flour, white sugar, jams, canned goods, refined vegetable oils, polished rice, etc.), **tooth decay was rampant**. In succeeding generations, the jaws of the offspring had narrowed and the facial structure lengthened, leaving insufficient room for the teeth to come in straight. These indigenous people and their children suffered greatly from this dental decay, all the more because, in these remote areas, there usually were no dentists available to ameliorate their distress. They also suffered from tuberculosis and other diseases.

Dr. Price attributed the physical degeneration he encountered to injuries caused by the deficient diet. The degeneration could occur at any time in a person's life. An adult raised on his native diet of whole foods had properly formed dental and facial arches, with plenty of room for all the teeth, and little or no decay. When that same individual switched to modern processed foods, they would then develop dental caries (cavities) and other health problems.

Degeneration also appeared in the offspring, from mothers and fathers having eaten the deficient diet. Dr. Price contends that the deficient diet causes an injury (or abnormality) to occur in the germ cells[6] prior to fertilization. This abnormality then leads to prenatal lesions in the children. The children, in addition to developing tooth

---

[5]In his book, Dr. Price refers to refined & processed foods as "the foods of modern commerce."

[6]Eggs and sperm are germ cells (germplasm).

decay, also showed a narrowing of the facial and dental arches, narrowing and lengthening of the chest cavity and narrowing and lengthening of the pelvic bones. Dr. Price calls this "disturbed" or "intercepted heredity," because when people adhered to their native whole foods diet, these defects in the offspring were not produced. Dr. Price even found instances where a particular family eating a native diet had children with no deformities, and then when, due to circumstances, they changed their diet to deficient modern foods, their subsequent children experienced degeneration. Later when the same family went back to eating their native foods, children, born after this change, again did not show degeneration.

Dr. Price goes on to make a connection between brain lesions or "incomplete prenatal development of nerve structures in the brain"[7] with anti-social behavior in susceptible people. Depending on the degree of prenatal injury, either a mongoloid (now referred to as Down's Syndrome), a mentally retarded person, or an individual with sexually deviant, criminal and/or aggressive tendencies could be produced. Dr. Price stated that mentally backward and delinquent individuals may be abnormal because of injury resulting from parental nutritional germ cell defect. Dr. Price cites various studies that were being conducted at that time. He also emphatically decries the unfairness of holding these injured individuals (those with criminal tendencies) **entirely** responsible for their behavior. He claims that society has some accountability because it allowed the food supply to be degraded, thereby causing these injuries to occur.

Dr. Price made the further observation that the pelvic bones of women in the United States and elsewhere were narrowing as a result of deficient diets, so that the necessity for cesarean sections was becoming more frequent.

RAW FOOD

Dr. Price does not distinguish between cooked and raw foods when he refers to native traditional diets. He does mention, sometimes in passing, that certain foods are consumed raw. From my understanding, due to the lack of fuel, food in many indigenous societies was cooked minimally, if at all. The lack of refrigeration also required that food be consumed fresh.

VEGETARIAN SOCIETIES

Most raw food or vegetarian books that have reviewed Dr. Price's work failed to mention one little detail. I mention it here, in fairness to his work.[8] Dr. Price stated that in his travels he did not find any strictly vegetarian society that was in good health. He surmised from this that animal food of some kind had to be included in people's diet to achieve optimum health. However, he does not elaborate as to what the vegetarians he did encounter were eating. I feel that just because he did not find strict

[7]*Nutrition and Physical Degeneration*, Dr. Weston Price. The Price-Pottenger Foundation 1945/1972.

[8]Many vegetarian books have favorably referred to Dr. Price's work without also mentioning his pro-meat stance.

vegetarian societies in good health doesn't mean that the vegetarian way is not conducive to good health. There could be any number of reasons for his findings. For example, he only studied 14 primitive groups, of which only a very small minority were vegetarian, too small a number from which to reach such a conclusion. Native societies have to deal with the limitations of what is available in their immediate surroundings. Many of them are not agricultural societies and do not raise their own food. Perhaps the vegetarians Dr. Price encountered did not have access to a sufficient variety of foods to stay in excellent health. Since his work was not primarily focused on this particular aspect (vegetarian vs. non-vegetarian), I do not feel that he gathered enough information to make this judgment. That he reported what he found, I do not dispute.

Other researchers have found vegetarian societies in various parts of the world living in good health. Dr. Charles T. McGee, for example, in his book *How to Survive Modern Technology*, describes several primitive societies in Ecuador which were primarily vegetarian, lived on native diets and experienced superb health.

In Dr. Price's book (which is still made available by the Price-Pottenger Foundation), documentation of his findings can be observed. This includes numerous photographs showing indigenous people following their traditional diets, who have perfectly formed dental arches and teeth with little or no decay. There is also photographic and documented evidence of indigenous people in the same geographic areas, who had been exposed to modern foods, that were suffering from rampant tooth decay and disease.

I urge you to get a copy of this book and study it.[9] Here is a well-documented, honest effort to learn the true cause of human physical deterioration authored by one of the pioneers in this field. And his studies were done more than 50 years ago. Why haven't we heard about them?

Maybe one day soon, Dr. Price's work will be made part of a required health study course that is given in every school in the nation. It certainly merits that; and maybe that's why it's been kept alive in reprints for so long.

---

[9]Since Dr. Price's book was written more than 50 years ago, some of its terminology has become dated or is now considered politically incorrect. This does not diminish the value of the work as the terms used just reflect the times in which they were written.

CHAPTER FOUR:
The Wonderful Rejuvenating Effects of Fasting

The body is self-cleansing, self-healing, and self-regenerating, if given the proper conditions, and it can maintain itself in a superb state of health.

Fasting is one of the valuable "tools" available to assist us in our internal cleansing. Americans understand the concept of exterior cleanliness and taking a bath or shower every day is considered normal; but the concept of interior cleanliness is less well known, understood or accepted.

When you fast, various body systems act like a large "sponge" soaking up toxins and impurities from wherever they are found in the body. Then the sponge gets squeezed out, and the toxins are expelled from the body in many ways. This is an ongoing process throughout the fast.

Many people who are unfamiliar with the mechanisms whereby fasting works doubt the veracity of this process. But by watching carefully what happens to your own body while you fast, you can easily prove it to yourself. Your tongue may become coated with a white residue. It stays coated until you are either cleaned out or you break the fast by eating solid food. This is one of the ways the "sponge" gets squeezed out and the toxins are released. It is good to remove this white residue by scraping the tongue with a spoon. However, while the fast is ongoing, the residue will reappear.

A headache is another symptom that may occur. It can be harsh or mild; it can last for a short while or longer. Headaches especially happen when one is detoxing from caffeine overload caused by ingestion of coffee, tea, cola and chocolate. I once observed Leigh (who had been drinking only one cup of coffee a day, and decided to quit) go through a detox by just abstaining from coffee drinking. He first experienced a harsh headache, which gradually decreased to a mild one, over a three-week period, until his body finally expelled the last of the caffeine. (Leigh was not fasting during this; if he had been, I think it would have shortened the time it took to eliminate the caffeine from his system.)

The development of a headache on a fast indicates that toxins and unwanted substances are being expelled into the bloodstream. As the blood circulates and recirculates through the liver, kidney, etc., the toxins are being filtered out of the body. Of course, until the toxins get filtered out, they are present in the blood which passes through the brain; hence the headaches. Toxins on their way out could also produce cramps, drowsiness, nausea, weakness, low energy, diarrhea, sweating, dizziness, fever and palpitations.

During fasting, you may notice some gooky white or gray build-up on the teeth and around the gums. This is also "sponge-squeezing" in progress. Just wash your mouth more often. Your skin may break out or develop rashes, white powdery residue or itching, which all clear up in a short time. You may notice unpleasant odors emanating from parts of your body. Someone close to you may even say that you smell or have bad breath. Don't get disturbed. Just know the cleansing is in progress. Hallelujah! Nature is working its miracle.

During the fast, you may also expel mucus from your chest, throat and nasal passages, causing sneezing, wheezing and coughing. On the seventh day of a coconut water fast, I eliminated so much mucus from my chest that I lost my voice for a couple of days.

You may get irritable about stupid little things and you may feel emotionally on the edge. One minute you're laughing and the next minute crying. You may experience unwarranted fears, anger and even depression. This will pass.

You may get flashes of startling inspiration or insight. Your thinking may become clearer and you may feel like writing and putting down thoughts. I wrote this chapter while on a car trip from New York to Florida. During the trip, I fasted on the juice of pomegranates for 3 days (4 per day), plus 2 oz. of Essiac Tea[1] (diluted) per day. At the end of this short juice fast, I felt great. This fast was also (for me) a convenient way of handling the problem of what to eat while traveling on the road, where often you can find only greasy restaurant fare and NO organic food. ("What's that? You say you want organic?!!") I just took an ice chest with me, the Essiac Tea, my organic pomegranates and a small hand orange juicer (which is also good for juicing pomegranates). If you want to fast on other juices, take the fruit or vegetables with you in the ice chest, and of course, take a juicer. I've criss-crossed this country many times, juice fasting all the way. (Juice fasting is also known as a liquid diet.)

Toxins also get expelled into the lymph system, which passes through the lymph nodes in its own process of purification. That's why you may notice that your lymph nodes, some of which are located behind and slightly below the ear, under the armpits and in the groin area, may be swollen and painful when you press on them.

There are numerous other effects that may occur. For further information consult a fasting book (*see* Bibliography).

Now, you may ask, if I might get all these unpleasant effects, why go on a fast at all? Why put myself through it?

---

[1]Essiac Tea is a combination of herbs, excellent for expelling toxins from the body. It consists of Sheep Sorrel, Rhubarb and Burdock Roots, and Slippery Elm Bark.

Here are some good reasons . . .

1) Fasting or juice fasting is the quickest route to rejuvenation. By expelling all this toxicity, you unload the results of years of abuse of your body in a very short time. You feel and look lighter, younger, cleaner, clearer. How long it takes depends on your previous lifestyle. You may need to do several short (3 day) or medium length (7 day) fasts.

Please undertake longer fasts only with the supervision of a health care professional who is knowledgeable about fasting. **If you feel uncertain or uneasy about fasting, or have a disease condition, then consult with a professional even for shorter fasts.**

2) If you endeavor to rid yourself of the toxins NOW, before any ill effects show up, then you probably won't develop symptoms further down the road. According to the teachings of Natural Hygiene, all disease stems from toxicity (with malnutrition occurring as a result), so if you deal with this before ill health forces you to do so, you may never have to deal with disease itself. And you can probably live to a ripe old age, in good health, with all your faculties in good order, and with a physical body that belies your chronological age. In the words of Dr. Stanley S. Bass: "These toxins being discarded are saving you from more serious disease which will result if you keep them in your body too much longer—possibly hepatitis, kidney disorders, blood disease, heart disease, arthritis, nerve degeneration or even cancer—depending upon your hereditary and structural weaknesses."[2]

3) Fasting may help you get in touch with your spiritual nature. In the fast-paced and frenetic, very physical world we live in, we oftentimes forget we are spiritual beings. Fasting helps you get in touch with this reality. You may experience periods of extreme clarity, flashes of insight, inspiration and revelation. You may remember your dreams more clearly and begin to understand some of them.

4) Fasting puts you in tune with what is going on in your body and mind. You become more aware of your physical, mental and spiritual needs. When you look at yourself, you will see changes taking place right before your very eyes. Your skin clears and tones up, your eyes clear up, your hearing improves, and you gain mental clarity and spiritual awakening. Many other positive things start happening.

5) You regain a good appetite for the simplest of foods. An organic apple, pear or carrot will really taste good to you.

---

[2]*Discovery of the Ultimate Diet: Testing Nutritional Theories on Mice, Vol. 2,* by Dr. Stanley S. Bass, N.D., D.C., Ph.D.

TYPES OF FASTING

It has been stated by some experts that if you are drinking juice, you are not fasting. For them, a true fast allows only the drinking of water. My definition of fasting, however, includes **any abstinence from eating solid food by which you effect a cleansing and elimination of the toxic waste matter of the body.** Juice fasting meets this criterion, and so I believe it to be a form of fasting. Three to four glasses of fresh juice a day, with plenty of fresh water in between, would be sufficient. If you are new to juice fasting, then you may need more juice in the beginning.

Another way to fast is on the water of fresh green water coconuts. I emphasize the word **fresh** because freshness is so important with coconuts (*see* Glossary). A fresh green water coconut may have more than a pint of water (sometimes called juice or milk) in it. Just open one and drink the water whenever you feel the need. It is very refreshing and energizing. On the islands, people use a machete to open coconuts by hacking off the end. I learned how to use a machete in Puerto Rico at the Ann Wigmore Institute, where these green water coconuts are made available to the guests at all times. (For reasons of safety, the Ann Wigmore Institute recommends drilling a hole into the coconut with an electric drill.)

Here at home, we devised an easier and safer way to open the green water coconuts. First, the cocos must be young and fresh. Take a large sharp knife and just slice off a chunk of the husk on one side (not the end). Then cut a hole through the inner skin and pour out the water. If the coconuts are old, you cannot slice into them because the husks will be too tough. The husk of a coconut begins to petrify as the coconut ages and then finally becomes hard as a rock! **Remember, when opening green water coconuts, always be extemely careful.**

The brown coconuts are easier to open. Always buy the lighter brown as opposed to the dark brown ones, because the lighter color indicates they are younger and fresher. There are three indentations or "eyes" on one side of the coconut, and you will find that one of these indentations is soft enough to punch through with a flathead screwdriver. Widen the hole a little, then pour out the water. **Caution:** Young coconuts from Thailand are also available, which have a light brown shell, but I do not use these coconuts for fasting because the water is too sweet; it contains a lot of sugar. (Yes, it's unrefined sugar, but I believe it's just too much for fasting purposes.)

IMPORTANT PREPARATION PRIOR TO A FAST

It is wise to prepare your body for a fast by eating a light diet for at least a week, or even a few weeks, before you fast. A light diet consists of lots of organic raw salads, raw vegetables, sprouts, fresh juices, *Dr. Ann's Energy Soup* (see page 198) and fruit. This allows the body to release some toxicity and acclimate itself to the deep cleansing which will be endeavored with a fast. The light diet gives the body a period of transition until, at the end of the preparation period, you remove all solid food and have just juice and water.

COLON MANAGEMENT DURING A FAST

During a fast you may become constipated because of a lack of fiber. Some practitioners advise having enemas or colonics at this time. You could also add a teaspoon or more of fiber, in a form such as flaxseed meal (freshly ground), into your juice. This will help create enough bulk to stimulate a bowel movement. Colon therapists report that they have seen much old rubbish expelled from the colon during a fast. Many years of impacted "goo and glue" (from flour products and foodless foods) become loosened enough to be expelled with the aid of enemas or colonics. I have seen pictures of some of this waste and it looks like long pieces of black rubbery material. When I was at the Optimum Health Institute, a colon therapist there recounted how she saw a client expel waste of many different colors during a colonic. Later examination of the material showed the presence of crayons, which the person had been carrying around in her colon since childhood! (Children have been known to eat crayons.)

Even though enemas and/or colonics help to cleanse the body of toxic waste material that has accumulated over years, they can also remove some important things that the body needs to function properly. If you do choose to have enemas and/or colonics, I would recommend that you restore the electrolytes immediately afterwards with a wheatgrass juice implant. Also, be sure to reestablish the predominance of friendly bacteria in your colon by doing a course of probiotics, or by drinking Rejuvelac, or eating sauerkraut or other fermented foods.

Some good books to read on colon cleansing are *The Colon Health Handbook* by Robert Gray and *Tissue Cleansing Through Bowel Management* by Dr. Bernard Jensen.

WHEN IS A FAST COUNTERPRODUCTIVE?

A fast could be dangerous if a person is in an extremely toxic state, such as often exists in various disease conditions. A fast could release too much toxicity too fast, and thus impede a safe healing. A fast carried on for too long could create deficiencies in the body which may not show up right away. The staff of the Ann Wigmore Institute of Puerto Rico feels that a diet consisting of *Dr. Ann's Energy Soup, Rejuvelac, Wheatgrass Juice* and blended raw/living foods provides a much safer and slower way to detox than fasting; while at the same time it builds up the body's reserves. They also believe that a fast should only be undertaken under the care of a knowledgeable physician.

> **The purpose of a fast is to cleanse, purify and rejuvenate the body. If a body is too toxic, it is wise to detoxify in small incremental steps, so as not to worsen conditions or endanger health.**

BREAKING THE FAST

Most fasting experts agree that breaking a fast **correctly** is the most important part of the whole experience. This is because by fasting you have initiated profound changes in your body. If a fast is broken with the wrong foods, you may lose all the benefits you have accrued, and even do some damage to your newly cleansed tissues. The best way to break a fast is by eating the same light foods that you consumed in preparing for the fast. (*See* IMPORTANT PREPARATION PRIOR TO A FAST above.) Depending on the length of your fast, eating fresh fruit for one to several days is appropriate. At the Optimum Health Institute in San Diego, a short three-day juice fast is broken with freshly prepared applesauce, followed by watermelon the next morning and salad, sprouts, and some fermented foods for lunch and dinner.

IF I EAT CLEAN, ORGANIC, RAW AND LIVING FOOD ON A DAILY BASIS, WOULD I STILL NEED TO FAST?

My answer to this very logical question is yes, you would still benefit from fasting occasionally.[3] This is because, in today's world, a toxic environment impacts upon us. We absorb toxins which are in the water when we take our showers and baths, from questionable chemicals in our soaps, shampoos, toothpaste, deodorants and cosmetics; and, if we don't eat organic food, from numerous combinations of chemical fertilizers, pesticides, herbicides and fungicides. We have become very indifferent and blasé about these dangers of modern life, but **"cide"** means **"to kill"** and we are killing ourselves every day through our feeding systems and through what is considered "normal, everyday living." We also absorb toxins from the chemicals in our mattresses (which by law are required to be there), from the chemicals put into our rugs, which give off vapors for years (this is called out-gassing), from furniture made from pressboard (which also out-gasses), from wearing clothes that have been dry cleaned with tetrachloroethylene, from using cleaning products in our homes and offices that are made with dangerous chemicals, from coming in contact with arsenic-treated woods (decks, playsets, picnic tables), from breathing chemical air fresheners and from using perfumes. As a result of living in our industrialized society, we absorb toxins from the acid air we're forced to breathe in our cities, from car exhausts, from the exudations of our manufacturing plants, from deadly pesticides sprayed on commuities to control mosquitoes or other insects and from the radiation given off by nuclear power plants all over the world. It doesn't matter from where this radiation escapes; it affects us all because the air currents travel everywhere.

Vaccinations also deliver an assortment of toxins to the body, such as aluminum, mercury, antibiotics, formaldehyde, drugs, GMOs, among other chemicals, and cells from monkeys, horses, dogs, pigs and aborted fetuses. Many parents are rethinking the wisdom of vaccinating their children. Researchers have made a connection between childhood vaccinations and the increasing rate of autism.

And, as if that is not enough, there are numerous other sources of toxins we absorb just by going about our normal daily routine.

Periodic fasting is an excellent way to clean all this out of your system.

---

[3]After an initial clean-out fast tailored to your own specific body needs.

CHAPTER FIVE:
Is Aging Inevitable?

IS AGING NATURAL, NORMAL AND INEVITABLE OR IS IT JUST A SYMPTOM OF SOMETHING THAT HAS GONE TERRIBLY WRONG WITH NATURE'S PLAN?

I do not think aging is natural, normal or inevitable, but rather is a result of choices we make in our lives.

> "We do not degenerate because we grow old . . .
> We grow old because we degenerate!"
> –Ross Horne

At any moment in time, you are either aging or rejuvenating. There is no standing still. You are either going one way or the other **depending on the choices you make:**

- **Food choices—do you eat vibrant live food or processed dead food?**

- **Do you make the effort to drink clean water and breathe clean air?** In former times we could just take it for granted that the air and water were clean but today the situation is different.

- **Do you have a grateful attitude towards life in general; about the life that you are living, in particular; and about all the potential truth and beauty it can unfold?** And if not, are you willing to cultivate a grateful attitude?

- **Do you choose to think life affirming, life sustaining, uplifting thoughts or negative, pessimistic and life depriving thoughts?** Thoughts, feelings and emotions create chemicals in the body just as surely as the food you eat does. Depending on the impact of the specific thoughts or emotions, the chemicals created can be beneficial or damaging to the body. Inharmonious thoughts and feelings create an acid condition in the body.

- **Have you allowed yourself to be burned out by life's troubles (challenges)? Or do you still face each new day with the expectation and fresh hope of uncynical youth?**

- **Exercise and breathing choices—do you find a way to include physical activity in every day or are you sedentary?** And when you do exercise, is it done perfunctorily or with exuberance and fun? Do you find time each day for deep pranic breathing to offset the shallow superficial breathing we engage in most of the time?

- **Do you get out into the sunshine regularly and let the natural light enfold and caress you with its healing brilliance?** Sunshine and natural light are tonics to the body.

- **Lifestyle choices—do you choose clean living with no addictions to smoking, drinking and drugs, no bingeing on food and no "burning the candle at both ends?"**

- **Do you surround yourself with positive, uplifting people or negative people who bring you down and sap your energy?**

- **Do you choose to worry about situations or, confidently and delightfully, visualize what you want to occur?**

- **Do you choose to be happy or unhappy?** Happiness is not something that happens to us but results from an attitude we consciously or unconsciously adopt.

- **Are you happy or unhappy in your chosen work or profession?** And if you're unhappy, do you have some hobby or a vocation you regularly engage in, which brings you joy, satisfaction and fulfillment?

- **Can you depend on yourself and on your word or do you let yourself and others down a lot?**

- **Do you hold a clear and pleasingly youthful image of yourself in your mind's eye, or do you find fault with your looks and put yourself down?** If we see ourselves as youthful we move towards youthfulness; but if we see ourselves as getting old, we inevitably move towards that.

> "Whatever thou seest, that too become thou must;
> God if thou seest God and dust if thou seest but dust"

is a quote that has fascinated me all my life. I don't know who said it. I just believe it to be the way all things work in our lives.

- **Do you choose love (or at least tolerance) over hate?**

- **Do you choose admiration over envy?**

- **Do you follow through on the things which are really important to you, the goals you set for yourself; or do you let them fizzle out?** When you don't follow through, unfulfilled goals and unfulfilled longings become as debris in the body.

- **Do you act on the knowledge and wisdom you have acquired in life or do you try to ignore it, living as if you did not know?** It's been said "Ignorance is bliss," and the reason this is so is because once you know something, once you truly believe something to be true and you then go against that belief by your actions and your words, your body and soul are adversely affected. Along with the acquisition of knowledge and wisdom comes responsibility.

- **Do you take advantage of life's invariable opportunities to cultivate a sense of humor? Do you choose to see the light side of things and not take yourself so seriously?** Laughter is a great healer.

- **Do you choose to find joy in each day of your life or are you waiting for everything to be perfect first?**

ALL of the above impact our rate of aging.

Why would these things contribute to our rate of aging? Because when you're on the positive side of all the above, you are nourishing yourself in diverse ways. Food is nourishment, yes, and the primary subject of this book, but we also receive (or fail to receive) nourishment in many other ways too.

In our world, it seems verboten to go against the established norm of believing in a progression of aging. Most people believe aging is inevitable and so the process of aging becomes a self-fulfilling prophesy. It is difficult to break out of the prevailing mind-set. But you are by now (hopefully) eating "high-raw"[1] . . . and so you've already broken through a few barriers. Harnessing the mind then becomes easier for you.

AGING AND THE ACID/ALKALINE BALANCE

A youthful, healthy body is alkaline. A diseased body is acid. The foods we eat must contribute to the alkaline state of the body. Consume 80 percent alkaline forming foods and 20 percent acid forming foods. If you adhere to this 80/20 principle, and minimize negative emotions, you'll be on your way.

When a body is in an acid state, what neutralizes the acid? Alkaline compounds neutralize acid. That's why you see all those ads on TV and elsewhere advertising products to neutralize acidity. Because they do not deal with the CAUSES of acidity, but only the symptoms, these products do not work in the long run. The Standard American Diet (*see* Glossary) is acid forming. Meat, poultry, fish, wheat, cola and dairy are acid forming. Stress is acid forming. Anger and negative emotions are acid forming.

The issue of acid/alkaline balance can be a little confusing because each organ of the body, as well as the blood and skin, has optimum pH levels that are different. The blood, for example, is slightly alkaline at pH 7.37 to 7.45. In order for the blood to be constantly maintained within this narrow corridor, the body engages in heroic efforts. If the blood gets too acidic, calcium from the bones is dissolved and utilized to adjust the blood's pH. Could this have anything to do with the high incidence of osteoporosis in this country?

---

[1]When you eat 85-100% raw/live foods, you have achieved "high-raw."

The skin has a slightly acid pH because one of the avenues the body uses to expel acid waste is through the skin. Interestingly, the "acid mantle" thus created then protects us by killing bacteria and viruses on the skin.

Other pH values are 1.5 for stomach juice and 8.8 for pancreatic juice.[2] Some authorities say the urine should be acid and others say that the urine must be slightly alkaline. Is it any wonder we are confused?

The waste products created from the body's own process of metabolism are all acid. Protein metabolism produces sulfuric acid and phosphoric acid. Carbohydrate and fat metabolism produce acetic acid and lactic acid. These acids are poisonous and must be washed out of the system on an ongoing basis. First however, they have to be neutralized by carbonic salts, which are composed of alkaline mineral compounds. We must have a reserve of these alkaline minerals available at all times to assist the body to do its work efficiently. This is why a high alkaline diet of fruits, vegetables and sprouts is so important to our health and well-being.

Nobel Prize-winning biologist and surgeon Dr. Alexis Carrel did an experiment in which he kept parts of a chicken heart alive for 28 years in a saline solution which contained a full spectrum of minerals. The solution was changed every day to clean out the wastes. **As long as waste products are disposed of, cells appear to be virtually immortal and cell renewal can go on indefinitely.**

---

[2]From *Acid & Alkaline* by Herman Aihara. Oroville, CA: George Ohsawa Macrobiotic Found.1986.

CHAPTER SIX:
It's a Matter of the Tongue

When switching to a more natural diet it may take time for the tongue to catch up to the new taste. This is because the tongue has been **"pickled"** by all the heavy salt, refined sugar, corn syrup, white vinegar, MSG,[1] nitrates, saccharin, Nutrasweet™, and other chemicals you have been ingesting. It takes approximately two to three months away from all of these things to get the tongue back to normal. Once you get through the initial phase, then you will start to appreciate the **true flavors** of the fresh fruits, vegetables, sprouted nuts, seeds, legumes and grains you are eating.

In the beginning, you may find you have to add a lot more seasoning to the foods to even taste anything. Over time, however, you will add less and less as your tongue normalizes. After you get over the first hurdle, you will be pleased to discover that when you again taste anything "chemicalized," you will be acutely aware of it and you will then recognize the difference between real food and "factory food." A good tongue and sense of smell are your best insurance against eating something not beneficial to you.

I am reminded here of the many times I have fed my cats fresh raw chicken, which they would normally eat. Even though this chicken was meant to be eaten by people, and the animals were hungry, they sometimes rejected it as unsuitable for their consumption. Obviously their sense of what food is fit to eat and what the producers (of chicken) are offering to the public are two different things. However, between these two, I always trust the instincts of the animals. **I am not, however, advocating consumption of meat, raw or otherwise, in a human diet.**

From eating a high-raw diet, you will become so sensitive that you will be able to distinguish, just by taste, which produce was grown with chemicals and which was not. I refer here to fresh raw produce. Once food is cooked and masked with salt, MSG and other chemicals, you will no longer be able to discern the difference, because these additives, particularly MSG, disrupt the normal functioning of your tongue. An **UN**pickled tongue will help bring back your natural instincts.

---

[1]MSG is monosodium glutamate (*see* Glossary).

In switching to raw, the initial phase is the hardest because of several factors. First, the tongue, because it cannot yet appreciate **un**adulterated flavors, impedes your ability to accommodate to a more natural way of eating. It may seem to be telling you "I don't like this," "I don't like that," etc. But if you persevere, you will find that your tongue will change. There will come a day when you will actually start to enjoy these foods **more** than the cooked foods you were formerly accustomed to.

Second, during the transition, you may be detoxing and this brings with it a whole array of symptoms. You may think at first, "This food is not agreeing with me!" But the real story is that YOU are not agreeing with the food. **The raw food is just doing its job, which is to clean up the body systems**. Once these systems are clean, no further symptoms should occur. Remember, the seemingly negative effects of eating raw food actually result from the poor condition of the eater. Once the raw eater has achieved health, the only effects to expect will be incredible energy and a sense of well being.

You may also experience mental and emotional effects as you detoxify, and you may temporarily feel out of sorts and become very emotional. The good news is that all of these effects and symptoms pass away, leaving your body in a much cleaner state than before.

CHAPTER SEVEN:
Vegetarianism and Ecology

It's been said that a plant-based diet is the most compassionate, least destructive way we humans can live upon this planet. Making the changeover, however, is not easily accomplished for most of us who were not raised as vegetarians. It takes belief, dedication and commitment to tread lightly upon the earth. Our present society does not make it easy; we're often made to feel that there is something wrong with us, or that we're too extreme. **In fact, it is the behavior of the civilized world, which has been corrupted by the economics of unbridled, unlimited growth—even to the point of destroying the natural environment—that is too extreme.** We vegetarians are just trying to live wisely and peacefully within it, and to make changes where we can— beginning with ourselves.

A mostly vegetarian planet would resolve so many problems: water problems, land problems, problems of insufficient food for the worldwide population. Yes, other problems would be created in their stead, primarily economic hardship during the time of transition. But once through the chaos, what a beautiful world it would be. I don't know if I'll see this happen in my lifetime, but I hold the vision for future generations.

Historically, many countries have been primarily or largely vegetarian. China and India come to mind. Sometimes the people in these societies are led to believe that an improved standard of living and increased wealth will allow them to obtain the so-called "better things in life"—like meat and processed "luxury" foods. These are things they didn't consume before, because they were economically unable to obtain them. Looking forward to such consumption and considering it an improvement, however, is a false ideal; because with increased consumption of these products, the health of the people deteriorates. This has happened in many societies. So what has been gained?

In his book, *Nutrition and Physical Degeneration*, Dr. Weston Price documented the many ways native people's health deteriorated after the introduction of refined and processed (deficient) "modern" foods into their communities. (*See* Chapter 3, "Some Significant Studies".)

Mother Earth, the planet that feeds and nourishes us, and permits life to even exist, is being systematically destroyed, in large measure today, by multinational corporations whose bottom line does not take into consideration the preservation of the resources which sustain them, and all the rest of us, in the first place. The forests are disappearing; desertification is overtaking our lands; the air and water are clean no longer.

Natural marine animals are being reduced in numbers by our poorly conceived fishing practices, which include mining of the oceans. In the search for a particular fish, nets stretching for miles, which trap everything, are spread out upon the waters. The other sea dwellers, which are caught in these nets, are just tossed away; most of them killed in the process.

Natural animals on land are dying of starvation because we have disrupted their natural habitats. We have taken over the land without making provision for a continuation of their natural environments, even if diminished in size.

Natural animals are also being pushed out by our predilections for the hamburgers of McDonald's and Burger King fame. Forests of all kinds are being cleared to raise the beef for these addictions. And with the forests go the natural animals (becoming extinct), as well as the oxygen we need for our survival. The forests are the lungs of our planet. As verified by analyses of oxygen bubbles trapped in amber, the atmosphere in ancient times contained 38 percent oxygen. In our modern world, the atmosphere contains 20-21 percent oxygen; but in many of our polluted, industrialized cities, could it be lower? Or is it that industrial pollution interferes with our absorption of it?

Natural animals are dying in droves because we carelessly dump all manner of petroleum products and poisons of all kinds into and onto the earth. We are losing species at an alarming rate. Whenever a species is permitted to disappear from the face of our planet, we all become impoverished and die a little. If just **one** species of life of any kind were to be detected in any of the other planets in our solar system, it would create worldwide front page news headlines, **big time**. And yet, the rapid disappearance of numerous species on our own earth appears hardly worthy of mention, except by the environmental organizations struggling valiantly to stem the decimation.

A man in touch with his mother, the earth, could not, would not, do this to her.

And yet the mother is not passive. Metaphysical teachers suggest that the earth is fighting for her life; that the movements of the earth, such as earthquakes, floods, tornadoes, etc., which we term "disasters" because they can destroy the unnatural things we have constructed on its surface, are a way for the earth to right itself, and to cleanse and heal itself. Metaphysical teachers suggest that the great increase in these natural movements of the earth in recent times are related to man's management . . . or more accurately, mismanagement, of the earth.

ANCIENT GUARDIANS OF THE EARTH

Indigenous Indian peoples are the most ancient guardians of our earth; and even into present times, their ancient beliefs in protecting and honoring the Earth Mother are very strong. Those of us who are becoming conscious of environmental issues would do well to align ourselves with native peoples in their continuing struggles to maintain what remains of their tribal lands. Their objectives—to maintain and preserve, or where lost, to reclaim, their ancient cultures (deprecatingly referred to as subsistence economies by Westerners) are right in line with our environmental objective—to put things right in the natural world once again. In recent years, many of the major environmental organizations have also come to recognize that an alliance with Indian causes is in the interest of protecting the earth. Where Indian traditional cultures survive, so there also, the earth survives.

Many Indian Nations and communities have not been traditionally vegetarian; nevertheless, indigenous Indian peoples all over the world share a consciousness of humanity's sacred connections to Mother Earth and of the sanctity of the land, forests, waters, air and creatures. In their way of life, they took from the earth only what they needed for their own survival, and no more. They did not produce surpluses, and if there happened to be a surplus for some reason, it was cause for a celebration or a feast, which would quickly take care of the surplus. When an animal was killed, they used every part of it, so that there was no waste. They did not hunt for sport.

In America, before the arrival of the colonists, millions of buffalo roamed. The flora and fauna were lush and abundant, and the soil was fertile, rich and productive. The waters were clean, and the forests intact. In traditional Indian cultures, all things were shared; there was no individual ownership of land or of any of the gifts of nature. They could not understand how you could own something that the Creator put here for the benefit of all. There were no crimes that they could not deal with, judging by their lack of prisons. There were no hospitals; medicine men capably took care of any health problems. There were no homeless. No one starved (under normal circumstances). An observer would be hard pressed to know that 25 million[1] native people lived here peacefully (for the most part) because they were so well integrated with their environment. Some of the numerous tribes had been here for 5,000 to 40,000 years. The Spanish, French and English, who had battled for possession of this "empty" land, thought of them as ignorant savages; there was even debate about whether they possessed souls.

Just a few hundred years later, the whole panorama of America has changed. Westerners have dug up, cut down and paved over the natural world. The Indians say we have stripped her of her skin. Westerners have stolen most of the Indian lands and murdered most of the Indians. Indians in other parts of the world have not fared well either. While that history is bad enough, **my plea here is for the restoration and preservation of our Earth Mother. What all native peoples believe—so deeply and unwaveringly, about our sacred connections to Mother Earth—these connections must be reawakened in the soul of all people.**

---

[1]"Widely dispersed over the great land mass of the Americas, they {indigenous people} numbered approximately 75 million people by the time Columbus came, perhaps 25 million in North America." Ref: *A People's History of the United States* by Howard Zinn, page 18.

Modern technology on its present course has no respect for nature or for the creatures living in it. Modern technology wants to disconnect us from the umbilical cord which fuses us to the very core of life.

CHAPTER EIGHT:
Irradiated Foods

The plans to irradiate our food supply leave me ALMOST speechless! They are ludicrous. I wish I could just leave the issue there; but I do feel impelled to say more. The technology is not just going to go away quietly, and consumers need to be aware and vigilant to ensure that its use does not become widespread.

In recent years I've noticed that whenever we hear about the uncleanliness of the food supply, whether it is about salmonella poisonings, E. coli, or the various bacterial contaminations (often resulting in massive recalls) of meat, cheese and even produce, the next thing we hear are the proponents of food irradiation stating how this technology will take care of the problem.

BUT WHY CAN'T WE CLEAN UP THE FOOD SUPPLY BY PRACTICING CLEANLINESS? WHY SHOULD PRODUCERS OF FOOD BE ALLOWED TO CONTINUE TO OPERATE IN FILTHY CONDITIONS WHICH LEAD TO CONTAMINATIONS IN THE FIRST PLACE? CLEAN CONDITIONS PRODUCE SAFE, CLEAN FOOD; FILTHY CONDITIONS PRODUCE CONTAMINATION. THAT'S THE BOTTOM LINE. WHAT'S SO HARD TO UNDERSTAND?

WHY ARE THE PRODUCERS OF MEAT ALLOWED TO FEED FARM ANIMALS, WHO ARE BY NATURE HERBIVORES, THE BODIES OF OTHER ANIMALS AND EVEN ANIMALS OF THEIR OWN SPECIES, THEREBY TURNING THEM INTO CANNIBALS?[1] THESE ARE THE CIRCUMSTANCES THAT LED TO BOVINE SPONGIFORM ENCEPHALOPATHY (BSE). THIS DISEASE OF CATTLE IN ENGLAND WAS IMPLICATED IN THE DEVELOPMENT OF nvCJD (CREUTZFELDT-JAKOB DISEASE), A SIMILAR BRAIN-WASTING DISEASE IN HUMANS, WHICH CAUSES HOLES TO DEVELOP IN THE BRAIN.

---

[1]A year after the British Mad Cow fiasco came to a head in 1996 (after percolating for more than ten years), our own FDA mandated a ban on feeding ruminant animal protein to other ruminants. The ban didn't go far enough however, because it excluded blood meal. As stated by Howard Lyman in *Mad Cowboy*, "Instead of making our cattle into full-fledged cannibals, we are now merely turning them into vampires. Spray-dried blood products, which have undergone little or no processing to remove infectivity, are used increasingly in the feed industry."

WHY ARE THE PRODUCERS OF MEAT ALLOWED TO FEED ANIMALS WASTE PRODUCTS, SUCH AS FECAL MATTER?

While filthy conditions and inappropriate feeding practices will always lead to contaminations, a new equation has been added. The beautiful, pastoral farms of our yesterdays have become transformed by agribusiness into the mechanized, assembly line, factory farms of today. Within such factory farms, animals are treated as commodities—mere merchandise (like coal or paper clips)—rather than as the feeling, sentient beings they actually are. The practice of viewing animals with such arrogant disrespect fosters attitudes that sanction our depriving them of any semblance of a quality life and allows us to subject them to all manner of horrendous gross indignities. For example, chickens have their beaks and toes cut off as a matter of course, are kept under fluorescent lights, crowded into wire cages where they can barely move, and forced to breathe ammonia fumes from their own waste. Conditions are deplorable. Then, in an effort to ameliorate the diseases that invariably result, these birds are fed diets laced with antibiotics, sulfa drugs, hormones, arsenic compounds, etc. Can we really expect chicken produced in this way to nourish anyone? **AND ISN'T IT POSSIBLE THAT THE E. COLI, AND OTHER BACTERIAL INFESTATIONS WHICH ARE BECOMING RAMPANT, ARE BEING PRODUCED IN THE BODIES OF THE ANIMALS THEMSELVES AS A RESULT OF THE OBSCENE WAY THEY ARE MISTREATED AND TORTURED?** It is very well known within the industry that these animals are riddled with disease. And while I've used chickens as an example, the same applies to all animals destined for the food market. Factory farming is the norm today. (For more information on the subject, refer to *Diet for a New America* by John Robbins and *Mad Cowboy* by Howard Lyman.)

We don't need food irradiation. We just need a Food and Drug Administration willing to protect the health of the people. Instead, the FDA and the USDA (United States Dept. of Agriculture) are cooperating with and even getting behind the push for this technology. The FDA has approved food irradiation for spices, meat, poultry, fish, fruits and vegetables . . . for practically all food except shellfish. While irradiation is not being carried out on a large scale at present (except for spices), unless the public actively protests, it will only be a matter of time before everything we eat is irradiated.

According to an article in *The Food and Water Journal:*[2]

"Food is irradiated using radioactive gamma sources, usually cobalt 60 or cesium 137[3] or high energy electron beams. The gamma rays break up the molecular structure of the food, forming positively and negatively charged particles called free radicals. The free radicals react with the food to create new chemical substances called 'radiolytic products.' Those unique to the irradiation process are known as 'unique radiolytic products' (URPs).

---

[2]From "Nuclear Lunch: The Dangers and Unknowns of Food Irradiation," *Food & Water Journal*, Fall/Winter 1997/1998. To contact Food and Water, *see* Source Index.

[3]Byproducts of the nuclear energy industry.

"Some radiolytic products, such as formaldehyde, benzene, formic acid, and quinones are harmful to human health. Benzene, for example, is a known carcinogen. In one experiment, seven times more benzene was found in cooked, irradiated beef than in cooked, non-irradiated beef. **Some URPs are completely new chemicals that have not even been identified, let alone tested for toxicity**. {Emphasis added}

"In addition, irradiation destroys essential vitamins and minerals, including vitamin A, thiamine, B2, B3, B6, B12, folic acid, C, E, and K; amino acid and essential polyunsaturated fatty acid content may also be affected. A 20 to 80 percent loss of any of these is not uncommon."

Up until now, the public has been unwilling to accept food irradiation. The labeling for irradiated foods was bold, prominent and conspicuous, requiring the Radura emblem and inclusion of the words "**Treated with Radiation**" or "**Treated by Irradiation**." Recently, in response to pressure from the food industry, two bills were fast-tracked through the House and Senate. These bills, which passed without so much as a hearing, have effectively eviscerated the labeling requirements. The indication that food has been irradiated is now required to be no larger than the lettering used for listing ingredients. This allows the disclosure of irradiation to **hide out** in tiny print, with the Radura emblem no longer a requirement. In addition, the FDA requires labeling only when whole food is irradiated and then sold unchanged. If that same food is processed in any way or if another ingredient is added to it, then no label disclosure is required.

SAFETY STUDIES WERE FLAWED

According to the "Nuclear Lunch" article:

"The FDA reviewed 441 toxicity studies to determine the safety of irradiated foods. Dr. Marcia van Gemert, the team leader in charge of new food additives at the FDA and the chairperson of the committee in charge of investigating the studies, testified that all 441 studies were flawed.

"The government considers irradiation a food additive. In testing food additives for toxicity, laboratory animals are fed high levels (in comparison to a human diet) of potential toxins. The results must then be applied to humans with theoretical models. It is questionable whether the studies the FDA used to approve food irradiation followed this process. In fact, the FDA claimed only five of the 441 were 'properly conducted, fully adequate by 1980 toxicological standards, and able to stand alone in support of safety.' With the shaky assurance of just five studies, the FDA approved irradiation for the public food supply."

Isn't that incredible! And the authors of this article go on to say . . .

"To make matters worse, the Department of Preventative Medicine and Community Health of the New Jersey Medical School found two {of these five} studies were methodologically flawed. In a third study, animals eating a diet of irradiated food experienced weight loss and miscarriage, almost certainly due to irradiation-induced vitamin E dietary deficiency. The remaining two studies investigated the effects of diets of foods irradiated at doses below the FDA-approved general level of 100,000 rads. Thus, they cannot be used to justify food irradiation at the levels approved by the FDA.

" . . . 12 studies carried out by Raltech Scientific Services, Inc. under contract with the U.S. government examined the effect of feeding irradiated chicken to several different animal species. The studies indicated the possibility of chromosome damage, immunotoxicity, greater incidence of kidney disease, cardiac thrombus, and fibroplasia . . . Studies of rats fed irradiated food also indicate possible kidney and testicular damage and a statistically significant increase in testicular tumors. One landmark study in India found four out of five children fed irradiated wheat developed polyploidy, a chromosomal abnormality that is a good indication of future cancer development."

Aside from the direct threats to our health posed by ingesting irradiated foods, there are other dangers associated with this technology. Setting up irradiation facilities all over the country poses serious public health risks to both workers in this industry and to the surrounding communities and increases the chance for accidents to happen. More radioactive materials will then be out on the roads of America, going to and from facilities. Such vehicular accidents as would inevitably occur would increase the risk of high radiation affecting our communities.

And all kinds of accidents have already occurred.

"Workers in irradiation plants risk exposure to large doses of radiation due to equipment failure, leaks, and the production, transportation, storage, installation, and replacement of radiation sources. The Nuclear Regulatory Commission (NRC) has recorded 54 accidents at 132 irradiation facilities worldwide since 1974. But this number is probably low since the **NRC has no information about irradiation facilities in approximately 30 'agreement states'** which have the authority to monitor facilities on their own."[4] {Emphasis added}

Irradiation does not even achieve the goals that its advocates espouse. Quoting again from "Nuclear Lunch":

"Irradiation poses serious risks, and it still does not ensure safe meat. Although it kills most bacteria, it does not destroy the toxins created in the early stages of contamination. And it also kills beneficial bacteria which produce odors indicating spoilage and naturally control the growth of harmful bacteria.

"Irradiation also stimulates aflatoxin production. Aflatoxin occurs naturally in humid areas and tropical countries in fungus spores and on grains and vegetables. The World Health Organization (WHO) considers aflatoxin to be a significant public health risk and a major contributor to liver cancer in the South.

"In addition, irradiation will likely have a mutagenic effect on bacteria and viruses that survive exposure. Mutated survivors could be resistant to antibiotics and could evolve into more virulent strains. Mutated bacteria could also become radiation-resis-

---

[4]From aforementioned article.

tant, rendering the radiation process ineffective for food exposed to radiation-resistant strains.

"Radiation-resistant strains of salmonella have already been developed under laboratory conditions, and scientists at Louisiana State University in Baton Rouge have found that one bacteria occurring in spoiled meat and animal feces can survive a radiation dose five times what the FDA will eventually approve for beef. Scientists exposed the bacteria, called D. radiodurans, to between 10 and 15 kilograys (kGy) of radiation for several hours—enough radiation to kill a person several thousand times over. The bacteria, which scientists speculate evolved to survive extreme conditions of dehydration, survived the radiation exposure."

Personally, what really offends me most about this dubious technology is that it deprives me of my God-given right to use my senses of smell, taste and sight to determine whether a food is fresh, and therefore suitable for eating. When irradiated, food may look fresh but it could be old and rotted. Nature, through her great magnificence, gave me the ability to judge by my senses what is good and whole, pure and fresh. Misguided legislation now wants to take this right away from me.

I hope I have convinced you to oppose this dangerous technology.

Food and Water is an organization that works valiantly to defeat food irradiation and other technologies detrimental to human health and environmental integrity. They can't do it effectively, however, without our **active** assistance. Their **Statement of Purpose** reads:

"Food & Water (F&W) is a national nonprofit, educational organization formed in 1986 by Dr. Walter Burnstein. After more than 25 years as a family physician, witnessing extraordinary increases in degenerative diseases, Dr. Burnstein founded F&W as an extension of his commitment to the prevention of both disease and environmental degradation. F&W educates the general public about various threats to the nutritional integrity of the food and water supply. F&W researches and publicizes environmental and health impacts of food irradiation and other food treatments, before and after harvest. F&W exposes the critical interconnections between health and environmental problems, and challenges the need for technologies, processes or additives that threaten both."

All quoted material was used with permission from Food and Water.

More information on food irradiation can be obtained from the following organizations:

THE CENTER FOR FOOD SAFETY
660 Pennsylvania Ave. SE #302
Washington DC 20003
202.547.9359
Website: www.truefoodnow.org/campaigns/food-irradiation

ORGANIC CONSUMERS ASSOCIATION
6771 So. Silver Hill Dr.
Finland, MN 55603
218.226.4164
Website: www.organicconsumers.org/irradlink.cfm
Website: www.organicconsumers.org/irrad/alternatives.cfm

PUBLIC CITIZEN
215 Pennsylvania Ave. SE
Washington, DC 20003
202.546.4996
Website: www.citizen.org/cmep/foodsafety/food_irrad

CHAPTER NINE:
Frankenfoods: Biotechnology and Genetically Engineered Seeds

Biotechnology is a vast and passionately controversial subject, very much beyond the scope of this book. I would be remiss, however, if I did not address some of the issues because they impact so dramatically and negatively upon organic and sustainable agriculture and also upon the inherent rights to our own genetic material. The most important aspect of this issue, which I believe to be the unconscionable allowance of the patenting of life forms by our government and other governments, began in 1971.

Life forms were endowed with life by their Creator, not by humans, so if anyone should be allowed to hold a patent on them it should be their "true" Creator. **Altering or shuffling a gene or any number of genes in a pre-existing life form is not equivalent to creating a new form of life**. This is because genetic engineers have used the already pre-existing life to supposedly "create" something new and novel. "Biologists who claim patents on life declare that 95 percent of DNA is 'junk DNA,' meaning that its function is not known. When genetic engineers claim to 'engineer' life, they often have to use this 'junk DNA' to get their results."[1] By using such terminology, they demean a process that they little understand, interposing upon it their own version of creation. If altering a gene configuration creates life, then let them try to create life without this so-called genetic debris. It is not the gene itself that is important, but it is the inherent life process of the organism that contains and empowers the gene. The gene can do nothing without the life process of the organism, and the organism only uses the gene in its own development. Biologists are also discovering that it is not solely a one-directional influence of the gene on the organism, but that the organism also interacts with and adds to the gene.

Genetically engineered seeds are being developed to take the place of hybridized seeds, which in their turn displaced heirloom or non-hybridized seeds. Why? It's strictly for profit. You see, it's very simple. With heirloom or non-hybridized seeds, the

---

[1]*Biopiracy - The Plunder of Nature and Knowledge* by Vandana Shiva, Boston, MA: South End Press, 1997.

farmer can collect his own seed each year for replanting the following year. This requires no outlay of cash, except for the cost of labor to collect the seed. This is what has been done for thousands of years. Today, over 1.4 billion people worldwide depend upon saved seeds for food security.

With hybridized seed, on the other hand, a farmer may collect the seed (assuming it is a variety that even produces seeds), but chances are slim to none that this seed will produce a productive plant similar to its parent. So a farmer who plants hybridized seed is forced[2] to buy new seeds every year for planting. A renewable resource has been turned into a nonrenewable resource by the dubious beneficence of technology.

With the recent introduction of genetically engineered seeds, the picture is altered even more. With no testing required by our government because somebody (no doubt, a team of "industry paid" scientists) designated these seeds to be "substantially equivalent" to normally produced seeds, this technology has moved forward with astonishing rapidity in the last four years. Today, it is estimated that fully 60% of all foods offered in the American marketplace contain genetically modified organisms. And, with no labeling requirements, the public has not been given the option to decide against being the guinea pigs in this dangerous experiment. Genetically engineered seeds have consequences in many areas, including:

- **Irrevocable damage to the natural world (nature's natural systems)**

  The results of independent research that is just coming to light, have shown that Monarch butterflies, bees, ladybugs, insects and other wildlife have been killed by ingesting pollen or produce from genetically engineered seeds.

  Pollen from genetically engineered seeds drift over into other non-genetically planted fields, including organic farms, and contaminate the gene pool. The organic farms cannot then sell their crop as organic. Genetic drift has the potential to wipe out organic farming.

  Some genetically engineered seeds have been engineered to have Bt toxin (a naturally occurring insecticide found in the soil) expressed in the plant, so that when insects bite into any part of the plant, they die. These plants are actually registered as insecticides. As is the case with normally produced insecticides, insects develop resistance to them after a few years. The insecticides then have to be reformulated into more lethal brews, or other insecticides have to be substituted. Does this mean the engineered plant's insecticide levels will be increased even further? And what about us poor humans who have to eat a plant that is now a potent insecticide? How about the effects on our body tissues? Have any studies been done on this? The government says no, because of the concept of "substantial equivalence." Most reasonable people understand that there is no equivalence—not by the furthest stretch of the imagination—between seeds which have been evolving and developing spontaneously over millions of years and seeds that have been artificially manipulated in a laboratory.

---

[2]I do mean forced because the seeds that are being offered by the multinational corporations, who now own most of the seed companies worldwide, are almost exclusively hybrid.

Some plants, such as Monsanto's Round-up Ready soybeans, are engineered to withstand much higher dosages of insecticides, which—well, what do ya know—Monsanto also sells, in the form of glyphosate. The legal limits for this insecticide had to be tripled when glyphosate came on the market. Was this a decision made with the health of the people in mind, or was it made to accomodate Big Business Interests? When spray from these potent insecticides drifts over into neighboring farms not planted with the resistant seeds they can kill the plants. The pollen from Round-up Ready soybeans can also contaminate wild relatives, creating super weeds.

- **Damage to human and animal health**

Dr. Arpad Pusztai, a well-respected researcher at the Rowett Research Institute in Scotland, conducted a study feeding rats genetically engineered potatoes for ten days. Two control groups were also employed in this study. After the ten days, tests showed that the rats fed the altered potatoes had damaged immune systems, and the weight of all their organs, including kidneys, heart, liver, etc., had decreased. Forty-eight hours after announcing these findings on a television program, Dr. Pusztai was relieved of his position.

Dr. Marc Lappe, in an independent study, found that phytoestrogen levels were greatly reduced in GM soybeans as opposed to non-GM soybeans. (Ref: Alterations in Clinically Important Phytoestrogens in Genetically Modified, Herbicide-Tolerant Soybeans. Journal of Medicinal Food, 1999, Vol. 1, No. 4)

- **Endangering indigenous peoples' food security, worldwide**

The livelihood and food security of native farmers and indigenous peoples all over the world are threatened by patents on seeds. In addition, there are terminator technologies being developed in which seed is programed to kill its own progeny.

- **Concentrating the world's seed supply into fewer hands**

This devastatingly damaging and irrevocable technology is being promoted solely for the purpose of concentrating the world's food supply into a few hands. Seeds are being genetically manipulated in a laboratory and all kinds of abominations are being perpetrated. To these "scientific minds," the transferring of genes across species lines (such as putting virus, bacteria or animal genes into fruits and vegetables) is just "business as usual." Genetically engineered seed can be legally patented so that farmers are prevented from collecting and replanting this seed, under the threat of prosecution. And farmers are also denied access to open-pollinated seeds because they are no longer made available.

SELF-DETERMINING LIFE FORMS

Seeds and the plants they grow into are self-determining, self-organizing life forms. No one tells them how to grow or form or live or breathe or whether to fruit or not or how to adapt to changing environmental conditions, or how to heal and repair themselves. They do all those things (and much more) on their own. No one created them in a laboratory. They were produced by the Creator of our earth to be as free as the air and the oceans, the rivers and the forests. By providing freely reproducing seeds, Nature is taking care of her own. Her intent is to provide all things of the earth freely for the use and sustenance of the earth and its creatures (humans included). Indigenous peoples in their native cultures have known and lived in harmony with the earth for many thousands of years. That's why private ownership of land was such an alien concept to them. To patent a life form is like putting a meter on our intake of air, which, at least for the present, is free for the breathing!

Genetically engineered seed is being pitched to the farmers as this great new, advanced seed, which will resist insect infestations and produce grandiose harvests beyond anyone's wildest dreams. This is the same hype pitched during the Green Revolution, but with potentially more dangerous outcomes. While the misnamed "Green Revolution" produced in its wake a poisoning of the earth with its accelerated use of pesticides and chemicals, the unchecked and unwise push forward with biotechnology may result in a barren earth. We have no way of knowing the outcome without judicious research, which has been pushed aside in the lightning rush for financial gains. (Sales of patented products can be made at whatever price the market will bear, with no fear of competition from others.)

We just don't know what the future effects of genetically altering life forms will be. Monsanto has genetically engineered a resistant strain of soybean to increase sales of its herbicide, Roundup. This soybean is overtaking the market right now.

In the natural world, Nature has placed constraints against cross-breeding—biological barriers which prevent most species from interbreeding. Could it be that in Nature's wisdom, these restrictions are essential to maintaining life's integrity and balance? Much of the genetic altering being done is across species lines, such as inserting a fish gene into a tomato or a moth or pig gene into a potato. For the great "advantage" of having a potato plant glow in the field when it needs water, jellyfish genes have been spliced into potatoes. (Why not just stick your finger into the soil to see if it's dry?) Nature has never done anything like this and on the rare occasions that remotely similar things have occurred in nature, freaks have been the result! We are tampering with things that we have no way of putting right, should the experiment fail. Once a genetically engineered organism is released into the atmosphere it will freely and spontaneously mix with wild species and then those will be unalterably changed forever, as far as we know. And for what? So someone can charge yearly for this seed? So someone can charge a royalty or "technology fee" for use of the patent, in addition to the cost of the seed? So a corporation can sue a farmer for infringing on its "patent," if the seed is planted for more than the one crop for which it was licensed? And what about our right to live as a vegetarian, if we so choose? It seems that this right is being usurped, because we are no longer able to recognize an altered plant product containing animal genes from a normal one.

The very sanctity of life on earth, as we know it, is being threatened. While I have only mentioned briefly the transgressions being perpetrated on the life of seeds, the same genetic manipulations are being visited upon all forms of life, from viruses and bacteria on up to cows, pigs, goats, sheep, and humans. Is this what we, as a people, really want? Have we become so disconnected from the natural world that we cannot see that this ominous interference in the very processes of life is like a toddler playing with a loaded gun? To quote the eminent biochemist, Erwin Chargaff, "I consider the attempt to interfere with the homeostasis of nature as an unthinkable crime."[3]

As I write these few lines, fields planted with genetically altered seeds are being burned in Europe, India and other parts of the world. Who is doing the burning? People who have taken the law into their own hands because the law is not lawful. We cannot let the greed of our market economy, whose bottom line is always profits, dictate the destruction of a heritage that belongs to us all, including future generations. I'm not advocating burning fields, but we can start by demanding that all genetically engineered foods be clearly labeled, in **LARGE PRINT**, no hiding the facts. We can become part of the solution by not purchasing any genetically altered produce or any products (like some supplements) which contain them. Two-thirds of all cheese at the present time is processed with genetically engineered organisms and one-third of all the milk is from cows that have been fed the genetically engineered hormone, rBGH. And of course, we can write letters to our leaders in Washington. Hopefully, some of them are still conscious, and will respond in a positive way to the will of the people, as opposed to the swill of the multinational corporations.

MEDDLING AND TAMPERING WITH THE PROCESSES OF LIFE CREATION SHOULD NOT BE IN THE HANDS OF PRIVATE CORPORATE INTERESTS.

IS ALL OF THIS TECHNOLOGY DETRIMENTAL?

There may be some positive advances, non-threatening to the earth, which could be gleaned from **certain aspects** of biotechnology. But the sane way to proceed is with **slow** and wise research. The Five (later six) Nations of the Iroquois Confederacy, as well as other indigenous peoples, demonstrated a reverence for life when they based their decisions upon the impact that these decisions would ultimately have on the seventh generation ahead. This is wise; this is taking care of our children, and grandchildren, and great grandchildren, their children, their grandchildren, and on into the seventh generation. If we could also do that, we could go back, perhaps not to a simpler life, but at least to a course of action which is based upon the sacredness of all life, upon caring for our progeny and for the earth which supports us all.

NEW INFORMATION UPDATE: 2002

In order to speed up the scanning process at the checkout counter, a system utilizing sticky labels has been devised. Sticky labels on fruits and vegetables, and soon to be on herbs, dried fruits and nuts, carry information. And lucky for us this information includes whether the produce is organic, genetically engineered or conventionally grown. It is called a PLU code.

---

[3]*Heraclitean Fire* by Erwin Chargaff, Rockefeller University Press, 1978.

For conventionally grown produce, the PLU code on the sticker consists of 4 numbers. Organically grown produce has a 5-number PLU prefaced by the number 9. Genetically engineered produce has a 5-number PLU prefaced by the number 8. So, a conventionally grown banana would be 4011, an organic banana would be 94011, and a genetically engineered banana would be 84011.The numeric system was developed by an affiliate of the Produce Marketing Association in Newark, Delaware. Their phone number is 302.738.7100 and website www.PLUcodes.com

Jeffrey Smith, a leading author, activist and speaker on the genetic engineering of foods says that there are no government regulations in place to require a producer of GE foods to place their food in the GE category of the PLU code.

GE companies are not stupid and they know that in numerous polls 80% of the people want GE food to be labeled and they also know that once labeled, people will reject this food in the marketplace, as they have done in Europe.

More information on biotechnology can be obtained by contacting the following organizations.

INSTITUTE FOR RESPONSIBLE TECHNOLOGY
641.209.1765
Website: www.responsibletechnology.com

THE CENTER FOR FOOD SAFETY
660 Pennsylvania Ave., SE, Ste. 302
Washington, DC 20003
202.547.9359
Website: www.truefoodnow.org

INTERNATIONAL CENTER FOR TECHNOLOGY ASSESSMENT
202.547.9359
Website: www.icta.org

THE ORGANIC CONSUMERS ASSOCIATION
6671 So. Silver Hill Dr.
Finland, MN 55603
218.226.4164
Website: www.organicconsumers.org

**NW RAGE
NORTHWEST RESISTANCE AGAINST GENETIC ENGINEERING**
P.O. Box 15289
Portland, OR 97293
503.239.6841
Website: www.nwrage.org

THE ALLIANCE FOR BIO-INTEGRITY
2040 Pearl Lane #2
Fairfield, IA 52556
206.888.4852
Website: www.biointegrity.org

GREENPEACE WORLDWIDE
Website: www.greenpeace.org/usa/ campaigns/genetic-engineering

MOTHERS FOR NATURAL LAW
Website:
www.safe-food.org/welcome.html

ETC GROUP
431 Gilmour St., 2 Fl.
Ottawa, ON Canada K2P OR5
613.241.2267
Website: www.etcgroup.org

THE COUNCIL FOR RESPONSIBLE GENETICS
5 Upland Road, suite 3
Cambridge, MA 02140
617.868.0870
Website:
www.councilforresponsiblegenetics.org

CHAPTER TEN:
Supplements—Yes, No, or Maybe?

The very word "supplements" implies they are to be viewed as supplemental to something else. After experiencing raw/live foods for yourself, I hope you will perceive supplements only as adjuncts to a basic raw/live food diet. The optimum diet comes first; then if you have extra funds to spend, you could add some wisely selected supplements. Of course, if you have known deficiencies, an appropriate supplement would be indicated. A much better solution, however, would be to find the reason for the deficiencies and then seek to remedy the situation at its source.

Contemporary thinking has a different perspective on supplements. Its skewed reasoning goes something like this: Eat anything you like, and then for insurance, to make sure you're not missing any important nutrient (or to compensate for eating too many "junky, foodless foods"), take a synthetic daily multiple vitamin-mineral tablet. This pattern of thinking is similar to the way people have been conditioned to think about drugs. Have a pain? Obliterate it with a pill, at least temporarily. (Pain or any other symptom should be viewed as an advance warning of something gone awry in the body; something to be looked into rather than suppressed.) **You can't make your eating habits right by taking pills, even those based on whole foods**.

Ideally, every nutritional element that our bodies need should be contained in the food we eat, or should be produced by the body itself. There has been much talk lately within health circles about the diminishing quality of our food supply. Generally, our soils are deficient in minerals, and so the foods grown on them are also deficient. The nutritional picture is much better for organically grown foods, produced under optimum conditions.

There are other reasons why our bodies become depleted of nutrients. Living or working under fluorescent lights makes us deficient in Vitamin A. Stress burns up pantothenic acid (one of the B-complex vitamins), which is needed by the adrenal glands. Antibiotics put into foods, such as fish and dairy, kill off beneficial intestinal bacteria, thereby allowing candida and other less than friendly strains to predominate. Any foreign materials not intrinsic to naturally grown food (such as pesticides and fungicides) use up Vitamin C and other antioxidants. These are just a few examples. When you clean up your diet and your lifestyle, much of this will no longer occur.

WHAT KIND OF SUPPLEMENTS ARE COMPATIBLE WITH THE RAW/LIVE FOOD LIFESTYLE?

Most supplements are formulated from chemical ingredients instead of from whole, raw foods. The word "natural" is meaningless when it comes to choosing quality supplements. You must dig deeper, read the fine print and ask questions if you want to get something that is worth putting into your body.

> The way to choose a food supplement that is compatible with the raw/live eating style is to first be sure it is derived from an organically grown, whole raw or live food. Then confirm that it is processed at low heat, in such a way that its enzymes and other naturally occurring factors are preserved intact.

The most beneficial way to add supplemental vitamins, minerals, phytochemicals and enzymes to the diet is to drink one or more glasses of **fresh**, organic vegetable (or fruit) juice or a bowl of *Dr. Ann's Energy Soup* each day. Fresh wheatgrass juice, juice from sprouted greens or green leafy vegetables and fresh herbal juices are wonderful also and rich in chlorophyll, which delivers oxygen to the body. Nutrients obtained through these freshly made raw juices and whole blender soups are readily absorbed by the body because they are in their optimum organic form; much superior to vitamin and mineral tablets. Juices are foods, of course, and not generally thought of as supplements. But if you want to supplement your diet, I believe juices are a better choice than synthetics.

A convenient alternative to fresh green juices (but definitely a second choice) is the low-heat processed, dried green powders that have become readily available, such as chlorellas, spirulinas, blue-green algae, wheat, barley and other grasses, etc. Make sure they are processed in such a way so as to retain their life force and enzymes.

Edible weeds make beneficial substitutes for vitamin pills. They can be dried thoroughly, then ground and stuffed into vegetable capsules (made from cellulose).

Vitamin C is a wonderful nutrient with many beneficial effects. It is found abundantly in all fresh fruits, vegetables and sprouts. If you feel you need more of it, there is a supplement made of low-heat processed acerola cherries that is available. It is a powder that can be stirred into carrot and other juices. A 1.5 tsp. serving provides 270 mg. of naturally occurring, non-toxic, highly absorbable vitamin C. It is the only supplement of its kind that I have found, and it is available from Healthforce Nutritionals (*see* Source Index).

Most vitamin C supplements, even though they may have a token amount of some natural ingredients added, such as acerola cherries or rose hips, are made primarily with synthetic and/or isolated ingredients. (An isolate is a single factor that has been separated out, thus isolated.) **Synthetic vitamin C mixed with whole foods is not the same as vitamin C contained IN whole foods.** Even though the dosage of the synthetic may be high and concentrated, it is still a fractionated product. Natural foods do not exist as isolates. Nature puts things together as complexes, with a myriad of factors working together synergistically. The C family of vitamins is a complex which includes a large group of compounds known as bioflavonoids.

B-complex vitamins are a large family found in a wide variety of foods, including brightly colored fruits and vegetables, green leafy vegetables, bee propolis, sprouted and unsprouted grains, seeds, nuts and some roots. Bee pollen and royal jelly are rich in pantothenic acid (Vitamin B-5). Pantothenic acid is a substance that gets used up in our bodies when we are under stress. Because of the stressors of modern life, it could be said that most of us (who do not learn to control or alleviate stress) are deficient in pantothenic acid at certain times or to some degree. Royal jelly is also rich in niacin (Vitamin B-3). Niacin helps alleviate irritability, and mellows the personality. For those who are not totally vegan and can tolerate bee products, they serve as a rich font of absorbable pantothenic acid and niacin. Find a source that is low-heat processed. Some health food stores and herbalists carry them fresh and refrigerated.

Lactobacillus acidophilus, bifidus, bulgaricus and other strains of friendly intestinal bacteria are sometimes useful as supplements. Purchase those that are kept refrigerated. These are the **active** cultures. Many things can upset the bacterial balance in the intestines and tip the scale in favor of negative bacteria (such as candida albicans). We all have some candida, but its proliferation means that there is an imbalance. You can assist your body to colonize the friendly bacteria (which keep candida in check) by adding these supplements as well as live sauerkraut, seed cheeses and/or *Rejuvelac* (*see* page 227) to your diet. When a good colony of friendly bacteria is present in the gut, your digestion and assimilation improve. These friendly bacteria produce B-complex vitamins too, including B-12. They also produce vitamin K.

Another way to supplement your diet when you think you need more of a particular vitamin, mineral or amino acid, is with herbs. Herbs are Nature's Pharmacy and, with the exception of culinary herbs, edible weeds and some others, I only recommend them for short-term application. I believe that herbs, however, are a better choice than synthetic vitamins and minerals. For example, if you need iron, yellow dock root or nettles contain organic iron. Oat straw is rich in silicon and calcium; chaparral contains potassium and sodium; safflower contains vitamins F and K. To find the appropriate herbs compatible with your body chemistry, kinesiology[1] is suggested.

Seaweeds or sea vegetables are foods rich in minerals. If you cannot cultivate a taste for them, you could take them in supplement form.

Exposing your skin to some natural sunlight every day serves as a supplement too, free for the taking. Sunlight helps our bodies synthesize nutrients, such as vitamin D. Contrary to popular opinion, the sun is not our enemy. Sunlight is beneficial to our health. People are being programmed to believe, without foundation in fact, that sunshine causes cancer. Sunlight may bring cancer to the surface of the body (as believed by Natural Hygienist T.C. Fry) but it does not cause cancer. The cancer rate has accelerated to an unprecedented degree only in the last 100 years. Sunlight has been around for eons. Former civilizations did not get cancer from the sun, and neither do we.

---

[1]Kinesiology or Muscle Response Testing technique is outlined in the book, *The Ultimate Healing System*, by Dr. Donald Lepore, N.D. Provo, UT: Woodland Books, 1988.

ARE ALL SYNTHETICALLY PRODUCED VITAMINS AND MINERALS WITHOUT VALUE?

NO, NO, NO; I AM NOT SAYING THAT! How could I go against the zillion studies that prove the value of vitamins and minerals? Too much research has shown these to have their appropriate application.

I **am** saying that the **OPTIMUM** supplements are whole food based, low-heat processed, additive free, and therefore compatible with the raw/live food lifestyle. We could, however, prevail upon manufacturers to give us what we want in a supplement by persuading them to produce more products that meet these standards.

UNDESIRABLE ASPECTS OF SOME VITAMIN/MINERAL SUPPLEMENTS

1) Following the pattern of the drug industry, the manufacturers of many "natural" supplements include synthetic fillers and other additives in their products. These come in the form of binders, lubricants, diluting agents, plasticizers, aromatics, hydrocarbons (such as paraffin or wax), dyes, flavoring matter, etc. These include, among others too numerous to list here, magnesium and calcium stearate, lactose (milk sugar), titanium and silicon dioxide, shellac, hydroxy propyl cellulose and methylcellulose, talc, sucrose, sodium benzoate, BHT, BHA, hydrogenated cottonseed oil, sorbic acid, cornstarch, etc., etc., etc.

2) Gelatin capsules are almost exclusively used. They are made out of boiled dead animal cartilage, bones, hoofs, horn and skin, usually from a cow, bull or pig. Gelatin is highly processed and decolorized with sulfurous acid. Glue is an impure form of gelatin.

3) Increasing numbers of supplements may be made or processed with genetically engineered organisms. A few years back, L-tryptophan, a naturally occurring amino acid, was banned from the marketplace because a genetically engineered version of L-tryptophan caused 37 deaths. This tragedy also permanently disabled 1,500 people and left thousands more very ill. To know for sure whether your favorite supplement contains or is processed with genetically engineered organisms, write to the manufacturer.

4) Full disclosure of all ingredients on the label is not a legal requirement. To obtain full disclosure, you must write the manufacturer and request it.

According to Canadian author Dr. Zoltan P. Rona, "Although it is true that most healthy people will have no obvious side effects from ingesting the small amount of toxins found in cheap vitamins, the long term consequences of continuous, daily intakes are potentially dangerous . . . Based on all this information, the best advice would be to purchase supplements in vegetable capsules, naturally compressed tablets, powders or liquids that contain the fewest possible additives."[2]

---

[2]From "Hidden Hazards of Vitamin and Mineral Tablets" – Website: www.srvitamins.com

CHAPTER ELEVEN:
A Little Controversy...

DISAGREEMENTS WITHIN THE MOVEMENT; OPPOSING VIEWS

In every system of health maintenance there is always some controversy. Remember however, that while the controversies may rage on and on, you, as an individual, can decide what works best for you. People become confused when they hear opposing viewpoints; one says black, the other says white, yet a third advocates gray. My advice is to pass all information (including mine) through the filter of your own intelligence and reach your own conclusions. You do not have to wait for the final word to proceed. Following are some pros and cons (as well as other ideas) regarding some of these issues.

ARE HERBS AND SPICES BENEFICIAL?

Some proponents of raw and living foods suggest that there is something wrong with herbs and spices; that somehow they are not compatible with the live foods eating style and philosophy. They say that if you cannot make an entire meal of some item, then it shouldn't be eaten at all. While it's true you cannot eat an entire meal consisting of herbs[1] and spices, I still do not think this is a good enough reason to discard them. Who made this rule, anyway? I believe nature put these wonderful things here for our health, pleasure and delight.

These same teachers suggest that we learn to appreciate the flavor of different foods on their own. For example, we should learn to savor and enjoy the flavors of vegetables such as zucchini, corn, or cabbage, without enhancement.

I understand this point of view and agree that we can learn to appreciate these foods on their own, but for me, doing so does not preclude the use of herbs and spices. After all, herbs and spices also originate from nature and have been used since antiquity to enhance or bring out the flavors of foods. Since we're not cooking the food,

---

[1]With the exception of edible weeds, which are sometimes referred to as herbs.

very little is needed, but this is an individual preference. Some people like more, some less, some none. An organic cucumber eaten straight out of my garden tastes wonderful to me; but when I bring it in, slice it up thin and put a sprinkle of dill or cumin on top, it tastes wonderful again, but in a different way. I like variety, and the use of herbs and spices gives me a **world of variety** in my menus. It keeps me interested and satisfied and makes me want to adhere to the lifestyle more faithfully. Again, this is a matter of individual choice and preference. Please find what works best for you.

Spices are derived from the fragrant or pungent parts of plants, which include bulbs, barks, rhizomes, stigmas, flower buds, fruits and seeds. Spice seeds are the tiny aromatic fruits and seeds of herbaceous plants. Herbs are usually considered to be the fragrant leaves of plants.

Some plants are both an herb **and** a spice. Cilantro (a leafy green herb) and coriander seed (the spice) are the same plant, harvested at different stages of development. Dill weed (the herb) and dill seed (the spice) are another example of both an herb and a spice derived from the same plant.

I believe culinary herbs and spices are beneficial to the body in ways that are just now being rediscovered. In ancient times, spices were used both in medicine and for preserving foods. I believe non-culinary herbs have their place also, but only for short periods of time and in response to specific bodily needs or conditions.

Turmeric is a spice with a long tradition of use in India and China. It is one of the main ingredients in curry powder. Now, I see it sold in health food stores, encapsulated, and promoted as an antioxidant. It's said to improve liver function, alleviate gastrointestinal complaints, eliminate parasites, and is also used to treat inflammations. It has proven effective for treating viral hepatitis, eliminating jaundice, relieving pain and reducing the size of diseased livers.

Fenugreek Seed, also used in curry powder, has great phlegm-expelling properties, and in the form of fenugreek sprouts, is used as a liver detox in many health spas. According to herbalist Maria Treben, in her book *Health Through God's Pharmacy*, ground fenugreek, combined with yarrow tea, has been used successfully for atrophy of the bones, osteomyelitis and bone growth.

Cayenne Pepper was used extensively by Dr. John Christopher, a renowned herbalist in the early part of the 20th century. Dr. Christopher used cayenne as a life saving remedy for people suffering heart attacks. He also used cayenne to improve blood circulation, and to stop both internal and external bleeding.

Horseradish is known for its mucus-dissolving properties and for alleviating sinus congestion. Try eating just a little bit and you'll experience its powerful effect.

Ginger is a spice that is good for the circulation. Ginger gets things moving. A one-inch piece, juiced, may be added to certain other juices to give them zing. Ginger is very warming to the body, and good for people who say they don't like to eat raw foods because they're too cold. Use a little ginger where appropriate, and you won't be cold.

Ginger has also been used to alleviate nausea and motion sickness. Some people who rev themselves up with coffee might try using ginger instead.

Ginger tea is wonderfully stimulating. You can make it by pressing one, two or three pieces of fresh ginger through a garlic press to get the juice, then add hot water (don't boil), and enjoy. Set aside a special garlic press just for ginger, because you don't want your ginger tea to taste like garlic, unless you're making garlic and ginger tea, which is also very good. Don't put honey in your ginger tea even if you like it sweet, because it takes a lot of honey to sweeten a cup of tea. Put the honey into a teaspoon instead, then sip the tea and lick the honey; sip the tea, lick the honey. It's just as satisfying and you won't be ingesting so much concentrated sugar.

Basil aids digestion and has calming properties.

Anise, Fennel, Dill and Caraway Seeds are useful for, among other things, alleviating gas and indigestion, and they increase the quantity of a mother's milk.

Sage, on the other hand, decreases mother's milk.

Numerous other herbs and spices come to mind, many of which are now finding their way into supplements that support or benefit health. But why not obtain these same benefits more gently, through your daily food consumption? (*See* Chapter 10, "Supplements—Yes, No, or Maybe?")

NOT ALL SPICES ARE FOR ALL PEOPLE

We are each biochemically unique, so what may offer the greatest benefit for one might be less advantageous or even detrimental to another. With experimentation, you can find the spices compatible with your own particular body chemistry. Dr. Roger Williams wrote a number of excellent books on the subject of biochemical individuality (*see* Bibliography).

DO HERBS AND SPICES INCREASE YOUR APPETITE?

Another opinion frequently voiced about herbs and spices is that they titillate your appetite and thereby cause you to eat more than is desirable. You won't know when to stop eating. In my experience I have not found this to be true for most people. The people who don't know when to stop eating are either those whose "appestats"[2] aren't telling them when they're full, or those who are using food as a sedative. After eating a high-raw diet for some time, their bodies will become more fully nourished. They will then find that the craving to overeat decreases and gradually disappears.

---

[2]For suggestions on normalizing your appestat and easing emotional overeating *see* Chapter 16, "Looking For A Better Way."

Why make the elimination of herbs and spices an ironclad rule for everyone when herbs and spices do not affect everyone in the same way? If you find that they stimulate your appetite, and you're eating more than is comfortable for you, then you can adjust your recipes accordingly. On the other hand, I have found that people who are dealing with health challenges, and who need to maintain their weight because they are getting too thin, will eat more if the food has flavor for them, than if it is bland. They are then better able to keep up their weight. Flavorful food also stimulates the secretion of digestive enzymes, which are necessary for good digestion.

In some cases, the absolute elimination of certain spices is essential for recovery. Dr. Max Gerson, a medical doctor who devised a nutritional approach for the healing of cancer with great success (back in the 1940s), worked with many herbs and spices. He found that while some were OK, others interfered with healing. In The Gerson Therapy, the herbs and spices allowed in very small quantities were allspice, anise, bay leaves, coriander, dill, fennel, mace, marjoram, rosemary, sage, saffron, tarragon, thyme, sorrel and summer savory. Chives, onions, garlic and parsley could be used in larger amounts.

OVEREATING ON COOKED VS. RAW FOOD

It's much easier to overeat on cooked food than on raw food because cooked food, being mushy and of soft consistency, doesn't seem to require much chewing. Raw foods, on the other hand, by their very nature, must be masticated in order to get them down. When consuming raw and living foods that have been juiced, puréed or made into a paté, we must make a conscious effort to masticate in order to release the digestive enzymes in the mouth and mix them with each bite of food.

The problem of insufficient chewing is a major impediment to trouble-free digestion. Every time I think of the customary bolting of food that goes on when people eat junk or fast foods, or really any kind of food, I always hear (in my mind) Lalita, a teacher and co-administrator of the Ann Wigmore Institute in Puerto Rico, saying "we must chew, chew, chew and chew and chew and chew." And I see her sweet, angel face demonstrating for the entire class the importance of chewing for optimum digestion and assimilation. You can just imagine the expressions on the faces of her students, most of whom have never been exposed to this idea before. Chewing each bite 30 to 50 times[3] can seem quite bizarre until you understand the reasoning behind it! Foremost in importance is breaking the food down to an emulsion, which gets mixed with enzymes that are secreted in the mouth. This is the first stage of digestion. Thorough chewing also releases the cellulase enzyme from the cellulose fiber that coats all fruits and vegetables. Releasing the cellulase enzyme is absolutely essential, since cellulase is not produced by the body. When food goes down the throat in a soupy form,

---

[3]Horace Fletcher popularized chewing, which he termed "fletcherizing," in his book entitled The ABZ of Our Own Nutrition (out of print).

with enzymes intact, it becomes much, much easier for the body to extract nutriment from it. Digestion is then faster and more efficient.

Mollie and Eugene Christian, who wrote *Uncooked Foods & How to Use Them* in 1904, state "From memory we made an inventory of the quantity of food consumed by one of the most advanced disciples of French cookery; and according to our best calculations if the same quantity of material had been eaten in its elementary state and thoroughly masticated it would have taken about thirty-one hours' continuous chewing to have disposed of the cargo." This means that when you eat raw food, you need **much less food** to nourish yourself and be satisfied.

Dr. Ann Wigmore created her famous "Energy Soup" to solve several problems, both for herself and for her students. First, because she was a busy woman, she wanted to optimally feed herself without spending the 1/2 to 3/4 of an hour necessary to chew everything thoroughly. (You must still chew the soup to mix it with the salivary enzymes, but not as much as with a salad, for example.) Secondly, some people don't have the teeth to chew well, and the blended Energy Soup solved this problem as well. For people with "health challenges," the soup is easily assimilated, without taxing the digestive system. Energy Soup simultaneously cleanses and nourishes the body without compromising valuable vitamin and mineral reserves that are sometimes lost during a water or juice fast. At the Ann Wigmore Institute in Puerto Rico, where I have been a guest on numerous occasions, Energy Soup is always available. During my visits, I have witnessed many people recover their health in very short periods of time.

I love to chew, but when I'm having a hectic day, it's either *Dr. Ann's Energy Soup* or *Green Power Soup* for me! (*see* Index).

The bottom line is: When you eat raw, you need much less food to satisfy both your natural appetite and the body's nutritional needs. In the beginning, however, while making the transition to raw, it may seem that you're eating more, and indeed you may be. For a period of time, while the food is doing its work repairing the body and bringing its systems to their normal state of health, you may be hungry all the time. But once the body cells become fully nourished, this condition passes.

RAW FOOD VS. LIVING FOOD

As defined by the Ann Wigmore Institute in Puerto Rico, Living Food consists of fresh, organic vegetables, sprouts, nuts and seeds whose enzymes have been activated by soaking, sprouting and/or fermenting. These foods are **easy to digest**. Some examples are soaked, blended almonds and sprouted seeds. A nut or seed in its raw state contains enzyme inhibitors. These inhibitors allow the nut or seed to remain in a dormant state until conditions are right for it to sprout. When you soak seeds and nuts in water, you remove the enzyme inhibitors. The peeling of nuts, such as almonds, removes tannins that are concentrated in the skin. Soaked and blended nuts then become easier to digest. Another example of a living food is veggiekraut, which is made from raw cabbage, carrots, and beets. Cabbage consumed in its raw state may cause the production of gas in the digestive tract, which is discomforting. Properly fermented cabbage and vegetables are rich in enzymes which enable the body to digest and assimilate nutrients efficiently, without forming gas. Friendly bacteria (e.g., acidophilus and bifidus cultures), which facilitate the veggiekraut fermentation process, help to maintain a healthy colon and a strong immune system. According to the teachings of the Ann Wigmore Institute, a combination of raw foods[4] and living foods provides a wonderful balance of vitamins, minerals, and enzymes that the body needs to function optimally.

I've heard other teachers make a distinction between raw food and living food, by saying that living food is superior. What they mean by living food is **sprouts**, because sprouts are still sprouting (thus living), as you eat them. Sprouts are very excellent food, superior in many ways. But I wouldn't want to limit myself to just sprouts, when nature has provided such a **gloriously bountiful feast**. Why forgo all the other delicious vegetables and fruits just because they don't sprout? (Actually, anything that contains a seed or any root vegetable is capable of sprouting also. You would not want to eat roots that have sprouted, however, as their sprouting indicates that the roots are past their prime.)

What is really being addressed here is the concept of life-force. To contain a vibrant life-force, fruits and vegetables must be as fresh as you can get them. Their nutritional value **really does** begin to **decrease** soon after they are harvested. Ideally, produce should be picked, prepared and eaten within a few hours. In our modern society, this seldom occurs. Suppliers say they cannot do it; that it is not practical. What they are really saying is that they do not want to be bothered to design a new method or system for bringing food to us, fresh from the fields. **It can be done and it will be done as soon as enough of us request the changes.** Eating locally grown produce cuts a few days off the transit time needed to get food to the market.

For optimum nutrition, try to buy your produce from an organic vendor at a farmer's market, as the produce here has just been harvested. Or shop at a food co-op, as food usually moves fast at co-ops. At least find out what day the produce comes in at the supermarket, so you can buy it on that day.

Best of all, of course, is to grow your own or part of your own produce organically, and with heirloom type seeds. Nothing can compare with going to your own garden and picking the ingredients for a fresh, delectable salad. If you don't have space for an outdoor garden, you could grow indoor greens such as buckwheat lettuce, sunflower greens, wheatgrass and herbs.

OILS—YES OR NO?

Some live food advocates reject the use of oils in the preparation of their food. They say we can get all the oil (fat) we need, in its natural state, from nuts, seeds, avocados, etc., and they are correct. We can get all we need this way and it is prime. Using

---

[4] raw fruits and vegetables ready to eat straight from the orchard or garden.

genuinely cold-pressed oils, however, will give you a little more flexibility in preparing some of your meals.

From a health perspective, most of the oils being offered to us are worthless and detrimental. Chemical solvents, such as gasoline, benzene and carbon tetrachloride, are used to extract oil from seeds and grains. The oil is then boiled to remove the solvents, but traces remain at 10 ppm.[5] Further processing is done to clarify the oil and remove fatty acids. The majority of oils on the market are also bleached, degummed and deodorized, after which synthetic antioxidants are added.

Oils labeled "cold-pressed" are mechanically extracted, but are heated WAY above 115° F. The **critical** point at which most foods start to lose enzymes and change from a living, vibrant food to a dead food is between 105° F and 118° F.

I suggest that you take great care in shopping for oils. If enough information is not available on a particular oil, call the company and ask questions. When you find **genuinely** cold-pressed (low-heat), unprocessed oils, they are a great plus, not only in enhancing the flavor of some of the dishes but in benefiting your health as well. Dr. Johanna Budwig of Germany has written extensively about the health-promoting benefits of flaxseed oil. Recently some of her writings, such as *Flax Oil As a True Aid Against Arthritis, Heart Infarction, Cancer and Other Diseases*, have been translated into English.

We are living at a time now when a lot of people are rejecting the inclusion of any kind of fat in their diet. They have been so overloaded in the one direction for so long, consuming saturated and processed fats, that now the pendulum is swinging too far the other way. This is contrary to good nutrition, however, because **"essential fatty acids" are a necessary and very important part of an optimum health program.** This is why they are called **ESSENTIAL**. Without them, we cannot process oil-soluble vitamins; our skin dries out; our nerves and glands suffer; and many other detrimental effects occur.

To maintain the varied ethnic flavors of the different dishes, it would be great if you could use the oils traditionally used by those cultures. For example, you may want to use peanut and sesame oil in Asian dishes, corn oil in Mexican food, olive oil in Mediterranean cuisine, sesame oil in Indian, etc., **BUT, DO NOT USE AN INFERIOR OIL PRODUCT FOR THE SAKE OF SUCH TRADITION.**

Sometimes I specify native oils in the recipes, but you can always substitute olive and/or flaxseed oil. In order to get peanut, sesame, corn and other oils that are **GENUINELY** cold pressed, you would have to make an extra special effort, or even order them by mail. For this reason, in most recipes that call for oil, I have used olive or flaxseed or a combination of the two. You can generally get these two oils in their optimum unprocessed form in a good health food store. However, if you do find other oils in this state, please feel free to use them instead. Flora, Arrowhead Mills and Omega put out a wide variety of GENUINELY cold pressed oils (*see* Source Index), but I do not mean to exclude other suppliers, as there are a few more who may also provide

---

[5]parts per million

truly cold-processed oils. (For more information on oils, *see* "Cold Pressed" in Glossary.)

CANOLA (RAPESEED) WASN'T SAFE FOR PIGS SO NOW WE FEED IT TO HUMANS (see "Canola" in Glossary)

HONEY VS. MAPLE SYRUP

I opt for raw, unheated honey instead of maple syrup because maple syrup is a boiled product. Maple syrup may also have tripe fat added during the boiling process. Unheated honey is full of life; teeming with enzymes, pollen, propolis, minerals and many other factors. Still, because it's a concentrated sugar, it is best to use honey sparingly.

Strict vegans may object to the use of honey. One suggestion for them is to use a date purée made from soaked and blended dates. A fruit syrup can also be made by soaking any dried fruit in filtered water for 24 hours in the refrigerator. Raisins, currants, dates, figs, and apricots (singly or in combination) work well for making a sweet syrup.

HULLED VS. UNHULLED SESAME SEED

THE PROBLEM:

Hulled sesame seed is more likely to be rancid, as it is usually not found refrigerated. Removing the hull takes away the seed's protection and thus hastens the changes that cause rancidity. Hulled sesame seeds, even when mechanically processed, may also have been pre-treated with chemicals to soften the hull.

Unhulled sesame seed contains oxalic acid in its hulls and is not as good tasting. It has a slightly bitter flavor that people don't like.

THE SOLUTION:

Use unhulled sesame seeds that have been soaked overnight in filtered water. This reduces the oxalic acid and improves the flavor of the seed, which then becomes milder. If you choose to sprout, do not sprout for more than one day because, after a day, the sprouts tend to get bitter.

MONO DIET

A Mono Diet consists of eating only one type of food at a meal. Breakfast may consist of grapefruit; lunch of tomatoes and dinner, avocados. A Mono Diet could also consist of eating one food, let's say papaya, for a day or a week or even longer. This is certainly an easy and simple way to go; but I don't think it will satisfy most people in the long run. I also do not believe that many of the people who eat this way will want to make a meal of greens or squash or roots or any number of other foods which call for a little dressing to make them palatable for most of us. And I believe it is very important to consume these greens and other foods, so our bodies can obtain a wide variety of nutrients and protective substances.

ANOPSOLOGY—ANOPSOTHERAPY—INSTINCTOTHERAPY—INSTINCTIVE NUTRITION

Anopsology, Anopsotherapy, Instinctotherapy and Instinctive Nutrition are different terms that refer to a diet in which only a single food is eaten—until its flavor changes. A comprehensive book on the subject is *Instinctive Nutrition* by Severen L. Schaeffer.

Eating one food at a time until the flavor changes, because of its simplicity, seems to be a very effective tool for reestablishing the health of the body. Proponents of this system say the body itself will tell you when you've had enough of a (raw) food. Its formerly good flavor will become unpleasant once your body has met its needs. If you are still hungry when the flavor changes, then you must look for another single food which appeals to you, but no mixtures are permitted. The "taste-change response" is not triggered when eating foods that are cooked, chopped, ground, frozen or mixed.

I believe Anopsotherapy has merit and applicability in certain situations for the short term. My reservations are the same as for the Mono Diet.

PEANUTS AND AFLATOXIN

Aflatoxin (Aspergillus Flavus) is a mold that may form on peanuts and other crops under certain conditions. Aflatoxin is usually most prevalent where plants are under considerable stress. The stress can be from excessive heat, extremely dry situations, excessive moisture and/or combinations of these conditions.

Valencia peanuts (small, round peanuts with a red skin) have a very good flavor, even when raw. Ninety percent of all Valencia peanuts grown in the United States are from New Mexico and West Texas. This area of the country provides a favorable climate with warm days, cool nights, and very little humidity. The cool nights and very low humidity help to deter the formation of aflatoxin.

Aflatoxin can also develop if peanuts are stored improperly, such as in an excessively wet environment.

The United States Department of Agriculture inspects every trailerload of peanuts that goes to a plant for processing. After processing, the USDA pulls samples from every bag and again tests for aflatoxin. The USDA's acceptable level for aflatoxin mold is 15 ppb (parts per billion).

Aflatoxin, a mycotoxin (fungus), is suspected of causing liver cancer in both humans and animals.

FRUITARIANISM . . . A FEW RESERVATIONS

For a very long time I was perplexed by having met many, many fruitarians and former fruitarians who had either lost their teeth or were having a lot of trouble with their
teeth. I wondered why this was happening. At first, I thought that maybe there was
too much sugar in a strict fruitarian diet. Perhaps all those ripe, luscious fruits had
more sugar than a body could handle, and the excess sugar was causing the teeth to
break down. But then a knowledgeable dentist put the whole issue into perspective.
He told me that the damage to and weakening of teeth that some people experience
when they go on a fruitarian diet cannot be blamed on the fruit. Instead, it is due to
their former acid-producing diet and lifestyle and the resulting build-up of acidity in
the body. When these people make the switch to fruit, the fruit starts to remedy the
acid condition in the body. It swiftly sets into motion a process that, over time, converts the body's acid condition to an alkaline state. During this period, the constant
exudation of acid, especially from the tissues in the mouth, sometimes takes a toll on
the teeth.

What could temper this rapid exit of acid from the body? What could serve as
a buffer for it? In my opinion, the solution would be to become more **vege**tarian; to
add more vegetables, leafy greens, sprouts and mineral dense foods (such as sea vegetables) to the diet, and to lessen the intake of fruit for a period of time.

Another instance where a fruitarian diet may be counterindicated is in the case
of hypoglycemia. Increasing numbers of people are afflicted with either hypoglycemia
(low blood sugar) or tendencies towards it, both of which, ironically, are caused (in
most cases) by eating foods containing refined sugars and refined carbohydrates.
However, the sugar that produces tendencies towards hypoglycemia is **rarely** the
sugar from natural fruit (with the possible exception of overconsumption of either sugar
cane juice or unsoaked dried fruit). Rather it is the refined and processed sugar so
prevalent in our modern lifestyle. After someone has developed hypoglycemia or the
tendencies toward it have surfaced, their body may not be able to handle even the natural sugars in fresh fruit (at least until their condition improves). That is why some
of the institutes that teach the raw/live food lifestyle suggest that people with these
tendencies curb their intake of sweet fruit. "Vegetable-Fruits," such as cucumbers, tomatoes, squash, okra, eggplant, etc. are not generally a problem for hypoglycemics.

In our highly polluted cities, it is an absolute necessity that we supply an
abundance of oxygen to our body cells. Leafy greens, which are not generally included in a fruitarian diet, deliver the oxygen we need. For this reason and because of the
foregoing observations, I have reservations about a strict fruitarian diet.

CHAPTER TWELVE:
Implementing the Lifestyle

WHAT IF I'M NOT INTO FOOD PREPARATION? CAN I STILL DO THE PROGRAM?

More than half of this book is dedicated to tasty, delicious, raw/live food recipes. You might be the kind of person, however, who is not really into kitchen stuff. Would you still be able to practice this wonderful, healing lifestyle? **IF** you can adapt to and be satisfied with foods as they come from the earth, the answer is "yes." After all, nothing really needs to be prepared. You can just eat food as nature delivers it.

Fruit, of course, is very tasty on its own and easy to eat. Most fruitarians, however, do not include in their diet the vegetable-fruits, such as squash, okra, eggplant, cucumbers and other less sweet fruits, which I feel are necessary for the body to receive the full spectrum of nutrients, as well as to feel balanced. If you've read my section on fruitarianism, and do more research on your own, you may come to believe, as I do, that fruit alone is not enough. I believe that in today's polluted world, the body needs heavy doses of green, leafy vegetables loaded with chlorophyll (for oxygen delivery), phytochemicals and other as yet unidentified factors.

For most people, however, these greens need a little preparation to make them palatable. My recipes (*see* Index for *Marinated Collard Ribbons & Down Home Greens*) are very easy and take all of 10 minutes to prepare. Many other dishes are also very easy and take only a few minutes. It is best to cultivate a taste for a wide variety of foods and include them in the diet, instead of concentrating on just a few favorite items.

A TASTE CAN BE CULTIVATED FOR UNFAMILIAR FOODS

Sea vegetables (seaweeds) can be soaked until soft, drained, and then tossed with cubed avocado or dressed with a quick and simple dressing. Flaxseed oil, lemon juice and garlic come to mind. Sea vegetables are invaluable for both their mineral content and their alkalizing effect on the body.

A taste can also be cultivated for root vegetables, and once you have acquired this taste, you can eat them like apples.

It's obvious that appetites for various foods can be cultivated. What person has ever liked the taste of whiskey, for example, when they first tried it? Perhaps, you think, people learned to like it because of the way whiskey made them feel. Well, the same can be said for raw/live foods. After a while, you will just love the way they make you feel . . . energized, and feeling good all the time.

Once the raw/live food diet becomes more generally known and accepted, then more and more restaurants will want to include at least some raw/live food choices on their menus. It will then become easier for people who do not enjoy preparing food to purchase what they need, ready made. In most large cities, numerous salad and raw juice bars are available right now.

You could also get involved with raw and live food circles of people, raw food support groups and potluck get-togethers. People are usually happy to share food. You might even become motivated to make some of the easy stuff yourself; and don't forget to support restaurants and caterers that provide this type of food by patronizing them regularly.

CONVENIENCE—AT WHAT COST?

We are living in a world of convenience. We can easily pick up what passes for food everywhere we go. We can eat it as we walk down the street, grab a bite at our desks, or snack while driving our cars. We can bring it home and pop it into the microwave. We can certainly satisfy our immediate hunger; but there is a deeper hunger that prevails. And that is the hunger for a pain-free body, for endless energy to do whatever we have to do or want to do, without fatigue. It is the yearning deep within our souls for exuberance and vitality and youthfulness. And this hunger will not be satisfied with fast foods, junk foods and foodless foods. In our quest for "convenience," we overlook the fact that feeling ill or down or depressed is not convenient. Instead, we take it as a matter of course.

In our "convenient" life, we think it is normal to go to doctors, hospitals, and clinics, and to submit to examinations, prodding and vaccinations. In our society, drugs, chemotherapy, radiation and surgery are the tools of choice for bringing the body back to some semblance of "health." Health is typically described as the absence of any clinical signs of disease, but do most of us really feel good? In our "convenient" way of life, we take it for granted that we will end up in old age homes, nursing homes and convalescent homes, if we even last that long. I have yet to discover what is so "convenient" about that.

In our devotion to "convenience" we have forgotten that Nature's ways for attaining "true health" cannot be circumvented.

Some people say they "just don't have the time" to prepare raw/live food; their lives are toooo busy. But when they get sick, they'll be spending time at home feeling ill and they'll find the time to go to doctors and hospitals, if necessary. So it's just a matter of choosing where you want to spend your time. **The time WILL be spent . . . either in the kitchen or at the doctor. You choose.**

You **CAN** find a way to implement the lifestyle—it just depends on your interest and motivation, and how important it is to you to live in good health.

SUGGESTIONS ON GETTING INTO AND MAINTAINING THE LIFESTYLE

The following suggestions are based on the assumption that you will want to move towards a High-Raw Diet.

I'm convinced that if we are to advance to a system of raw eating in the near future and if this eating style is to become acceptable to a majority of people, the food will have to be, above all, flavorful and satisfying. Most people are emotionally attached, and even addicted, to some parts of their present diet. Making changes for them will not be easy. Their logical mind may tell them that raw and live food is the best way to go, and they may even know that they feel much better when they eat it consistently; but then they fall back into the trap of their old habits and fixations and return to their emotional comfort foods. I certainly did this for longer than I care to admit, until I weaned myself from these foods, one by one.

GO AT YOUR OWN PACE

I suggest that you go at your own pace, making changes as they feel right to you. Start by adding a lot more raw food and sprouts into your regular diet. Then decide what you want to get rid of, and find reasonably satisfying substitutes. One by one, e-a-s-y does it. If it takes a year, or even five, six or seven years—to come to a High-Raw Diet—that is a short time in the course of a lifetime. Changes made gradually, but consistently, may have a better chance of sticking. (My only exception to the idea of gradually pacing yourself into the program is in the case of serious illness, where it seems more appropriate to go 100% raw, at least until health is reestablished. Check with your health care provider.)

Viktoras Kulvinskas, a pioneer with Dr. Ann Wigmore in the modern day living foods movement, in his lectures, talks about trying to change overnight and how he then struggled with years of setbacks and bulimia. On the other hand, some people may take to the changes more easily. Charles J. Hunt III, in his book, *The Christ Diet*, states "I found quick relinquishment of cooked foods the best way for me to make the switch to living foods. In my case, I knew if I was to do it at all, I must do it all the way. And after all my research, I sincerely felt it was the best way to eat and saw no good purpose in putting it off." **We are all individual. In making transitions, what may work for one may not work for another.**

One thing for sure: Try to incorporate and develop a taste for more raw and living foods while you are well, rather than waiting for a disease condition to overtake you. When you are ill, it will be much more of a struggle. You will have to contend both with the changes that will invariably happen to your body by adopting a diet of this type as well as with the fear and uncertainty your illness engenders. More than likely, you will need to go to one of the institutes that teach this lifestyle in order to have the support you will need. Family and friends may discourage you because they don't understand that "weird" diet you're on. **Prevention is always the easier, though less traveled, road.**

When you go to visit family and friends, take some food with you, and take enough to share. This way you will always have something to eat since they probably will not prepare raw food, though they may offer a salad. But we raw fooders know we need more than salad to be satisfied.

When you go to a catered affair, always eat beforehand, unless you know for sure they will have raw salad or crudité and that this will hold you for the evening. Catered affairs usually serve glorified junk food, not worth the eating.

When you're invited to dinner, you have to decide whether you are going to eat the dinner offered. Sometimes it seems rude to refuse. But I always tell my host or hostess what I'm into beforehand, so I breed no misunderstandings. The host(ess) then usually offers to make a big salad and I offer to bring a main course dish, and I bring enough to share. I find that if I'm eating when everyone else is eating, the host(ess) is usually satisfied and feels his/her dinner was a success.

Restaurants are easy because you usually have some say in where you will be going and you can then make sure they have salad offerings. I've gone to Italian and French restaurants and had two different salads as an entree and then fresh strawberries or raspberries for dessert. Of course it's best to reverse the order and have the fruit first, but it depends on who you're out with, how outrageous (to them) you might appear and whether it matters to you. Mexican restaurants offer raw salad and guacamole. Chinese restaurants are workable if you can persuade them to give you the food *before* they sauté it in the wok. I haven't had much luck in Indian restaurants. American restaurants and coffee shops don't usually have very good salad offerings but I've been able to get fresh fruit like cantaloupe, honeydew melon or watermelon there. Of course, nowadays, there are salad bars in every big city.

Sometimes you can get trapped into a situation. This may occur when there are language barriers and cultural differences; like if you're in Outer Ghanistan[1] and the tribe wants to share an insect meal with you and they would not understand your refusal. You can't explain it to them because you don't speak the language. When you get trapped, just eat slowly, take tiny bites and smile. Remember the scene in Indiana Jones?

I envision that in the near future, restaurants will spring up in every city in the country to offer our growing community wonderful raw and living foods to feast upon. That will be a day for celebration! And it is not so far-fetched as it may sound. Now in most large cities, we **can** find fresh raw juice bars and a selection of raw vegetables and sprouts in salad bars. In the meantime, there are a few raw restaurants scattered about. (*See* "Raw Restaurants" in the Source Index, and for a more extensive list, go to www.rawfoodinfo.com and look in the Directories.)

---

[1]A fictitious place

STICK CLOSE TO NATURE—SHE'S NOT STUPID!

YOU DON'T HAVE TO BE AN EXPERT IN NUTRITION IN ORDER TO TAKE CARE OF YOURSELF EFFECTIVELY

Every day more and more information becomes available on the myriad of nutrients, antioxidants, phytochemicals, etc., which our scientists and researchers are discovering at an ever-accelerating pace. How do we "just plain folk" expect to keep up with all the latest information, and then make intelligent decisions regarding their application for our health? We really can't. Even as the experts make these discoveries, they merely see the tip of the iceberg, and not the vast bulk of knowledge (wisdom) hidden still in the complexities of Nature's masterpiece. These discoveries are only bits and fragments and, without all the pieces in place, cannot be cohesively organized in the foreseeable future in a way that benefits our health.

In the field of nutrition there will always be the latest discovery; the latest and best possible nutrient, phytochemical or other factor, which will resolve all or some of our problems (according to the advertising copy); only to be replaced in a few months or years by some other nutritional discovery, which then takes center stage. I am not denigrating these discoveries, as I believe them to be very important. But I don't feel that, based on our current knowledge, we can make intelligent choices as to which nutrient supplements to use.

The better bet is to just stay close to the "source." **Untampered-with Nature** is still the best source and the best teacher. Eating a WIDE variety of vegetarian foods, in their natural, live state, grown from open-pollinated seeds, is the best insurance we have that we will get all the "latest" nutrients, the already well known nutrients, as well as the still undiscovered nutrients into our bodies. Co-Q10, DHEA, selenium, folic acid, neuropeptides, proanthocyanidins, polyphenols, glycosides, catechins, carotenoids, lecithin, acetylcholine, picolinates, zybicolin, isothiocyanates, anthocyanosides, phytosterol, dimethylglycine: Who can keep track of all these and thousands of other factors, both identified and not? **Yet all of them are available to us in their prime, utilizable form in raw and live foods. No manufactured supplement[2] can compete with these foods. No manufactured supplement can do as much to reestablish our health.**

Don't doubt for a second that Nature is intelligent and that everything created in nature (and that includes us) is intelligent. Our bodies were not haphazardly put together with just a hope they would survive; they are magnificent, well-constructed creations, with superb capacities, many of which are still poorly understood. Do we know or realize how many functions each of our organs performs for us . . . so effortlessly, unconsciously, quietly? It's all directed by the supreme intelligence in each one of our 75 trillion cells. Trust your **self**.

---

[2]For information on suggested food-based supplements, *see* Chapter 10, "Supplements—Yes, No or Maybe?"

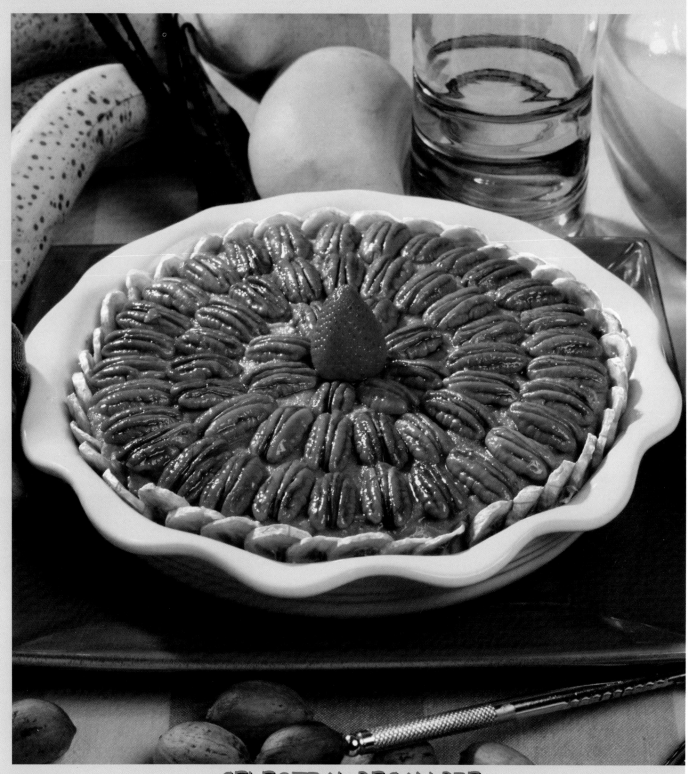

CELESTIAL PECAN PIE

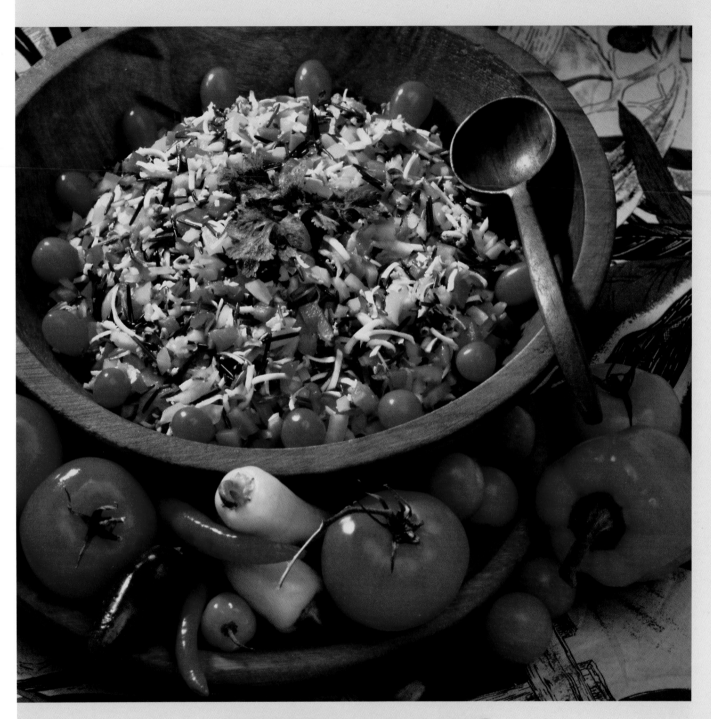

CARIBBEAN WILD RICE

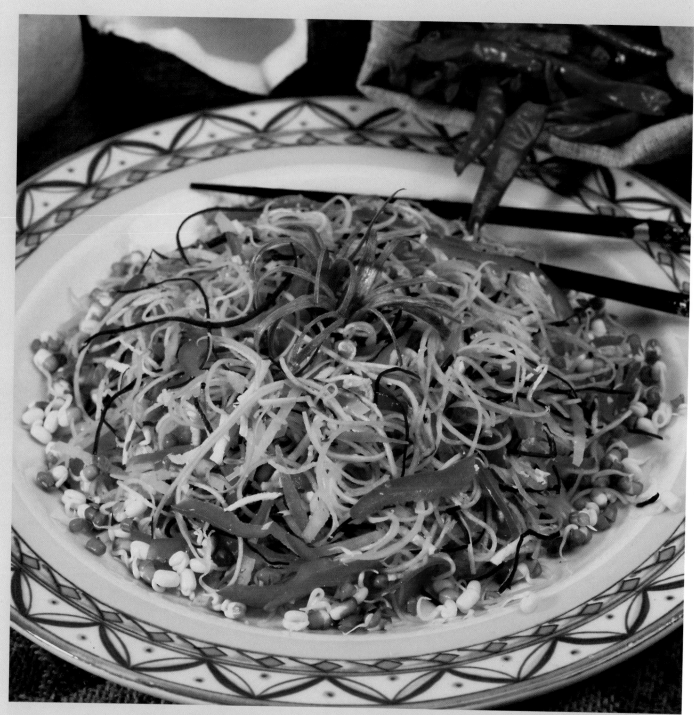

SZECHUAN-STYLE MOCK NOODLES

SUPER SALADS

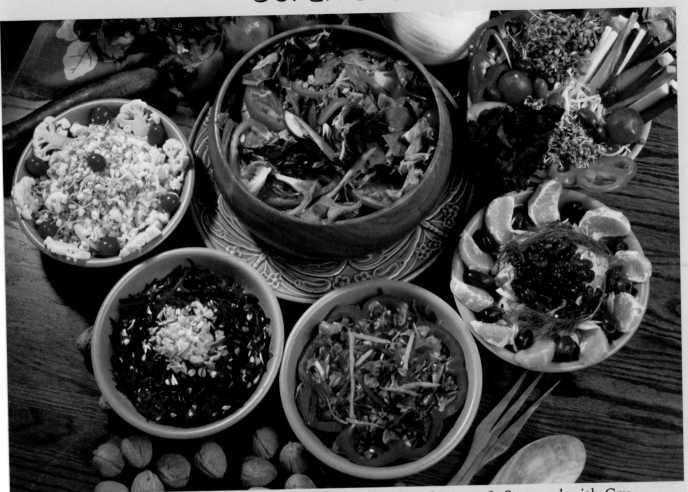

Gorgeous Greens in center salad bowl, then clockwise: Sprouts & Seaweed with Crudité, Fennel Salad with Cranberry Vinaigrette, Watercress & Red Bell Pepper Salad, Beet-Hiziki Salad, Cauliflower & Mung.

MAIN COURSES (and more)

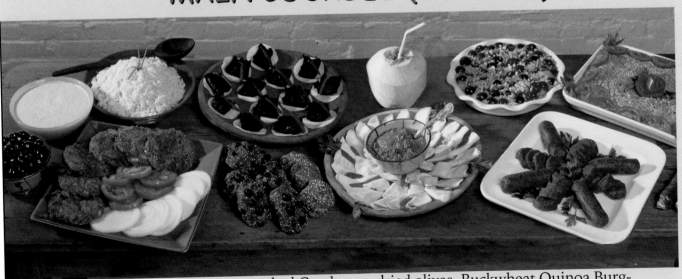

From left to right, bottom row: soaked Greek, sun-dried olives, Buckwheat Quinoa Burgers with trimmings, Blueberry Muffins, Fabioli with Pesto Sauce, Almond-Beet Nut Roll. From left to right, 2nd row: Pecan Gravy, Mashed "Potatoes," Dim Some, Thai Coconut, Leigh's Cherry Cobbler, Neat Loaf.

SOUP: FOOD FOR THE SOUL

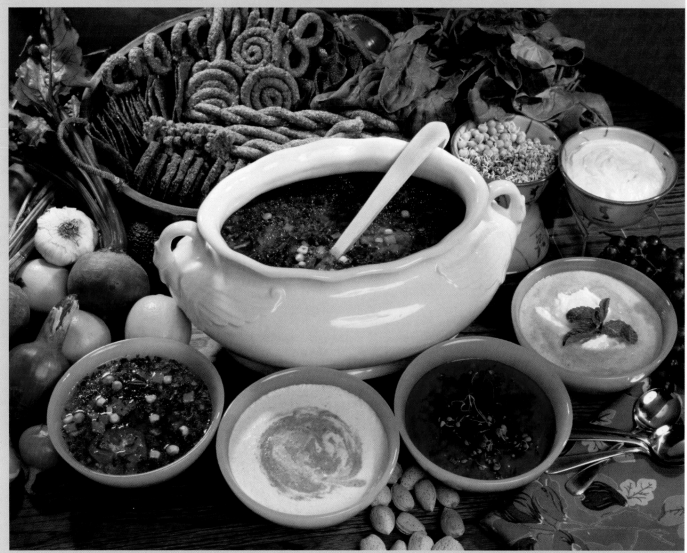

Minestrone in tureen, then clockwise: sprouts, Almond Yogurt, Refreshing Fruit Soup, Borscht, Creamy Spinach Swirl, Minestrone, Pretzels & assorted crackers.

DELECTABLE DESSERTS

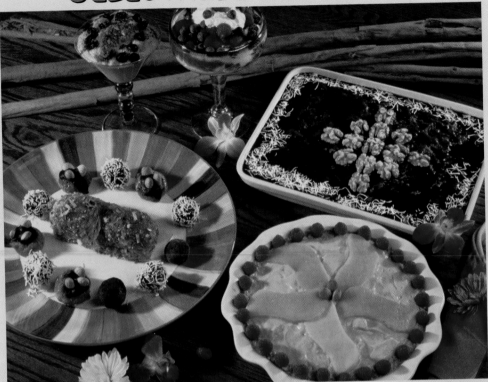

Platter with Coconut Almond Log in center, surrounded by Almond Roca and assorted treats, then clockwise: Connie's Spumoni Ice Cream, Berries & Cream, Fudge X Tasty, and Mango Pudding Pie.

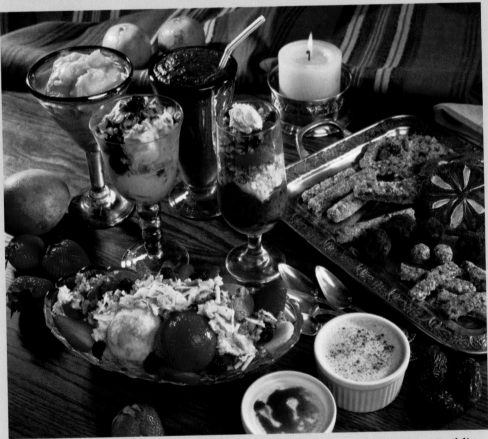

Counterclockwise from Banana Split: Creme Brulée, Sweet Brown Rice Pudding, platter of assorted cookies & sweet treats, Raspberry Frappé with Macadamia Cream & pistachios, Shake, Honey Vanilla Ice Cream, Orange Sherbert

HUNZA . . . LAND OF PARADISE

The people of Hunza, in the Himalayas, are among the healthiest people in the world. Unreachable by modern transportation, and outside food sources until recently, they have maintained optimum health and longevity eating a high-raw diet.

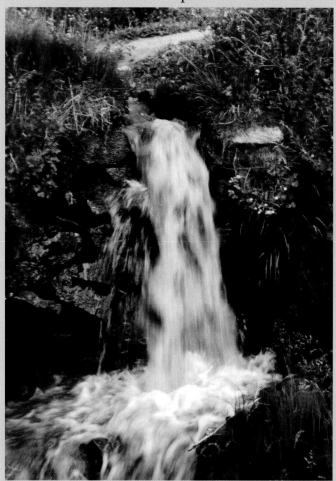

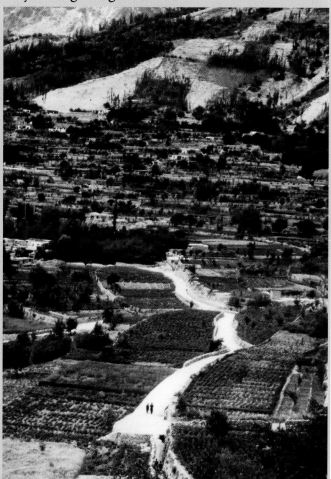

Unchanged by Modern Civilization:
Hunza Glacial Waterfall

The Fertile Hunza Valley

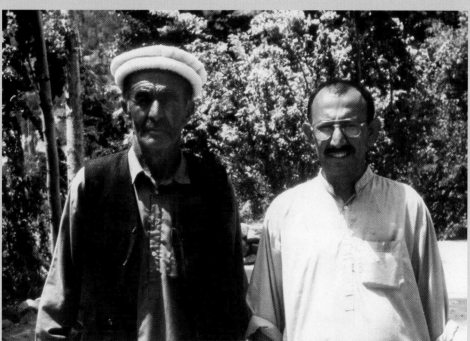

Traditional Hunza Citizen and Visitor

Hunza photographs courtesy of Dorleen Tong

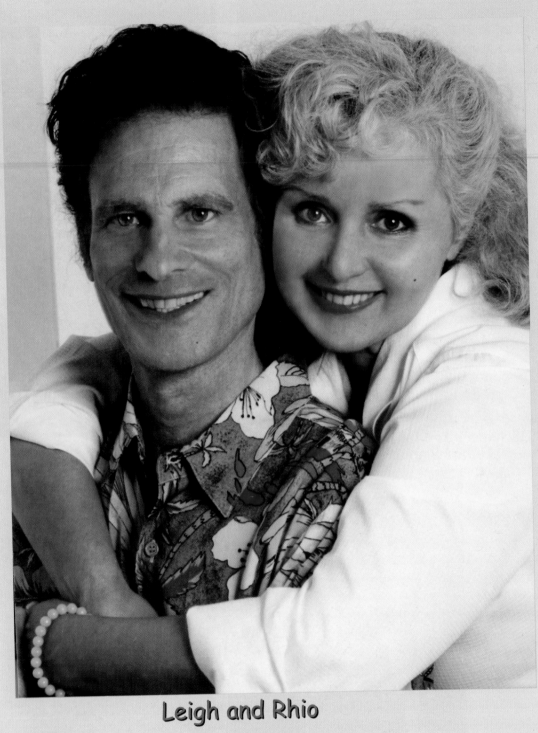

Leigh and Rhio

Part Two

CHAPTER THIRTEEN:
Sprouting is a Simple Affair

THE CONCEPT OF SPROUTING

Basically, sprouting is what nature does everywhere in its wondrous system of self-renewal. A seed falls from a plant or tree and rests in or on the ground. When the rains come, the seed gets soaked, the enzyme inhibitors are washed away, and the seed begins to sprout and create a new tree or plant. The cycle is eternal . . . never ending.

The sprouting of seeds for food has been going on in China for over 5,000 years. Sprouts, referred to as "pulses," were mentioned numerous times in the bible. The word pulse conjures up such an appropriate image. To pulse is "to vibrate or flow" and this is exactly what sprouts do. They are "pulsing" with life, and when eaten, will make your body and soul pulse with life. Using sprouts for food is an ancient practice that is increasingly being "rediscovered" here in the United States.

Researchers have found that when nuts, seeds, grains, legumes and beans are sprouted, several beneficial things occur:

1) First, the enzyme inhibitors are washed away. Enzyme inhibitors are substances put there by nature to protect the seed, grain, etc. from rotting and to keep the seed viable (alive) until conditions are right for it to be reawakened and grow into a new plant. Have you ever heard people say they cannot digest nuts and seeds, or that beans give them gas? Research has shown that it is not beneficial for us to eat the enzyme inhibitors, so soaking and sprouting is the perfect way for us to consume these foods. (Of course, chewing insufficiently may also interfere with optimum digestion.) Could it be that the squirrel is not just burying nuts to store them away for another day, but he instinctively knows that he needs to eat nuts that have been soaked and sprouted first?

2) Phytic acid (phytins) is a substance found in most legumes, beans, seeds and grains. It reportedly binds up calcium, iron and zinc, thereby making them unavailable for your body to absorb. Soaking and sprouting process the phytins by developing the phytase (phosphatase) enzymes which then make it possible for your body to absorb the minerals contained in the food. Further, as cited by Dr. Gabriel Cousens in his book, *Conscious Eating,*

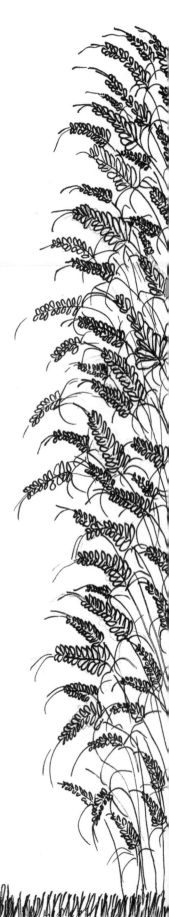

Once You Get the Hang of it

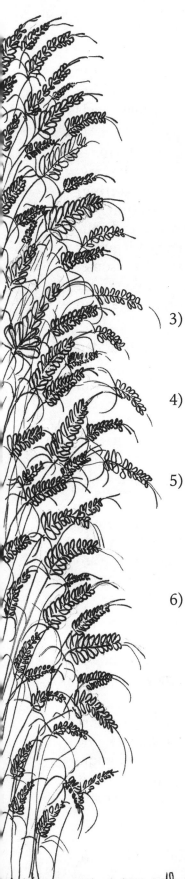

" . . . recent research has found that over time, the body begins to produce its own phytase enzyme for breaking down the phytates. According to Bitar and Reinhold in *Biochemica et Biophysica Acta*, the phytase enzyme produced in our intestines releases the calcium from the phytate binding so that the calcium can be absorbed into the system."

3) Nuts and seeds become easier for your body to digest and assimilate after they are soaked and sprouted. The oil (fat) content is reduced, as some of the oil is released into the soak water, and some more is used up in the process of sprouting.

4) Soaking and sprouting increase by many times the vitamin and enzyme content of foods (the amount of increase depending on the type of grain or seed) and actually creates Vitamin C where it did not previously exist in the dry seed or grain.

5) Sprouting changes protein into amino acids, starch (carbohydrate) into simple sugars, and fats into soluble fatty acids. By doing this work (which would otherwise be done by your digestive organs), sprouting relieves your digestive processes of the task. For this reason, sprouted food is considered to be pre-digested and very easily assimilated by the body.

6) Sprouts are loaded with vitamins, minerals, enzymes, bioelectrical energy, and other as yet undiscovered factors. Sprouts contain the **LIFE-FORCE**. Scientists have been able to reconstruct a grain of wheat in the laboratory, but when they try to sprout that synthesized grain, IT DOES NOT SPROUT—why? Because the **life-force** is missing. Yet grains of wheat found in 4,000 year-old tombs **have** sprouted.

SPROUTING—AN INTERESTING CHALLENGE

Learning how to sprout various seeds, beans and grains can seem daunting at first but once you know it, you know it. Because a significant part of the raw food diet utilizes sprouts, I encourage you to acquire this skill. Sprouting your own seeds is very rewarding and will also save you money.

Basically, in sprouting, the first step is to rinse the seeds, grains or legumes very well to remove any stones, damaged seeds or beans and other debris. Removing the damaged beans[1] helps to keep the sprouts from fermenting (and rotting) while you're in the process of sprouting them. Next, you introduce clean (filtered) water to seeds, grains or legumes and allow them to soak up the water and soften. Small seeds require less time for soaking (8 to 12 hours), while larger legumes and beans need a longer soaking time (24 to 36 hours). My soaking times are somewhat longer than those recommended by other teachers. I find that if you don't rehydrate the seed enough in the beginning, you will still get a sprout, but the bean or grain part itself may be too tough to chew.

I like to soak my seeds in glass bottles, or in bowls. The water added should be more than twice the volume of the seeds. The seeds will soak up the water and expand. If you do not put in enough water, then some of the seeds will not get sufficiently rehydrated. Change the water twice in the soaking process, except when soaking small seeds overnight. Seeds to be soaked overnight (8 to 12 hours) can be left in the same water. (In a tropical climate these seeds would only take 5 to 8 hours of soaking time.) If you leave them in water longer than 12 hours, then you must change the water because it will begin to ferment. Then the seeds start to spoil and won't sprout properly.

After soaking for the appropriate time, drain, rinse, drain again, and set the seeds out to sprout. Some people like to sprout in bottles, other people do it in baskets, some prefer wet paper towels, and still others use sprout bags. There are numerous methods to choose from. You can experiment and find the technique that suits you.

The method I use, which I haven't heard mentioned anywhere, employs bowls. I use bowls because when I travel, I can find them everywhere I go. Whether it's off to a friend's house, staying with family, or in a hotel, there are always bowls around, so all I have to do is buy or take my seeds with me, and I'm ready to sprout. The best bowls to use are the ones that taper out a little bit.

As indicated, after the soaking period, I rinse and drain the seeds. For rinsing, I use a restaurant type strainer with an extra long handle. (You can pick one up at a restaurant supply store.) I set the strainer on the sink. The long handle is very convenient because it allows the loop(s) on the front of the strainer to sit on one side of the sink ledge while the handle sits on the other side, with the main

---

[1]By damaged beans, I mean beans that are cracked or not whole and beans that may have little insect holes in them.

part of the strainer suspended in the middle, so I don't have to hold it up. I pour my seeds into the strainer, rinse well, let the water drain and then put the seeds back into the bowl. With my fingers I spread the seeds up the sides of the bowl a little bit. I let them sprout at room temperature, rinsing and draining twice each day, generally morning and evening. In hot and humid weather, three times may be needed. Soak the seeds initially in filtered water; but sink water is OK for rinsing.

Some teachers say you must keep sprouts in the dark. They may advocate covering them with a breathable cloth or screen, which also helps keep insects away. I find that the ordinary light in my kitchen is fine, although I don't keep the sprouts in bright light. I don't usually cover the sprouts, but I would if I was having trouble with insects. (Sprouts that I've planted in soil, I do keep in the dark for about three days—*see* below under Baby Greens.)

Some sprouts, like clover and alfalfa, need to be "greened up" after they are sprouted; that is, they need to be exposed to light near a window, so they turn green. The light develops chlorophyll in the leaves.

And that's all there is to it.

Pretty soon you'll get so good at it, you'll just snap your fingers and everything will SPROUT; and I'm **not** just a'kiddin! **OK, OK, that's not ALL there is to it**, but it is the basics.

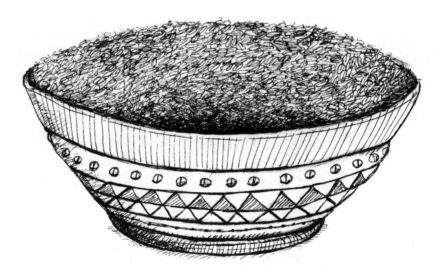

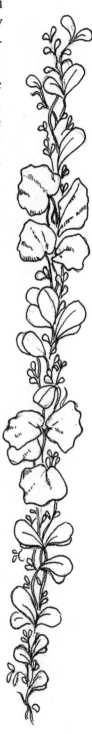

WHAT CAN GO WRONG?

When you are having trouble sprouting, there are only a few things that can go wrong. Generally, the problem is OLD seeds. This is the **number one** cause of failure in sprouting. Old seeds rot instead of sprout. This is not your fault. Find a source for **fresh** seeds. Don't buy seeds for sprouting from supermarkets or from tiny health food stores, which may have had those seeds sitting around for a long time. Find a place that sells and moves a lot of seeds; theirs will be fresher.

Another reason for failure is forgetting to rinse frequently enough. The purpose of rinsing is to keep the sprouts fresh. You don't want them to start fermenting or spoiling, because then they will not sprout properly. So rinse them in a **timely** manner.

Two other causes of sprouting trouble are putting the seeds either in the sun or close to a draft, which causes them to dry out; and failing to drain off the water well enough, so the sprouts sit in a puddle and start to rot. Those are about all the reasons I can think of for failure.

TINY SEEDS NEED A DIFFERENT METHOD

For very tiny seeds, like amaranth and teff, the bowl method doesn't work as well. (Tiny seeds are more difficult to transfer back and forth from strainer to bowl.) For growing these sprouts I prefer to use a sprout bag (*see* Kitchen Equipment). First, of course, soak the seeds overnight in a bowl or bottle. Then transfer them to a sprout bag, and rinse the sprouts by just letting water wash through the bag. I then hang the sprout bag over my sink, but you can hang it anywhere that is convenient with a bowl underneath. Two to three times a day, rinse the sprouts by placing the bag in a bowl of filtered water for five minutes. Then hang the bag again.

For alfalfa, clover, onion, broccoli, and cabbage sprouts, I use the bottle method. Put two tablespoons of seed into a wide-mouthed jar. Cover with water and let soak overnight. In the morning, put a double layer of cheesecloth over the top of the jar (cut to size) and secure with a rubber band.* Drain the water out of the jar. Pour fresh water into the bottle and rinse and drain the seeds well. Lay the bottle on its side and allow the seeds to sprout, rinsing twice a day. When the sprouts nearly fill the bottle, put them by a window where light comes in, so they can "green up."

*There are also special tops with screens that you can get.

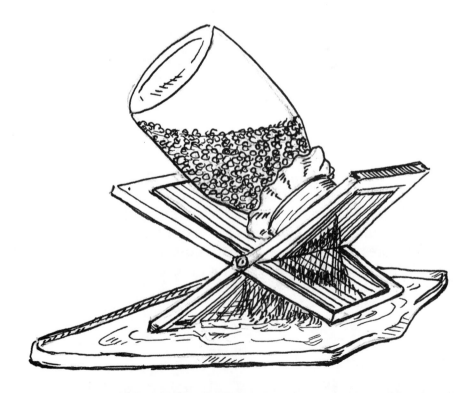

BABY GREENS ARE ANOTHER TYPE OF SPROUT. THEY INCLUDE:

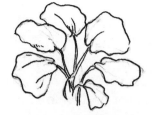

Buckwheat Lettuce
Sunflower Greens
Pea Greens
Wheatgrass, etc.

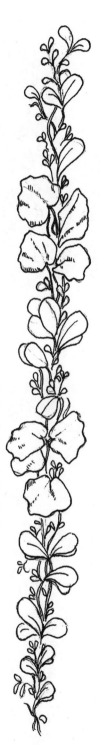

These sprouted greens are a little more difficult to grow and you will need the following:

> Some good organic soil
> Peat moss
> 10" by 21" plastic "Growing Trays" (or other size) with
> small holes on the bottom (these are also
> called nursery flats)
> Slightly larger trays with no holes
> 2 small soup bowls for each "Growing Tray"
> A plastic watering can
> Willard Water (optional, *see* Glossary)
> Sprouted unhulled seeds

1) Sprout seeds for your Growing Tray (*see* #3 below), before commencing. Mix the organic soil with peat moss. Three parts soil to one part peat moss is about right. If your soil is very heavy, use half and half. You mix peat moss with soil in order to create a lighter soil, loose enough for tiny roots to grow easily.

2) Spread the soil approximately 1/2 inch thick into the plastic tray with the holes. The holes are small enough to prevent too much soil from falling through them. This is your "Growing Tray." (You can easily obtain these trays from a nursery.)

3) On top of the soil in the Growing Tray, you will be spreading a layer of sprouted seeds, but first:

> **TO SPROUT SEEDS FOR YOUR GROWING TRAY**: Soak your seeds for 24-36 hours, changing the water once or twice. Then let the seed sprout for approximately 2 days or until you see the sprout start to emerge.

Next, spread a layer of sprouted seeds over the soil (in the Growing Tray) and water the seeds thoroughly. I usually do this over my sink so as to catch any soil which might come through the holes.

4) Put the two small soup bowls, inverted, into the larger tray with no holes. Set the Growing Tray on top of the inverted bowls and cover it with a third tray. (I use an empty tray with holes, inverted.) Then put the whole setup into a dark place with good air circulation. The idea is to keep the sprouts

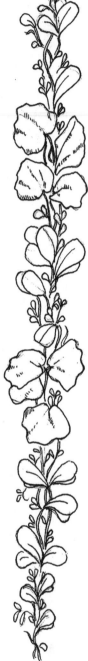

in the dark for two or three days. During this time, you do not need to water them.

5) When the sprouts are one to two inches tall, uncover the Growing Tray, water it and put it either into a greenhouse or by a window that allows light to enter.

6) Water twice a day. The bottom tray will catch the draining water while the soup bowls keep the Growing Tray high enough so the roots are not sitting in water. (If the roots do sit in water, your greens will rot or develop mold.) You may have to drain the bottom tray occasionally. Once during the growing process I water the sprouts with Willard Water. This is optional, but I like it because the greens get an extra boost of energy.

7) In approximately seven days, your greens will be ready to harvest. Cut them off a little above the roots with a sharp knife.

8) Wheatgrass can be juiced for drinking as a tonic. It is also known to be a powerful cleanser, neutralizing and expelling accumulated toxins from the body. The juice can also be used externally by applying to the skin as a mask, for cleansing the eyes, for snuffing up the nose, etc. The other baby greens can either be juiced or put in salads and in all kinds of dishes.

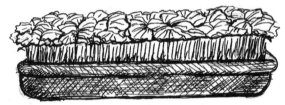
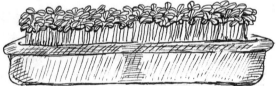

HOW LONG SHOULD YOU SOAK YOUR SEEDS, GRAINS, NUTS, LEGUMES AND BEANS BEFORE DRAINING THE WATER AND ALLOWING THEM TO SPROUT?

Generally, SMALL seeds like:

Alfalfa

Buckwheat, hulled

Clover

Fenugreek

Lentils

Pumpkin Seeds

Radish

Sunflower Seeds, etc.

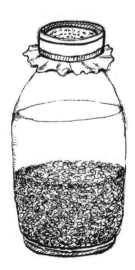

and most nuts[2] can be soaked overnight (approximately 8 to 12 hours). They can then be drained, rinsed, drained again, and set out to sprout. (Nuts that do not sprout, such as walnuts, pecans and Brazil nuts are soaked only.)

LARGER legumes, hard beans and rice need to be soaked in water for a longer period of time. The following do better when soaked for 24-36 hours (change the water once or twice). Then drain, rinse, drain again, and set out to sprout.

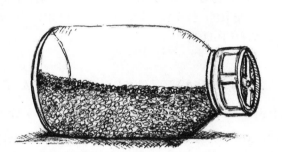

Aduki beans
Barley, hulled
Black beans
Buckwheat, unhulled
Chick-peas (garbanzos)
Mung beans
Oats,[3] hulled (oat groats)
Rye
Sweet Brown Rice
Wild Rice,[4] etc.

HOW LONG DOES IT TAKE TO SPROUT?

The length of time it takes to sprout different types of seeds, grains, etc. depends on many varied factors. Were the seeds, legumes or grains well–hydrated first? What is the weather like? In hot weather, things sprout a lot faster than when it's cold. I've seen many charts, and when I try to use them, it becomes obvious to me that no chart can be created that takes into account all the varied conditions under which sprouts are grown.

Living in the extreme conditions of New York City (very hot and humid in summer and very cold in winter) has made me flexible in my sprouting expectations. The same sprout might take two days to grow in summer, and four or five days in winter. If you live in a tropical climate or a dry climate, in each case it will be different again. So how long sprouting takes is something you will discover for yourself through a little experimentation. I have, however, included a chart with sprouting time **spans**, just to give you some idea of how far ahead to plan for your living foods dishes.

[2]Some nuts, like pecans and macadamias, lose a lot of their flavor when soaked too long; so I prefer to soak them for a minimal time (2–4 hours).

[3]Whole oats and wild rice don't actually sprout, but they soften up enough to become chewy. **Whole hulless oats obtained from Sunorganic Farms (*see* Source Index) do sprout.**

[4]Ibid.

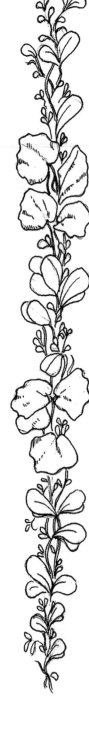

WHEN IS THE SPROUT READY TO EAT?

A general rule is that the sprout is ready to eat when the sprouted part (sometimes called the tail) is about the same length as the seed, legume, or grain itself. (But I find that sprouts are also fine to eat when the sprout tail is smaller.) This rule does not apply to all sprouts, however. For example, the almond sprout is very tiny; sometimes you can't even see it unless you remove the skin. Generally, almonds can be soaked overnight, and sprouted for one day and they're ready to eat. Pumpkin sprouts are also tiny, if you can see them at all. I like sunflower sprouts when they are just 1/4 the length of the sunflower seed itself; longer sunflower sprouts can turn bitter.

AN IMPORTANT VARIABLE: HOW THE SPROUT IS USED

There's Not Just One Right Way To Eat Sprouts

You can sprout them long, and you can sprout them short. It all depends on the purpose for which you are growing the sprout. If you are growing the sprout for a salad, then you probably want to grow it long and let it develop a couple of green leaves, so it will be more like a salad green. The same sprout, however, if used for a main course dish (generally speaking), would be ready when the sprout is very small, long before the leaves develop. As an example, a soybean sprout for salads is sprouted long like the ones you see in the Chinese markets, not starchy at all. With this type of sprout, you can hardly see the soybean anymore. However, if you wanted a main course bean dish, like my *Unbaked Beans*, you would sprout the soybean just a little (approximately 1/4 to 1/2 the length of the bean itself), so it still looks like a bean. This bean sprout is more starchy, suitable for main course dishes which are a little more concentrated than salads.

For more tips on individual sprouts check a good sprouting book (*see* Bibliography).

HOW TO STORE YOUR SPROUTS

Store your sprouts in the refrigerator. Most sprouts can be placed in a glass jar, with water covering the sprouts. Use filtered water, and change the water every second (preferred) or third day so as to prevent the sprouts from fermenting. This way most sprouts will last at least 5 days, except for sprouted brown rice, which turns bitter when kept too long. (Use brown rice sprouts within 2–3 days.) You will find that sprouts continue to grow in the water, too.

Some exceptions to storing sprouts in water. Do not store in water:

1) Sprouts grown to the stage where they have developed green leaves.
2) Tiny sprouts such as flaxseed, quinoa, amaranth, fenugreek, teff or even buckwheat.

The smaller sprouts do better when stored dry. However, to extend their life, you could rinse them with water every second or third day, then drain well before putting them back into the refrigerator.

The sprouts that store very well in water are the larger legumes, beans, and most nuts, seeds and grains. By storing them in water you will avoid altogether the problem of the hulls turning black. Some sprouts, like sunflower and soybean sprouts, have hulls (or skins), and the hulls of these sprouts, when stored dry, tend to turn black and cause the sprout itself to rot. When stored in water, the hulls do not turn black and will generally separate from the sprout. If you lightly rub the sprouts between your hands and put them back into the water, many of the hulls will eventually float to the top of the jar, making it easier to discard them when you drain the water.

You can eat the hulls, of course, along with the sprouts, as long as they haven't turned black. Some chefs like to remove them, but I find it takes too much time (although I sometimes do it for company). The hulls don't have much effect on the flavor of the dish anyway. Some of the teachers at institutes that teach this lifestyle will suggest you be more meticulous about removing the hulls if you have digestive problems.

By storing sprouts in water this way, you will always have sprouts on hand for all your recipes. If you become confused as to how long your sprouts have been there, and whether they should still be used, taste them. If they taste fermented, give them to the birds or put them in the compost. You could also put a sticker on the bottle, giving the date when you first put the sprouts into the refrigerator for storage.

Due to space limitations, I cannot go into extensive detail on all aspects of sprouting. For more information, *The Sprout Garden* by Mark M. Braunstein, is very comprehensive. Also, Steve Meyerowitz is a prolific writer on the subject (*see* Bibliography). There are numerous books by other authors as well; check at your local health food store.

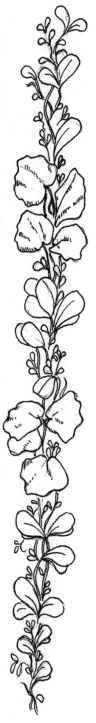

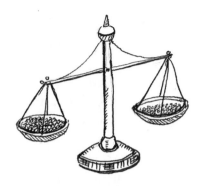

SOAKING/SPROUTING YIELD CHART

TO HELP YOU ASSESS HOW MUCH SOAKING AND SPROUTING INCREASES YIELD PLUS . . . SOAKING TIME AND GROWTH SPAN ESTIMATES

Remember, these are approximations.
Yield also depends on the length of your sprout tails.
Dried fruits, seaweed & some nuts are soaked only.

DRY MEASURE		SOAKING TIME IN HOURS	GROWING TIME IN DAYS	APPROX. YIELD WHEN SOAKED & SPROUTED
1 cup	**Aduki Beans**	24-36	3-5	3 cups
3 tbsp.	**Alfalfa**	overnight*	3-6	3-4 cups
1 cup	**Almonds**	12-15	1	1 3/4 cups
1 cup	**Amaranth**	overnight	2-3	3 cups
1 cup	**dried Apricots**	overnight		1 1/4 to 1 3/4 cups (depends on the variety)
1 tbsp.	**Arame**	10 minutes		1/4 cup
1 cup	**Barley, hulled**	24	1-3	2 cups

*Overnight is approx. 8-12 hours.

DRY MEASURE		SOAKING TIME IN HOURS	GROWING TIME IN DAYS	APPROX. YIELD WHEN SOAKED & SPROUTED
1 cup	**Brazil Nuts**	overnight		1 1/8 cups soaked only
1 cup	**Buckwheat, hulled**	12-15	1-3	2 3/4 cups
3 cups	**Buckwheat, unhulled**	12-15	2-3	6 1/2 cups
(for Buckwheat Lettuce: 2 1/2-3 cups sprouted unhulled buckwheat will plant one tray 10" x 21")			7-9	one tray
2 tbsp.	**Cabbage**	overnight	4-5	3 cups
1 cup	**Chick-peas** (Garbanzos)	24-36	3	2 1/2 cups
3 tbsp.	**Clover**	overnight	4-6	3-4 cups
1 cup	**dried Cranberry**	overnight		almost 2 cups
1 cup	**Currants**	overnight		1 1/8 cups
3 tbsp.	**Fenugreek**	12-15	1-3	almost 1 cup
1 cup	**Filberts**	12-15	1	1 1/4 cups
1/4 cup	**Flaxseed**	don't soak (spray to keep moist*)	3-5	2 3/4 cups
1 tbsp.	**Hiziki**	20 minutes		1/2 cup

*Flaxseed and all mucilaginous seeds need to be misted when sprouting. Because of their gelatinous quality, they will not sprout If you try to soak them. In order to sprout these seeds, spread them out in a large clay saucer (like the kind used to catch the water under a houseplant), and set the saucer into a larger pan which contains filtered water. The seeds will soak up the water as needed.

DRY MEASURE		SOAKING TIME IN HOURS	GROWING TIME IN DAYS	APPROX. YIELD WHEN SOAKED & SPROUTED
1 cup	**Lentils, French**	24	1-3	4 cups
1 cup	**Lentils, Green**	24	1-3	2 3/4 cups
1 cup	**Lentils, Red**	8	1	2 3/4 cups
1 cup	**Macadamias**	4 hours to overnight		1 1/4 cups soaked only
1 cup	**Mung Beans**	24-36	1-3	3 3/4 cups
3 tbsp.	**Mustard**	overnight	3-5	3 cups
1 cup	**Oat Groats** (Hulled Whole Oats)	24	1-3	2 1/4 cups
1 tbsp.	**Onion**	overnight	4-5	2 cups
1 cup	**dried Peaches**	overnight		1 1/2 cups
1 cup	**dried Pears**	overnight		1 1/8 cups
1 cup	**whole dried Peas**	24-36	2-4	2 1/2 cups
1 cup	**Pecans**	2-8		1 1/8 cups (soaked only)
1 cup	**Pine Nuts**	8	8 hours	1 1/4 cups
1 cup	**Prunes**	overnight		1 1/4 cups
1 cup	**Pumpkin Seeds**	12-15	1-2	1 1/2 cups
1 cup	**Quinoa**	12-15	1-2	2 1/2 cups

DRY MEASURE		SOAKING TIME IN HOURS	GROWING TIME IN DAYS	APPROX. YIELD WHEN SOAKED & SPROUTED
1 cup	**Raisins**	overnight		1 1/4 cups
1 cup	**Rice, Brown** (long grain or short grain)	24-36	3-4	1 1/2 cups
1 cup	Sweet Brown Rice	24	1-3	1 3/4 cups
1 cup	**Rye**	24	1-3	2 1/4 cups
1 cup	**Sesame Seeds** unhulled	12-15	1	2 cups
1 cup	**Soybeans**	24-36	3-4	2 3/4 cups
1 cup	**Sunflower Seeds** hulled	12-15	1-2	2 cups
3 cups	**Sunflower Seeds** unhulled	24	2	5 cups
(for Sunflower Greens: 3–3 1/2 cups sprouted sunflower seed is enough to plant one tray 10" x 21")			7-9	1 tray
1 cup	**Urad Dal**	24	1-2	3 1/2 cups
1 cup	**Walnuts, English**	overnight		1 1/8 cups (soaked only)
1 cup	**Wild Rice**	24-36	3-6	3 cups
1 cup	**Wheat, soft**	24	1-3	1 3/4 cups
3 cups	**Wheat, hard winter**	24	1-3	8 1/2 to 9 cups
(for Wheatgrass: 3 cups sprouted wheat is enough to plant one tray 10" X 21")			8-10 days	1 tray

CHAPTER FOURTEEN:
Kitchen Equipment

To facilitate the implementation of the raw/living foods lifestyle you will need to acquire a little equipment. If you cannot purchase these tools all at once (most of us can't), then use whatever equipment you have on hand and add more items as you are able.

The one most important piece is either a Champion, Green Power or Green Life Juicer because any one of these will provide you with great versatility. Instead of buying them new, you might consider used. I can't tell you how many "brand new" Champion juicers I've bought for $75, because they were just sitting around in someone's closet. (Many people, unfortunately, will purchase them and then lose interest in using them.)

A blender and food processor are easily acquired and inexpensive, unless you're going for the top of the line. I started with a $49 food processor and then, a few years later, finally acquired a Cuisinart. **Work with what's at hand** so you don't have to wait to get started. Most of the patés can be made in a food processor, although they don't come out as smooth as in a Champion or Green Power. In lieu of a food dehydrator, you could always set your oven to the lowest temperature and leave the door open. If you live in a sunny climate, you could dehydrate in the sun, with a screen placed over the food. If you don't own a juicer as yet, you could go to a juice bar to obtain your juices. You could even ask for the pulp, if you needed it for a recipe.

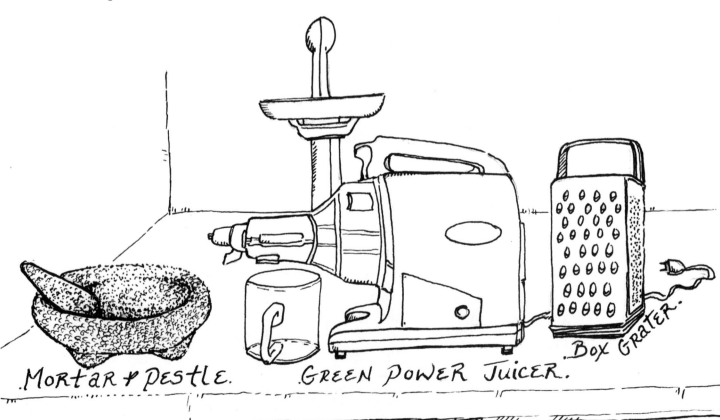

MORTAR & PESTLE.   GREEN POWER JUICER.   BOX GRATER.

Once the decision is made to go high-raw or even just to add a greater percentage of raw to your diet, the ways and means to do so will come to you.

BLENDER

Blenders are very useful for making nut milks, smoothies, purées, dressings and soups. Most of them work pretty well and are usually priced very reasonably, between $30 and $50.

CABBEC

A heavy-duty utensil that cuts hard vegetables into spaghetti-like threads. Expensive, but good. Refer to the Saladacco listing in this section for an excellent, low-priced alternative.

CHAMPION JUICER

The Champion juicer is a piece of equipment that is very versatile for this type of cuisine. First, of course, it makes juice. It is a masticating type juicer, which automatically expels the pulp, while continuously juicing. No intermittent cleaning is required, as with the centrifugal type juicers. It also has a blank screen (homogenizer) that you can install to make patés, nut butters, ice creams, and sherbets, and it will shred vegetables, such as carrots, beets and coconut, if you remove the blank. In addition, there is an attachment you can purchase separately to grind grain. The grain grinder, however, is made with aluminum parts and so is not recommended by this writer.[1] The

---

[1] Aluminum has been implicated in the development of Alzheimer's Disease because "Aluminum buildup is seen in all Alzheimer's sufferers (100%)" (Ref: *The Cure for all Diseases* by Hulda Regehr Clark, Ph.D., N.D., 1995.) Alzheimer's Disease is a deterioration of the brain, characterized by severe memory impairment.

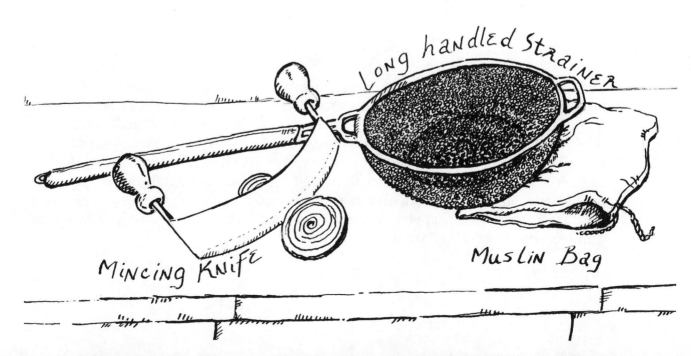

Long handled strainer

Muslin Bag

Mincing Knife

company that makes the Champion has been in business for almost 50 years. It is an American product, and I have found it to be well-made and durable. The Champion juicer is available in two types: a home model and a heavy-duty industrial model. The difference in price between the two is very small ($30-50). I would recommend the industrial model, although I've had both models and they are both very good and last for years.

CHEESE BAG
(aka Sprout Bag)

These bags, generally made of nylon, are used specifically to sprout seeds, beans and grains, and usually go under the name of Sprout Bags. **They can also be used to make the nut and seed cheeses in my recipes.** They are sold at the different institutes that teach the living foods lifestyle, such as the Hippocrates and Ann Wigmore Institutes and the Optimum Health Institute of San Diego. The institutes also make them available by mail order for a nominal price (*see* Source Index).

COFFEE GRINDER, NUT/SPICE MILL

A small electric coffee grinder or nut/spice mill is excellent for grinding dried herbs, spices, nuts, seeds and dehydrated vegetables into a powder. It is an inexpensive kitchen accessory.

COLANDERS & STRAINERS

Colanders and strainers are handy for draining and rinsing your sprouts, nuts and seeds. I like the large restaurant-type that has an extra long handle. This handle makes it very easy to free up your hands for rinsing sprouts. I set the strainer on the sink. The long handle allows the loop(s) on the front of the strainer to sit on one side of the sink ledge while the handle sits on the other side. The main part of the strainer is then suspended in the middle, so I don't have to hold it up.

DEHYDRATOR

I've used several dehydrators and I recommend the Excalibur. It comes in 4-tray on up to 9-tray sizes and has the heating element in the back, which blows warm air evenly over the trays of food. The round dehydrators that you see advertised on television don't dry food evenly because the heating element, which is on the bottom, only dries the first couple of trays and then you have to keep rotating the top trays to the bottom. It's not very convenient. Also, the round dehydrators generally do not have thermostats so you don't know at what temperature you are drying the food. The Excalibur has a thermostat that you can set to low temperatures. It is also well made and durable. (*See* "Excalibur" in the Source Index.)

GARLIC PRESS

A handy little tool for pressing garlic cloves. You just insert a garlic clove, press the two handles together and out comes finely mashed garlic. A garlic press can also be used to press small chunks of ginger.

GREEN POWER JUICER

The Green Power juicer is the first significant advancement in juicing technology in a very long time. This juicer has a number of advantages over the Champion. Like the Champion, it can juice fruits and vegetables. Unlike the Champion, it can also juice herbs, leafy greens and wheatgrass. (The Champion can juice some leafy vegetables, if they are put through along with harder vegetables.) The Green Power has a unique twin-gear triturating extraction system. It operates at a slow speed of 90 rpm. Because of this slow speed, there is less chance of the juicer heating up and damaging enzymes and other nutrients in the juice. Independent laboratory tests provided by the company show that the nutrient value of juice made in the Green Power is comparable to that of the Norwalk, which is the best (and most expensive) juicer on the market.

With the Green Power, you can create patés, sherbets, ice creams, nut butters, doughs (for Essene breads) and pretzels. It also includes attachments for making pasta. In experimenting with it, however, I was never able to create a pasta using sprouted grains because the pasta holes were too small and the raw ingredients gave too much resistance. (They didn't go through easily.) This attachment was obviously designed for making pasta from cooked grains.

The Green Power Juicer (as well as the Green Life) are also the only juicers on the market with magnetic rollers that magnetize the juice (or food), to delay oxidation. This is a revolutionary feature, which the company claims allows the juice to be stored for two or three days. Even so, I do not recommend storing juices more than one day, unless you are using a Norwalk. Another feature that I particularly like is that the Green Power operates quietly. Even though this is an excellent machine, be prepared to replace plastic parts from time to time as they tend to crack after a few years of heavy usage.

GREEN LIFE JUICER

This juicer is a redesign of the Green Power juicer and is sold by the same company. The Green Life has the same gear and motor as the Green Power. It is a little smaller and the front end of the machine was changed to be slightly stronger.

HAMMER

Because I use coconuts of all types in my kitchen, I find a hammer to be an indispensable piece of kitchen equipment. Use it to crack coconuts open, after draining the water. Also, use a hammer to crack open prune pits.

KNIVES

A variety of knives, each geared to a specific task, is very important and makes chopping and slicing faster and easier.

MANDOLINE

Mandolines are used by many restaurant chefs because they are heavy-duty utensils for grating and slicing vegetables and some fruits into various textures and shapes. They are made of stainless steel and are usually priced between $150 and $200. A low-priced substitute, under $40, is the V-Slicer (*see* below).

MEZZALUNA
(Mincing Knife)

This is a half-moon shaped knife, with a handle on both ends, which is very handy for quickly mincing vegetables and herbs. I've seen some Oriental chefs, who are very proficient in its use, mince things faster than a food processor. Well, almost! And you don't have to clean the processor afterwards. Since I'm not as fast as some of these professionals, I use this knife when I'm not in a hurry or for mincing small quantities.

MUSLIN BAGS

To make seed and nut yogurts and milks, I use small muslin bags. After the seeds and/or nuts are blended with water in the blender, I pour the liquid into a muslin bag. Then I squeeze the bag, releasing the milk into a bowl, until the bag is dry. The seed/nut pulp stays inside the bag. The pulp is discarded or saved for another use and the bag can be washed and reused.

These bags are not easy to locate, even in health food stores. (I guess not too many people are making seed and nut yogurts and milks yet.) The bags go by the name of "Salad Jelly Bags," because they are sold for storing salad vegetables and making jelly. They are available through my Website: www.rawfoodinfo.com

SALADACCO

The Saladacco is a low-cost utensil that cuts hard vegetables into spaghetti-like threads. Sometimes called a spiralizer, It also cuts vegetables into spiral shapes. The Saladacco is easy to use and easy to clean. It is available through my Website:
www.rawfoodinfo.com

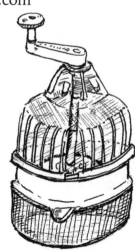

SALADSHOOTER®

The SaladShooter® Slicer/Shredder is a small, hand-held appliance, which very quickly slices or grates almost all vegetables, nuts, seeds and some fruits. It has various blades called "cones," that allow you to grate to a fine or medium consistency. You can also make chip shapes, both regular and crinkled. It is easy to use and quick to clean.

This handy piece of equipment is put out by National Presto Industries, Inc. It is very inexpensive and usually available anywhere small appliances are sold. There are two models available; one with a cord and the other, cordless and rechargeable. Having used both, I like the one with the cord better. (*See* "SaladShooter®" in the Source Index.)

SALAD SPINNER

A salad spinner is a handy tool for spinning leafy greens dry. You just place the washed greens or lettuces in the salad spinner basket, put the top on and keep turning the handle. The water is thrown out of the basket by centrifugal force. (Some salad spinners work by pulling a cord or pushing a large button but I like the type with the handle best.) It's a good idea to spin dry your leafy greens because the dressing will then adhere to the leaves better and the salad will be much tastier.

SCREWDRIVER

A flathead screwdriver is the tool for opening the "eye" of a coconut. Every brown coconut has three "eyes" in the shell and one of these "eyes" is soft. You can push through it with a flathead screwdriver and then widen the hole, which allows the coconut water to drain out into a large glass.

SPROUT BAG

(See Cheese Bag)

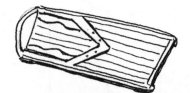

V-SLICER

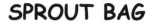

This is a low-priced plastic mandoline. The blades are very sharp, so you must exercise **extreme caution** in using it. It shreds and slices fruits and vegetables quickly and easily.

VITA-MIX

This machine is a heavy duty, high quality blender. It does not really make juice as it's touted to do, because it does not separate out the pulp. The company's advertising claims it makes a "total juice," which includes the pulp, but it is very thick unless you thin it out with water or juice. I believe the Vita-Mix is more suitable for making soups, but you must be careful you don't keep it running too long, because it will heat up the food. With the addition of a little liquid, you could use the Vita-Mix to prepare the ice cream and sherbet recipes. It does make very smooth and creamy patés, like *Hummus*. The drawbacks are that it is a little noisy (although I've heard the newer models are quieter), and it costs **a lot more** than a regular blender, but it is well worth the investment. A lot of people love 'em, including me.

WHEATGRASS JUICER

There are several brands of electrical equipment available that are specifically designed for juicing wheatgrass and leafy green vegetables. One popular model is the Miracle Wheatgrass Juicer. Some hand-crank models are also available. For a comprehensive review of the various wheatgrass juicers available, please refer to *Wheatgrass—Nature's Finest Medicine* by Steve Meyerowitz, published by Sproutman Publications, 1998.

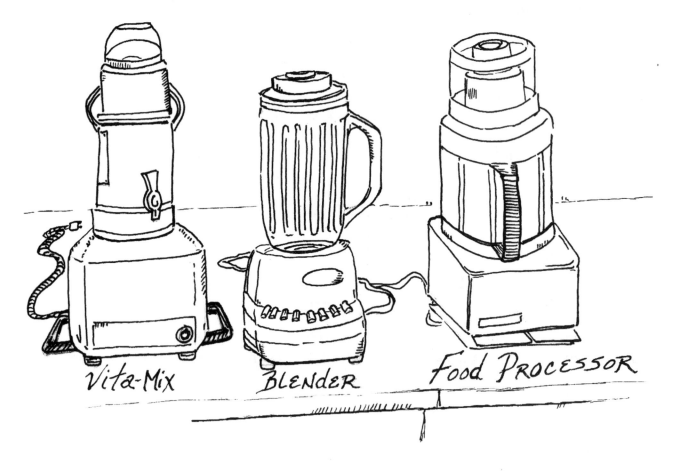

CHAPTER FIFTEEN:
Food Combining

Food combining has been devised as a system to help people better digest their food. According to food combining guidelines, if you separate certain foods and do not consume them together, then your digestion will improve and you will avoid creating gas, overacidity, insufficient acidity (lack of hydrochloric acid) and other digestive problems. Proteins are not to be combined with carbohydrates (starchy carbs). You can combine protein with vegetables or starches with vegetables but not both. You can combine certain fruits together, but not others. The acid, sub-acid and sweet categories of fruits are best consumed separately. Melons should be consumed alone. The rules can be confusing at times, and I wonder how the animals in nature keep it straight. They don't seem to worry about it though—but then, their diet is raw.

I do believe there is validity to this system, ESPECIALLY when applied to the eating of cooked foods. But I've come to have my doubts about the necessity for these rules in relation to a high-raw and living foods diet, AFTER YOU'VE STRENGTHENED YOUR DIGESTIVE SYSTEM SO IT FUNCTIONS OPTIMALLY. I can only go by my own experience here, and tell you I have had no trouble digesting raw foods, even when they are supposedly miscombined. Again, everyone is different and you may experience some discomforts, especially when first beginning to incorporate more raw and living foods into your diet.

If you have been food combining and it works for you, then please continue. You may have to adapt some of the recipes which don't conform, but that's what I'd like you to do anyway. Be innovative. Make these recipes work for you. Don't like garlic? Leave it out. Don't like something else? Substitute. Get into that kitchen and be creative. After all, you are creating your own future health.

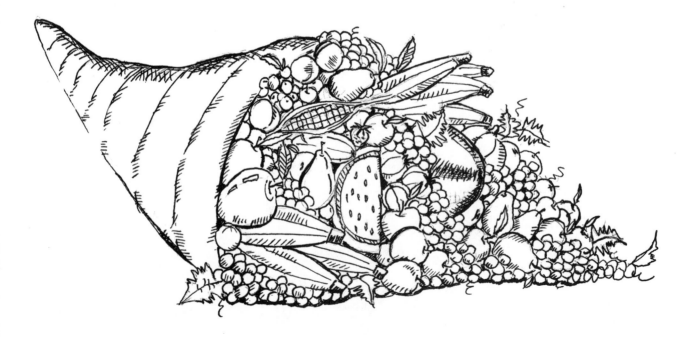

For people with *health challenges* or digestive problems to overcome, it is best to make food combinations as simple as possible. Follow the food combining guidelines as outlined in *Living Foods for Optimum Health* by Brian R. Clement[1] and Theresa Foy DiGeronimo.

Food combining principles tell us not to mix fruits with vegetables. Fruits should go with fruits, vegetables with vegetables, but how many of us think of a cucumber or bell pepper as fruit, or a tomato, or an eggplant? Or how about okra? Though usually classified as vegetables, these are, in fact, fruits. Sometimes the experts don't even agree as to what is a fruit and what is a vegetable. If it has a seed or pit inside, it's generally considered to be a fruit (the above-mentioned fruits all have seeds or pits), but where does that leave pineapple?[2] I've seen pineapple classified as a vegetable (no seeds inside), and indeed it does mix very well with the leafy green vegetables, as you will discover if you try *Dr. Kirschner's*[3] *Green Drink* (*see* page 244), but most of us think of pineapple as a fruit. What about corn? Is it a fruit? The corn kernels themselves are seeds. Or is it a vegetable or a grain?

In food combining, we are told not to mix a starch (or carbohydrate) with a protein, but how does that explain legumes, which are carbohydrate and protein beautifully combined by nature?

It seems to be a matter of degree; if a food is more protein than carbs, then it's classified as a protein food. If it's more carbs than protein, then it's classified as a carbohydrate. But how does this deal with the fact that carbs and protein are both there in the food? So how can these food combining principles apply? The food combiners say that you need one type of enzyme to digest proteins and another type of enzyme to digest carbohydrates and that the body cannot do the two at once. But since every raw plant food is not strictly a protein or a carbo-

---

[1]Brian Clement is the director of the Hippocrates Health Institute in West Palm Beach, Florida.

[2]Recently I learned that pineapples used to contain seeds, but hybridization has done away with them.

[3]Dr. H.E. Kirschner of Monrovia, Calif. became convinced of the powerful healing properties of medicinal herbs (sometimes called weeds), leafy vegetables, grasses and legumes and used them extensively in his medical practice. When he was put in charge of a ward of "hopeless" patients, he decided to supplement their starchy over-cooked food diet with one glass of juice per day. He mixed pineapple juice in a blender with leafy green herbs, such as malva, comfrey, filaree, lambs-quarter, chickweed, dandelion, etc. He also added in almonds, dates, sunflower seeds and kelp powder. With one glass of this wonderful healing drink a day, many of these patients, who hadn't been up and out of their hospital beds in years, became mobile. You can get the whole story in Dr. Kirschner's book entitled *Nature's Healing Grasses* (*see* Bibliography).

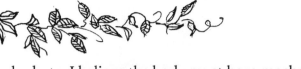

hydrate, I believe the body must have mechanisms that food combining parameters do not take into consideration.

The scenario goes something like this. A food, which contains carbohydrate, protein and fat, is chewed and mixed with enzymes that are secreted into the mouth by the salivary glands. Here the process of digestion begins. The Ptyalin (salivary amylase) secreted by the parotid glands work on the carbohydrates (starch). Protease, released by the submandibular glands, work on protein; and lipase, released by the sublingual glands, work on fat. In addition, cellulase, which digests the soluble parts of cellulose, is released from raw fibrous foods by thorough chewing. (Cellulase is not produced by the body.) Then the food moves into the upper stomach,[4] where enzymes from the raw food, as well as salivary enzymes, continue their work. The food stays in the upper stomach for approximately 30-60 minutes. Up to 60% of the carbohydrate (starch), 30% of the protein and 10% of the fat is digested even before the food moves to the lower stomach area. When the stomach secretes enough hydrochloric acid to lower the pH to below 3, the food moves into the lower stomach, where pepsin is activated and works upon the protein. Finally the food moves into the first part of the small intestine where "enzymes delivered to the duodenum in pancreatic juice continue the digestion of starch and protein. In addition, pancreatic lipase is responsible for the digestion of most of the dietary fat."[5]

Most plant, so-called, PROTEIN FOODS CONTAIN CARBOHYDRATES (as well as fats, vitamins, minerals, enzymes and unknown factors) and most so-called, CARBOHYDRATE FOODS CONTAIN PROTEINS in the form of amino acids[6] (as well as fats, vitamins, minerals, enzymes and unknown factors). Of course, I'm talking about whole foods here, not food artifacts.[7] Among artificial, factory manufactured foods, you can find all protein or all carbohydrate foods, but these do not occur frequently in nature.

Many of the food combining guidelines may not apply to people who have been eating a wide variety of raw and live food for an extended period of time. Depending on the state of your health when you first begin

---

[4]Dr. Edward Howell, preeminent researcher on enzymes, contends that the human stomach is divided into two parts. The upper part (predigestive stomach) functions as a place where enzymes in the food, plus salivary enzymes, begin digesting the food, before it moves to the lower stomach. In the lower part, hydrochloric acid initiates the activity of pepsin.

[5]*Structure and Function in Man* (4th ed) by Jacob Francone Lossow. W.B. Saunders Co., 1978.

[6]Ref: *SEEDS OF CHANGE The Living Treasure* by Kenny Ausubel, pgs. 109-112.

[7]Foods which have been processed by the food technologists into fractions of their component parts, sometimes called isolates. For example: isolated soy protein. Ref: *Smart Nutrients* by Dr. Abram Hoffer and Dr. Morton Walker (*see* Bibliography).

a high-raw diet, you may want to follow the rules. Then as your digestion and health improve, you could either ease up or continue food combining if it suits you. Of course, there are some obvious miscombinations we all could abide by—like PLEASE don't eat fruit directly after a main course meal. The fruit cannot get digested when it's consumed directly following a main course meal, and so it just sits there and ferments while creating gas and flatulence. Fruit digests very quickly, in as little as 1/2 to 1 hour. A main course meal will take longer: four hours or more. Since the fruit is sitting on top of the main course meal, it has to wait until the meal is digested first before its turn comes, but in the meantime it ferments instead.

Dr. Ann Wigmore innovated the combining of fruits and vegetables together in her healing energy soups with extremely beneficial results. The blending, I believe, makes all the difference. These soups are made mostly with vegetables, leafy greens and sprouts, but with fruits added in for flavor (*see Dr. Ann's Energy Soup—pg. 198*).

I realize I am out here on my own with some of these ideas. As a **seeker** of truth, I can only report from my own experience and observation. Please remember, what may be true and correct for me (and others) may not be for you. I encourage you to evaluate food combining, as taught by other teachers. Then try some recipes and reach your own conclusions.

RHIO'S PARAMETERS FOR OPTIMUM DIGESTION

What I find infinitely more important for attaining good digestion and assimilation are the following:

1) Eat in a spirit of gratitude for the beautiful food the earth has brought forth.

2) Eat only when really hungry.

3) Don't eat when overly stressed out, upset or angry. Don't eat out of boredom; find something interesting to do instead.

4) Eat moderate amounts. Don't stuff yourself. Listen to your body's signals that you've eaten enough.

5) Let one meal digest completely before eating another.

6) Don't eat fruit directly after a main course meal. Let at least an hour elapse, two is better. If you want, you can eat fruit 1/2 hour **before** a main course meal. It's best really to eat fruit as a separate meal. "But, Rhio," I hear you say, "this doesn't make sense to me. You say to eat fruit as a separate meal, but then you've combined fruits and vegetables in some of your recipes?" Good point. If fruit and vegetables are eaten together (and chewed well), they do not appear to

impede the digestive process or create a problem, as will tend to happen if you eat fruit directly after a main course meal.

7)   Don't eat on the run. Sit down to eat by yourself, or with good company, and eat slowly, chewing very well.

8)   Don't drink water with meals because it dilutes the digestive enzymes and interferes with their work on the food. If you get thirsty, drink **little** sips of water.

9)   Don't eat dinner and then lie down directly afterwards. Between the last meal of the day and bedtime, a few hours should pass. If you must eat, make it something very light, like fresh fruit.

10)   Don't choose mealtimes to discuss things that upset you. Try to make mealtimes as relaxed, pleasant, fun and loving as possible.

My advice on food combining boils down to this: Nobody knows your own body better than you do, especially when you start paying attention. So prepare some (raw) recipes, chew well when eating, and check out what happens. If you have no discomfort,[8] the combination works for you, no matter what any chart says.

A person following a high-raw/live food diet and related lifestyle will gradually cleanse their body of accumulated toxins. Eventually their digestion will become strong, resilient and effortless. At that point, food combining principles diminish in importance.

> Those who cannot or will not follow a high-raw program are advised to adhere to food combining guidelines.

---

[8]Remember though, when **beginning** these dietary changes (and raw foods are new to you,) you can expect some unpleasantness, usually due to toxicity release. (*See* Chapter 4.)

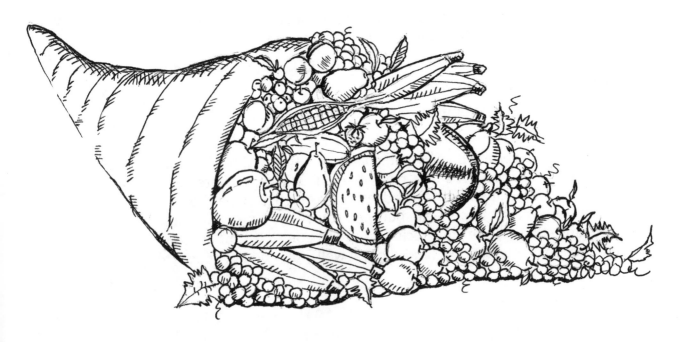

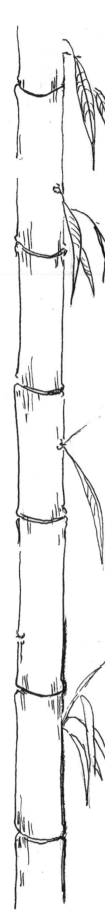

CHAPTER SIXTEEN:
Looking for a Better Way

If you are reading a book of this nature, I would imagine you are searching for a better, more excellent way to achieve and/or maintain glowing good health; or you may be trying to reestablish good health. I'm talking about the kind of health most people do not experience today, judging by the numerous commercials for pain killers, analgesics, headache potions, arthritis remedies, laxatives, etc., on TV and in magazines, not to mention the recent proliferation of prescription drug ads. A healthy populace would soon put the sellers of these products out of business.

Now, I'm not for putting people out of business, believe me, but they could switch to another field, and I'd like to help them do so, in my own small way. Such switching, however, does not seem imminent, because too many people (millions) seem to think they need these things to cope in today's world. Or could it be that they've been "programmed" to feel that the use of such products is normal? And once people are caught in the trap of these drugs, dependency and addictions to them can and do take hold. Most people in the United States exist in a kind of twilight zone between health and illness—they are well fed, but marginally nourished.

Just eating a high percentage of raw and living food regularly will, over time, strengthen your natural instincts for choosing (and preferring) them. Your body will start to recognize what it needs. This does not happen overnight, because you must first get over your addictions to sugar, salt, MSG, caffeine and whatever other chemicals you may have been ingesting. Over time, though, you will form new neuron pathways in your system and you will actually come to prefer raw food over any other.

When opportunities present themselves, try especially to eat these foods in a congenial atmosphere with other like-minded people. Eating has emotional connections, and if we surround ourselves with fun and loving situations with which this food becomes associated, then we speed the process of creating these new neuron pathways.

If you ARE looking for a better way to improve or regain your health, then give these raw and living foods a fair chance. If you do, then I feel confident your search will be over. I have seen it work for many, many people . . . why not for you?

BUT THIS FOOD DOESN'T FILL ME UP, YOU SAY!

Raw and living foods take little energy to digest, which is why you feel light after eating them. Because of how we are accustomed to feeling or have been conditioned to feel after eating a meal, we actually think that something is missing, that something is not right. We don't feel heavy. We don't feel as if we ate, and yet, think of it: What a wonderful way to feel! You won't be getting drowsy in the mid-afternoons anymore because all your energy is being diverted to your digestion—you'll feel energized but not weighed down. Digesting your food with the full complement of enzymes and other intrinsic factors intact is a much easier and faster process and is not taxing to the body. Uncooked foods digest in 1/3 to 1/2 the time of cooked foods. Admittedly, this light feeling takes some getting used to in the beginning.

If this light feeling is a problem for you, my suggestion is to eat (for lunch and dinner) a main course dish, **and** a salad, **and** some dehydrated crackers. If you get hungry again in two hours, eat some fruit, or some blender soup, a vegetable side dish, or a mixed sprout dish, but only if you really can't wait until the next meal. A sprouted mixture of legumes, grains and seeds is particularly filling. (Check out the *Masala Medley* and *Coconut Rice* recipes - *see* Index.) Many people, when they change to this way of eating, are very hungry in the beginning, but this should taper off gradually. Some teachers say the abnormal hunger occurs because the cells of the body have been deprived of optimum nourishment for so long, they can't get enough of it when it is finally provided.

FOOD IS INEXTRICABLY TIED TO LIFE EXPERIENCES AND EMOTIONS

Eating can be a very emotional experience because it's tied to so many other things that take place in our lives. Learning to give up foods we love in favor of foods we can eventually come to love is no easy thing, and it takes time. In my case, I had a real love for ice cream. Analyzing it one day, I realized it stemmed from a cherished childhood experience with my father. My father worked as a waiter for some very fancy restaurants, as well as for lavish banquets in Beverly Hills, while he was trying to fulfill his dream of creating a fantasy getaway resort in Mexico. These were places that catered to the stars. Daddy used to bring home lots of fancy food (not the best food, I now realize), which was left over from these events. One night I was awakened at about 1 or 2 in the morning, along with the rest of the family, because Daddy had brought home a huge ice cream cake. Can you imagine being awakened out of a sound sleep to have a luscious piece of ice cream cake, with the whole family gathered around? It was like a fantasy. And of course, this cake came from the party of a famous movie star, which made it even more delicious! We all felt very loved and pampered.

So ice cream became a comfort food for me. When I discovered that store-bought ice cream was tainted with so many chemicals, I learned to make my own.

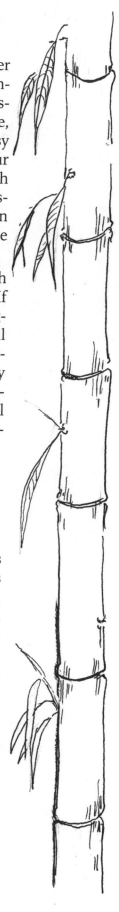

(You can read the labels, but be aware that not everything in the ice cream is listed, because of a little-known deceptive practice based on the "Standards of Identity"—*see* Glossary.) First, I made ice cream with milk and cream, and then, when I gave up dairy, with nuts and fruit. If you try some of the ice creams in the dessert recipes section of this book, you will realize that you are not really giving up anything. These are as rich and luscious as any store-bought ice cream made with dairy—but without the questionable additives. It's easy to convert. With some other foods, it may not be so easy, and adapting may take some time.

EASING EMOTIONAL OVEREATING

The "appestat"[1] tells you when your body has had enough to eat. Some people do not pick up these cues. To normalize your appestat, you must become more sensitive to signals from your body. A short, periodic fast (three days) shrinks the stomach a little bit. Then, after you begin eating again, if you pay attention to your body, you can usually pick up the signals that tell you when you've had enough. Another way to get in touch with these signals is to occasionally eat half as much as you normally would, or leave the table a little bit hungry. This will begin to make you aware of your true food intake needs. Most people can actually get along very well on much less food than they consume, and many studies have proven that health is better and life is longer when we consume less food.[2]

Sometimes you know you've had enough, but you keep on eating anyway. This has to do with emotional needs that you are attempting to stifle, smother, tamp-down, appease or cope with through consumption of food. This strategy does not address the underlying problem and usually leads to other problems, such as gaining too much weight. Sometimes people turn to food when they are bored, or when they get some bad news, or when they get some good news, or when they feel like celebrating, or when they're feeling emotionally overwrought, tired or overworked. Many times what you really need when you're feeling out of control regarding food is just some time for yourself; so make the time to nurture yourself as much as you need.

And keep eating High-Raw, because the foods themselves, over time, will normalize bodily and thus emotional conditions. Body, mind and soul are intertwined and interconnected, like tightly woven fibers in a fine tapestry. What affects one will always affect the others.

---

[1]"Appestat" is a word coined to describe a function of the hypothalamus, a part of the brain which controls appetite and satiety.

[2]*The 120-Year Diet*, Roy L. Walford, M.D. NY: Pocket Books, a Div. of Simon & Schuster, 1988.

Part Three: The Recipes

CHAPTER SEVENTEEN:
Raw/Live Food Preparation:
General Guidelines

SOME POINTS TO REMEMBER

All soaking of nuts, seeds, grains, beans and legumes, as called for in the recipes, should be in pure, filtered water. Sink water is OK for rinsing.

Unless otherwise stated in the recipes, measure all soaked and sprouted foods AFTER soaking and sprouting them. Refer to Soaking/Sprouting Yield Chart (*see* Chapter "Sprouting Is A Simple Affair . . ."). Or to make it simple, you could measure when dry, sprout, and then measure again for the recipe. Save the leftover sprouts to toss into soups or salads or to share with the birds.

For smaller portions, the recipes can be cut in half. For larger portions double the recipes.

When doubling the recipes, don't automatically double the oil content, if the recipe calls for oil. Most of the time you can get away with the same amount of oil or just a little bit more.

Some raw fooders object to the use of oil. They say that food oils do not exist in this form in nature. For those who don't want to use oil, I suggest you replace the oil in a recipe with a nut or seed yogurt. You will have to use more yogurt than the amount of oil stated in the recipe. I use yogurts to replace oils very often myself.

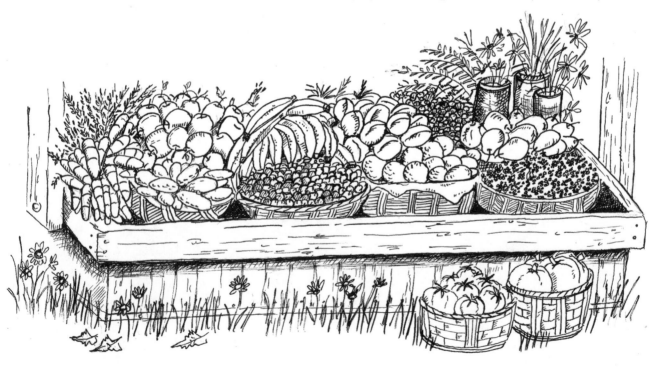

Store all oils, nuts and seeds in the refrigerator. They could easily go rancid at room temperature.

Most leftover patés can be shaped and dehydrated into crackers. Pulp left over from making seed and nut yogurts can be made into cookies, with the addition of soaked and blended dried fruit, cinnamon and/or vanilla and a touch of honey (optional). (*see Mommy's Almond Cookie Surprise,* page 260.)

Use only the freshest produce you can possibly find. The flavors of raw food, unlike those of cooked foods, cannot be masked. **You only get what you had to begin with**. So start with the very best, which in today's world means organically grown.[1] If you live in an area where organically grown food is not readily available, begin asking for it. If enough people ask, it will become available. By some estimates, organic food will comprise 10% of the American food supply by the year 2010. This represents tens of billions of dollars . . . **and it is our buying power making it happen**.

When available, buy produce grown from heirloom or open-pollinated seeds. Begin asking for this type of produce **specifically**. This is very important, because such produce is closer to what nature provided for us.

Buy produce in its own season as much as possible. Many fruits are held in cold storage for months. When you buy apples in the summer, for example, you are getting last year's crop. When the summer fruits come in, eat them at that time because they are then in their prime. In addition, their cooling qualities will help your body cope with the hot weather. Juicy summer fruits are also very cleansing to the body. When the autumn fruits, such as pomegranates, persimmons, passionfruit, fresh

---

[1]Organic food is grown without pesticides, herbicides, fungicides, etc., and without artificial chemical fertilizers. In addition, it is grown with seeds which have not been genetically engineered through biotechnology (no DNA tampering).

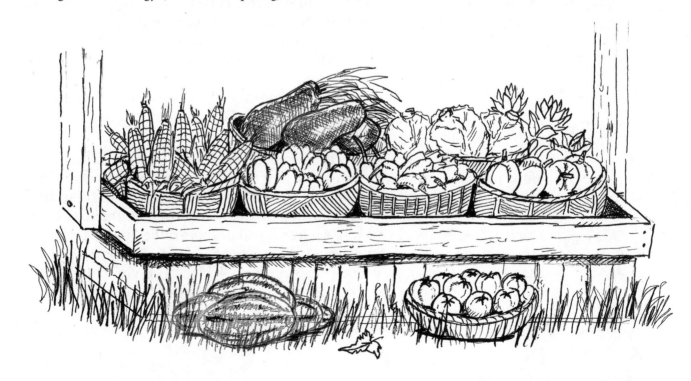

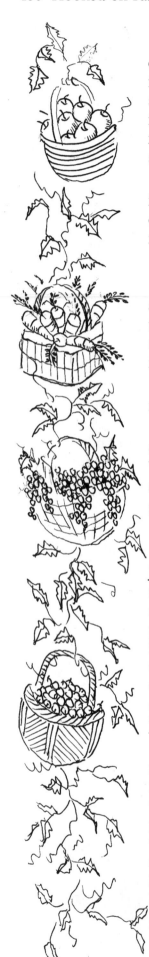

dates and figs, cranberries and others come in, go for them. Eating autumn fruits in their season is much more nourishing and satisfying than eating summer fruits out of season. When I've tried to put together summer-type fruit salads in the winter months, they are invariably disappointing. The summer fruits available at that time are usually pale and insipid ghosts of their summer counterparts.

For the most part, try to eat fruits when they are ripe (tree-ripened is best). Bell peppers and hot peppers are ripe when they are red, yellow or orange. Green peppers are those that have not ripened yet. Limes are ripe when they turn yellow.

Reject all genetically engineered food. (*See* Chapter 9.)

When making a recipe, always begin with **less** spice, adding more according to your own taste. You can always add later, but it's not so easy to take away what you have already put into the dish. (If you add too much spice, you can mitigate the damage somewhat by adding more vegetables, more grains and/or more of the main ingredients.)

After preparing a recipe, adjust the flavors to your taste. It may need more lemon, herbs, spices, Celtic sea salt, etc.

I've given a time frame for how long the dishes should last in the refrigerator, but please remember, it is best to eat foods when just freshly prepared. When consuming dishes that are two or three days old, pair them with salads freshly made. With the exception of fermented food, prepared foods progressively diminish in nutrient values the longer they are stored.

Store all prepared food in glass containers.

Three machines are available: the Champion Juicer, the Green Power Juicer and the Green Life Juicer, any one of which is indispensable for creating a variety of flavors and textures in this cuisine. Experiment with the equipment you have at hand. If you become convinced of the value of incorporating more raw and live foods into your diet, then you may want to look into acquiring either a Champion, a Green Power or a Green Life juicer. For the recipes, you can use these almost interchangeably. They all make juice, of course, but with these machines you can also create paté textures, ice creams, sherbets, and nut and seed butters. For more information on these juicers, *see* the Kitchen Equipment section.

If you do not have any of these machines, then you can substitute a food processor for making patés, but your final dish won't be as smooth. You may have to add a little water or other liquid to get the paté to blend better (but not too much, because you don't want it too loose). Without a Champion, Green Power or Green Life juicer, it will be more difficult to make either the nut and seed butters or the ice creams and sherbets. (Some sherbets can be made in a food processor using the "S" blade.) If you have a Vita-Mix, you can prepare ice creams and sherbets with the addition of a little liquid.

Some recipes are located within other recipes. So, for example, if you find the *Pine Nut Pesto* listed in the Index and go to that page, you will see that it brings you to a recipe called *Mock Black Ink Pasta with Pesto*. Within this recipe you will find the recipe for *Pine Nut Pesto*. This was done to save space so that more recipes could be incorporated into the book.

Some recipes call for raw peanuts, but if you prefer not to use peanuts because of concerns about aflatoxin, substitute almonds, filberts or pistachios.

Dried dates and figs are used in the recipes, unless otherwise specified.

Keep a small jar of soaked dates on hand. They last a couple of weeks in the refrigerator. (After that they will ferment.) Some of the recipes call for one or two soaked dates.

When preparing leafy salads, always use a salad spinner. The dressing you toss the salad with will stick to the leaves better if they are dry.

For cole-slaw type salads, use any of the nut or seed yogurts in place of mayonnaise. This is an easy and satisfying substitute.

Don't be afraid to change the recipes and make them your own. If there are some ingredients you don't like or can't get, make substitutions. Be creative, and you will start collecting a set of recipes which appeal to your own individual palate.

If you try a recipe and it is not to your liking, don't get discouraged. Try another, because there are recipes here for all tastes.

Most of the recipes are vegan. But there are exceptions: A few of the recipes call for raw honey. If you prefer not to use honey, substitute with blended dates or date syrup (water in which dates were soaked). You could also use the water in which raisins, figs, or currants have soaked for 24 hours.

Variety is very important. Different plants pick up different elements from the soil. What is missing in one food may be present in others, so rotate a wide variety of foods. Try not to get into a rut, where you eat the same dishes over and over (except for leafy greens, which you can eat to your heart's content).

Some people have said: "If soaking and sprouting are optimum and release the enzyme inhibitors, why do you have some ingredients in the recipes that are not soaked and sprouted?" As you can see, my students don't let me get away with anything! Ninety percent or more of nuts and seeds used in these recipes are soaked and sprouted. That's good enough for me.

Think of food preparation as a **healing alchemical endeavor**. Leave your stress, worries and cares at the kitchen door, put on some healing music and get into the beauty of your creations. You are truly creating your own future abundant good health and that of your family, so put all the love of your soul into it.

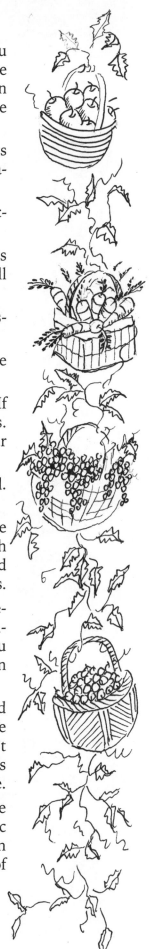

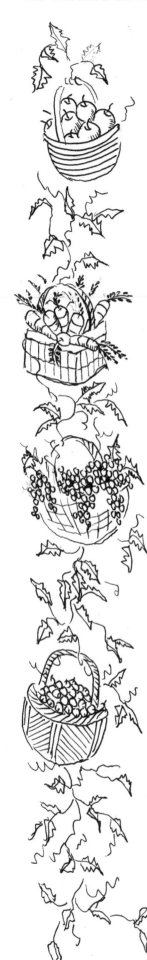

GETTING THE CHILL OUT

Eating cold food from the refrigerator is not pleasant (unless you're eating ice cream). In the process of preparing raw and living food, the food stays out and usually warms up to room temperature. If you are serving, let's say, a paté made the previous day, straight from the refrigerator might be too cold. Let it sit out for about 1/2 hour to get to room temperature.

If you're short on time, the next best way to warm up food is to use a double boiler. But PLEASE, read carefully how to do it or you may inadvertently . . . COOK! Put about an inch of water into the bottom of the double boiler and boil the water. Then turn off the flame, and put the food into the top part of the double boiler. Put the top part with the lid on, over the bottom part, and let sit for 5 or 10 minutes, stirring once or twice. The chill will be off with no loss of enzymes. I recommend a double boiler made of tempered glass (by the brand name of Visions). Next best is stainless steel.

YOU MAY WANT TO KNOW WHY THERE ARE NO RECIPES UTILIZING WHEAT, SPELT, TRITICALE OR KAMUT

With the exception of *Rejuvelac* and *Wheatgrass Juice*, there are no recipes in this book utilizing wheat (spelt, triticale and kamut are varieties of wheat). This is because I personally do not handle wheat well, and therefore could not work with it, as I would not have been able to check the recipes for flavor and digestibility. In my experience, I have found a large majority of people have sensitivities to wheat, whether they are aware of it or not, and therefore, wheat may not be the best food choice for a lot of people. With myself, I've noticed I gain weight, get congested, and create mucus. My lymph glands may swell and the wheat generally puts me right to sleep. I've noticed these same symptoms, to a greater or lesser degree, in other people. I've read that this happens because of an intolerance to the gluten in wheat. I have suspicions, though, that it has to do with the fact that all the wheat today has been extensively hybridized. In addition, we are overconsuming wheat. Dr. Bernard Jensen, in his book, *Vibrant Health From Your Kitchen*,[2] points out that almost one-third of the American diet is composed of wheat products. Just three foods—wheat, milk products and refined sugar—make up 63 percent of our nation's diet. This doesn't leave much room for eating all the other things needed to support our health! There is no gluten in *Rejuvelac* or *Wheatgrass Juice*. Oats, barley and rye also contain gluten, and some people are sensitive to these products as well.

---

[2]Published by Bernard Jensen Enterprises, Escondido, CA 1986

Occasionally, I do eat a sprouted wheat dish when someone else makes it, like if I'm out at a friend's house. After so many years on raw and live foods, I do not have the severe reactions to wheat that I used to get. It seems that by eliminating it from my diet for a long period of time, I have been able to clean up the toxins wheat ingestion produced in my system. Now I can tolerate wheat without any discernible effects. However, I wouldn't want to reintroduce it on a regular basis and take the chance of building up or accumulating these toxins or sensitivities again. **For me**, it's just not worth it, and I don't really miss it.

PLAN AHEAD

Plan for and think about food long before you become hungry, because, when hunger strikes, you'll just want to eat. And if you haven't planned for it, then you may not make the best choices. I admit that this does curtail freedom and spontaneity somewhat, but in exchange, you will always have something good to eat. You won't have to worry about being able to find decent food, when it seems that only crap is available. And best of all you will have boundless energy!

The most important principle to remember in making this lifestyle work for you is **P L A N   A H E A D**.

A BEAUTIFUL PRESENTATION

There is a seduction involved in food presentation. Most fabulous restaurants understand this and they present the food very beautifully and seductively. A tantalizing picture is created when the food and the plate become a palette of delectably pleasing colors and textures. As your eyes take in the beauty and aroma,[3] your digestive enzymes start flowing, preparing you to savor and enjoy the dish, while at the same time improving digestion.

To enhance the visual, use herb, vegetable or fruit garnishes. Use beautiful plates and silverware, cloth napkins, flowers . . . use your imagination. First, it's a feast for your eyes and then, a delight for your taste buds. Believe it or not, if it looks beautiful to you, it will taste better.

AND NOW TO THE RECIPES

---

[3]Raw foods emanate subtle aromas, not as overt as the aromas you experience when cooking food, but definitely there just the same.

CHAPTER EIGHTEEN:
Hearty Main Course Dishes

I have devoted a great deal of space to Main Course Dishes because I feel that there is a definite lack of these dishes in the raw/live food recipe books that are available. You can find an abundance of recipes for salads, soups, juices and desserts, but where's the . . . main course?

Authors of some of the more recent raw food recipe books, have also recognized this need and are trying to fulfill it through their tasty entrée recipes. Check out Juliano's *Raw, The Uncook Book*, Nomi Shannon's *The Raw Gourmet*, and Imar Hutchins' *Delights of the Garden*.

Raw/live food main course dishes can be delicious, filling and satisfying. After consuming them for a period of time, the pull back towards or attraction to cooked foods will lessen. If you can manage to stay completely away from cooked foods for at least 3 to 6 months, then when you again taste cooked foods, you will discover that the flavor is not as good as you remember. That is when you'll notice that something is missing in them that you were never able to discern before. And you would be right. The missing factor is . . . the Life.

You can choose to eat only raw/live foods or you can choose to incorporate more of these types of foods into your cooked menus. This choice is yours alone to make. Even if you choose the second option, your health is sure to improve and this may lead you to adhere even more faithfully to the raw food diet in the future.

Health is our heritage.

BON APPETIT!

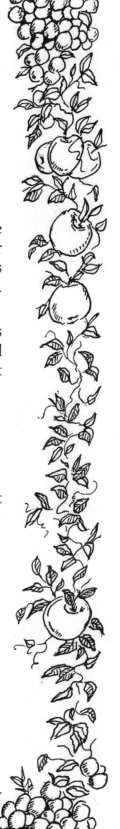

TOONA

3 cups walnuts, soaked overnight (or for at least 3 hours)
3 cups carrots (chop first, then measure)
1/4–1/2 medium onion
1 cup celery with leaves (leaves add good flavor)
1/2 cup parsley or cilantro
1/2 cup fresh basil (other fresh herbs, such as dill, can be used
    in place of basil for a slightly different flavor)
1–2 garlic cloves (according to your own taste)
2 oz. lemon juice
Nama Shoyu and/or Celtic sea salt, to taste

1) Drain and rinse walnuts. Cut the carrots into chunks and measure out three cups. Process walnuts and carrots to a paté through a Champion or Green Power juicer, with the blank in place. If you don't have one of these machines, process in a food processor until smooth. You may have to add a slight bit of water. Set aside in a bowl.

2) Cut the celery into 1-inch pieces so that you don't end up with long strings (to get stuck in your teeth), then pulse chop garlic, onion, celery, herbs and lemon in a food processor until well chopped. Add to the carrot and walnut paté and mix well. Add Nama Shoyu and Celtic sea salt to taste.

   Serves 6. Keeps for 2-3 days in refrigerator. Goes well with a crudité.

VARIATIONS:

- In place of celery, use fennel for a different taste.
- Use as a stuffing for nori rolls, adding in clover sprouts and matchstick-cut pieces of cucumber and tomato. Use in *Fabioli* (*see* page 136).
- This recipe also makes delicious dehydrated crackers.

WILD RICE MEDLEY

1 cup sprouted wild rice
1 cup diced tomato
1/4 cup minced onion
1/2 cup diced zucchini
1/2 cup diced green bell pepper
1 cup diced red bell pepper
1/2 cup *Chedda Sauce* (*see* page 210)

1) Mix all the ingredients together in a bowl. Serves 2. Best when eaten freshly made.

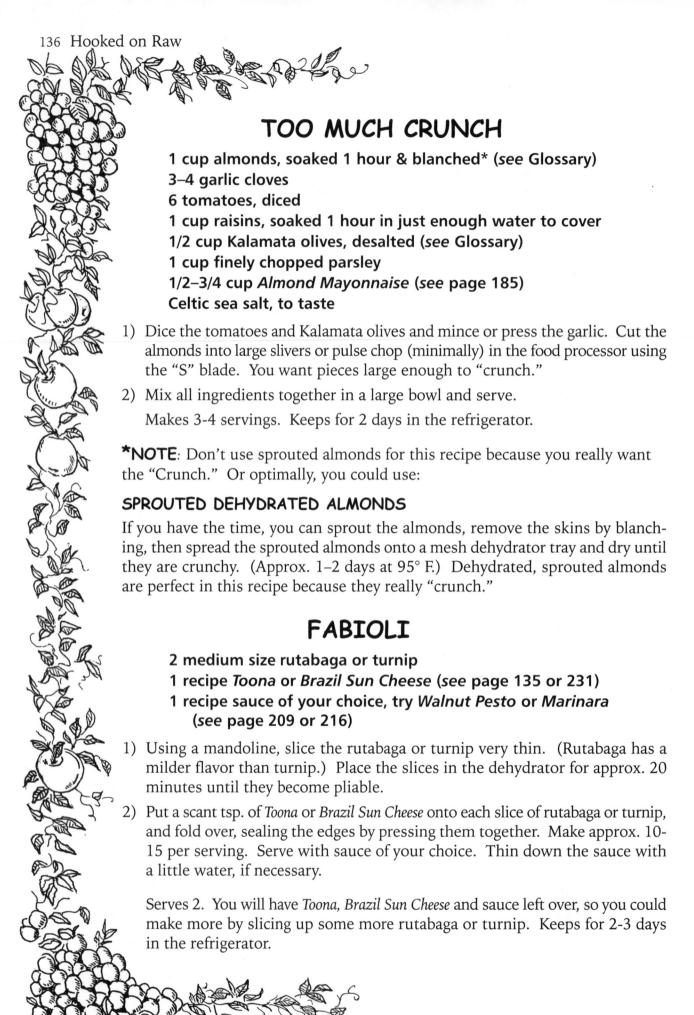

TOO MUCH CRUNCH

1 cup almonds, soaked 1 hour & blanched* (*see Glossary*)
3–4 garlic cloves
6 tomatoes, diced
1 cup raisins, soaked 1 hour in just enough water to cover
1/2 cup Kalamata olives, desalted (*see Glossary*)
1 cup finely chopped parsley
1/2–3/4 cup *Almond Mayonnaise* (*see page 185*)
Celtic sea salt, to taste

1) Dice the tomatoes and Kalamata olives and mince or press the garlic. Cut the almonds into large slivers or pulse chop (minimally) in the food processor using the "S" blade. You want pieces large enough to "crunch."

2) Mix all ingredients together in a large bowl and serve.

   Makes 3-4 servings. Keeps for 2 days in the refrigerator.

*NOTE: Don't use sprouted almonds for this recipe because you really want the "Crunch." Or optimally, you could use:

SPROUTED DEHYDRATED ALMONDS

If you have the time, you can sprout the almonds, remove the skins by blanching, then spread the sprouted almonds onto a mesh dehydrator tray and dry until they are crunchy. (Approx. 1–2 days at 95° F.) Dehydrated, sprouted almonds are perfect in this recipe because they really "crunch."

FABIOLI

2 medium size rutabaga or turnip
1 recipe *Toona* or *Brazil Sun Cheese* (*see page 135 or 231*)
1 recipe sauce of your choice, try *Walnut Pesto* or *Marinara*
     (*see page 209 or 216*)

1) Using a mandoline, slice the rutabaga or turnip very thin. (Rutabaga has a milder flavor than turnip.) Place the slices in the dehydrator for approx. 20 minutes until they become pliable.

2) Put a scant tsp. of *Toona* or *Brazil Sun Cheese* onto each slice of rutabaga or turnip, and fold over, sealing the edges by pressing them together. Make approx. 10-15 per serving. Serve with sauce of your choice. Thin down the sauce with a little water, if necessary.

Serves 2. You will have *Toona, Brazil Sun Cheese* and sauce left over, so you could make more by slicing up some more rutabaga or turnip. Keeps for 2-3 days in the refrigerator.

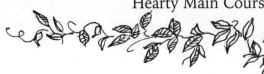

NEAT LOAF

2 cups sprouted hulled barley (sprouted for 1 or 2 days)
2 cups soaked walnuts (soaked overnight)
1/2 red bell pepper
1/2 stalk celery (cut into 1" pieces, so the strings won't
  get stuck in your teeth)
1/4 onion
1–2 garlic cloves
3/4–1 tsp. poultry seasoning*
Nama Shoyu and/or Celtic sea salt, to taste
garnish: 1 large tomato, sliced thin

1) Put barley and walnuts into a food processor and using the "S" blade, process for approx. 15 seconds. Set aside in a bowl.

2) Put the vegetables into the food processor and process well. Add to the barley-walnut mixture, add in the seasoning and mix well.

3) Pack into a glass loaf pan and cover with sliced tomatoes.

   Serves 4. Keeps in the refrigerator for 2-3 days. Serve with a large salad.

*Find a poultry seasoning combination that contains basil, rosemary, sage, marjoram, thyme, and oregano. The Spice Hunter is one such brand.

BROCCOLI WITH CHEDDA SAUCE

3 cups finely chopped broccoli*
1 cup *Chedda Sauce* (*see* page 210)

MARINADE: **1 tbsp. olive or flaxseed oil**
          1 lemon or lime, juiced
          1–2 tsp. Nama Shoyu or dash of Celtic sea salt

1) Toss the broccoli with the marinade until it is well coated. Cover and let marinate overnight in the refrigerator. The marinade ingredients help to "cold cook" the broccoli, which tames down some of the raw flavor.

2) Next day, mix the broccoli with some of the *Chedda Sauce*.

   Serves 2. Keeps for 2 days or longer in the refrigerator. *Broccoli with Chedda Sauce* can also be dehydrated for 2-4 hours at 95° F for those who still balk at eating broccoli raw.

*This recipe can also be made with thinly sliced Brussels sprouts.

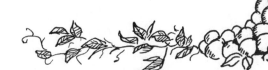

DEEP DISH PIZZA

**This is One of the Best Raw Pizzas I've Ever Tasted!
Created by Dennis Knicely, Former Director of
The Living Light House, Santa Monica, CA**

DENNIS' PIZZA CRUST:

1 cup (dry) buckwheat = approx. 2 1/2 cups sprouted
1 cup (dry) quinoa = approx. 2 1/2 cups sprouted
1 cup (dry) flaxseed
1–2 cups carrot pulp (optional)
season to flavor: Celtic sea salt or Bragg Liquid Aminos
fresh herbs: oregano, marjoram, basil, etc.

1) Soak dry buckwheat and quinoa overnight in filtered water (using separate bowls). Next day rinse well, and then sprout for 2 days, (rinsing twice each day).

2) Soak flaxseed for 2 hours in 1 1/2 cups filtered water.

3) Combine all ingredients, except flaxseed, in a food processor using the "S" blade and process until well mixed, adding seasoning and herbs according to your taste. Transfer to a bowl, add in the flaxseed* and blend by hand until a dough is formed. Roll out the dough between two Teflex sheets to 5/16" (or so) thick and place on a dehydrator tray, gently peeling off the top sheet. Instead of rolling the dough (which can be a little tricky), you could just spread the mixture onto a Teflex-lined dehydrator tray. Score 4" squares with the dull side of a butter knife and allow to dehydrate at 100° F for approximately 16 hours or until thoroughly dry. Halfway through, peel the crusts off the Teflex, turn them over and place them directly on the mesh dehydrator tray. At approx. 10 hours, the crust is soft and flexible, but if you want to store for use as needed, then dry until hard.

Thoroughly dried pizza crusts can be stored in a covered container at room temperature.

PIZZA PATÉ FILLER:

1 large or 2 small avocados
1 cup soaked pumpkin seeds (soaked 2-3 hours)
1 cup sprouted quinoa
1 or 2 small lemons, juiced (add to taste)
2 medium tomatoes
lots of fresh basil, oregano and misc. herbs
2 tbsp. olive oil (extra-virgin)
season to flavor: Celtic sea salt or Bragg Liquid Aminos

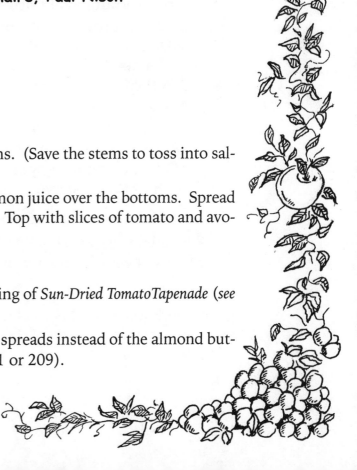

4) Put all paté ingredients into a food processor with the "S" blade and blend to a spread consistency.

PIZZA TOPPING:

>   **2 cups sun-dried tomatoes**
>   **olive oil**
>   **red & yellow bell peppers, diced**
>   **lemon juice**
>   **sun-dried Greek olives, chopped**
>   **Bragg Liquid Aminos**

5) Chop up the dried tomatoes and marinate in olive oil, lemon juice and Braggs overnight (or for 2-3 hours). Make sure all the tomatoes are coated.

6) When the crust is ready, break into individual sections. Spread with the paté, and sprinkle with the topping ingredients. This is ready to serve or you could dehydrate for an additional 2 hours.

Makes approx. 18 servings. Serve immediately.

*By keeping the flaxseed whole instead of ground, it has less chance of going rancid.

LAZY MAN'S PORTO PITZA

This Deceptively Simple Recipe was Shared by Raw Food Chef Extraordinaire, Paul Nison

>   **4 portobello mushrooms**
>   **1 lemon, juiced**
>   **raw almond butter**
>   **1 tomato**
>   **1 avocado**

1) Clean the mushrooms and cut off the stems. (Save the stems to toss into salads or dehydrate them.)

2) Turn the mushrooms over and squeeze lemon juice over the bottoms. Spread almond butter on the mushroom bottom. Top with slices of tomato and avocado.

Serves 2. Serve immediately.

SLOPPY JOES: Top with a generous slathering of *Sun-Dried Tomato Tapenade* (*see* page 271).

VARIATIONS: To vary the flavor, use other spreads instead of the almond butter. Try *Hummus* or *Walnut Pesto* (*see* page 211 or 209).

MASALA MUNG

2 cups sprouted mung beans (or lentils)
2–4 tbsp. freshly grated coconut
1 1/2 tbsp. sesame oil (or combination of sesame &
flaxseed oils)
1–2 tbsp. lemon juice
1/4 tsp. garam masala
1/8 tsp. ground brown mustard seeds
1/8 tsp. ground cumin seeds
1/8 tsp. cayenne pepper (optional)
dash of Nama Shoyu and/or Celtic sea salt

1) Put all the ingredients into a bowl and mix well together. Adjust flavors by adding more lemon juice, coconut or seasoning to taste.

Serves 2-3. Keeps for 2-3 days in the refrigerator.

MASALA MEDLEY

A Variation Of The Above

1 cup mung sprouts
1 cup lentil sprouts
1 cup sprouted wild rice (or oat groats or barley)
3 heaping tbsp. freshly grated coconut
1 1/2 tbsp. sesame oil (or combination of sesame &
flaxseed oils)
2–4 tbsp. lemon juice
1/4 tsp. garam masala
1/8 tsp. ground brown mustard seeds
1/8 tsp. ground cumin seeds
1/8 tsp. cayenne pepper (optional)
dash of Nama Shoyu and/or Celtic sea salt

1) Put all the ingredients into a bowl and mix well together. Adjust flavors by adding more lemon juice, coconut, or seasoning to taste.

Serves 4. Keeps for 2-3 days in the refrigerator.

NOTE: I've found that most sprouted seeds, lentils, mung beans and sprouted grains work well with this combination of oil and spices. If you have one, two or almost any combination of these sprouts on hand, you can whip up a quick and satisfying meal.

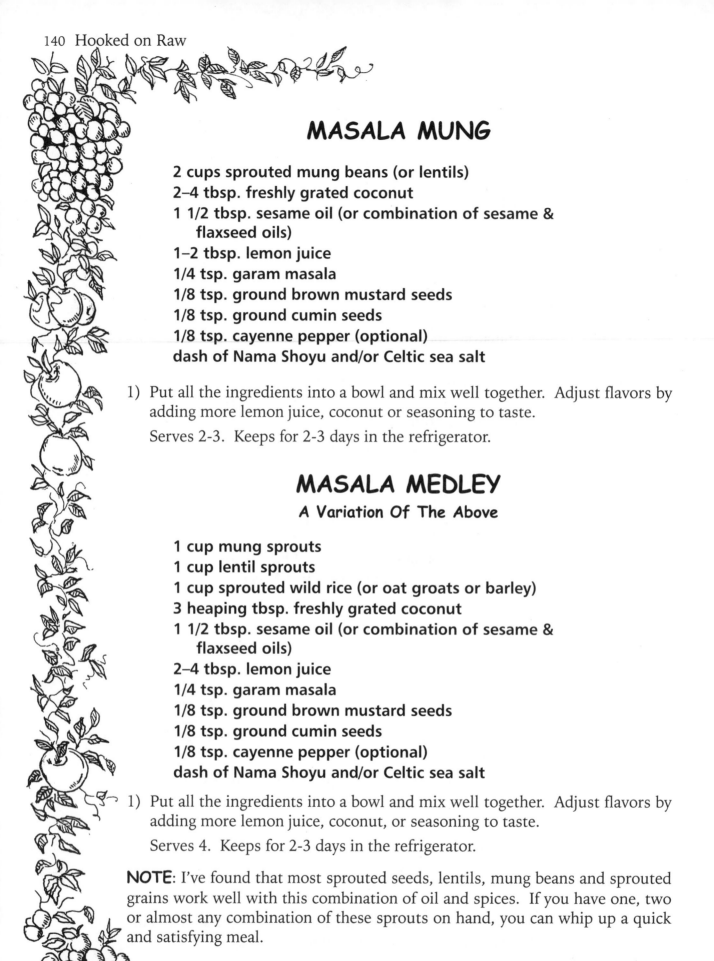

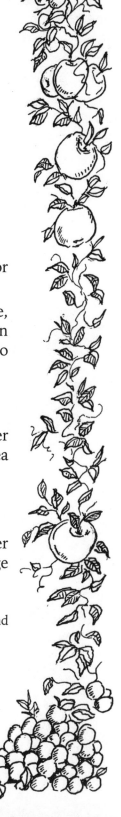

MASHED "POTATOES" AND GRAVY

Inspired by a Memorable Evening Spent at
the American Living Foods Institute, Glendale, CA

1 cauliflower
2 cups pecans, soaked 1 hour
2 cups filtered water
1/4 onion
2 tsp. poultry seasoning*
1 tbsp. olive oil (extra-virgin)
Celtic sea salt, to taste

"POTATOES":

1) Take the leaves off of the cauliflower and cut the core out. Save for salads or juicing. Cut the remaining cauliflower into small chunks.

2) Put the cauliflower chunks into a food processor, and using the "S" blade, process very fine until it kind of looks like mashed potatoes. Depending on the size of your food processor, you may have to do this in 2 or 3 batches (to process the entire cauliflower). Set "potatoes" aside in a bowl.

PECAN GRAVY:

3) Put the pecans, water, onion, poultry seasoning, and olive oil into a blender and blend to a gravy consistency. Taste and adjust flavors by adding Celtic sea salt if necessary.

4) To serve: Put one or two scoops of "potatoes" onto a plate, cover with gravy and ENJOY!

Serves 4-6. The gravy keeps in the refrigerator for 2-3 days. The cauliflower should be freshly prepared. Goes well with *Buckwheat-Quinoa Burgers* (*see* page 145), and a leafy salad.

*Find a poultry seasoning combination that includes basil, rosemary, sage, marjoram, thyme, and coriander. The Spice Hunter is one such brand (*see* Source Index).

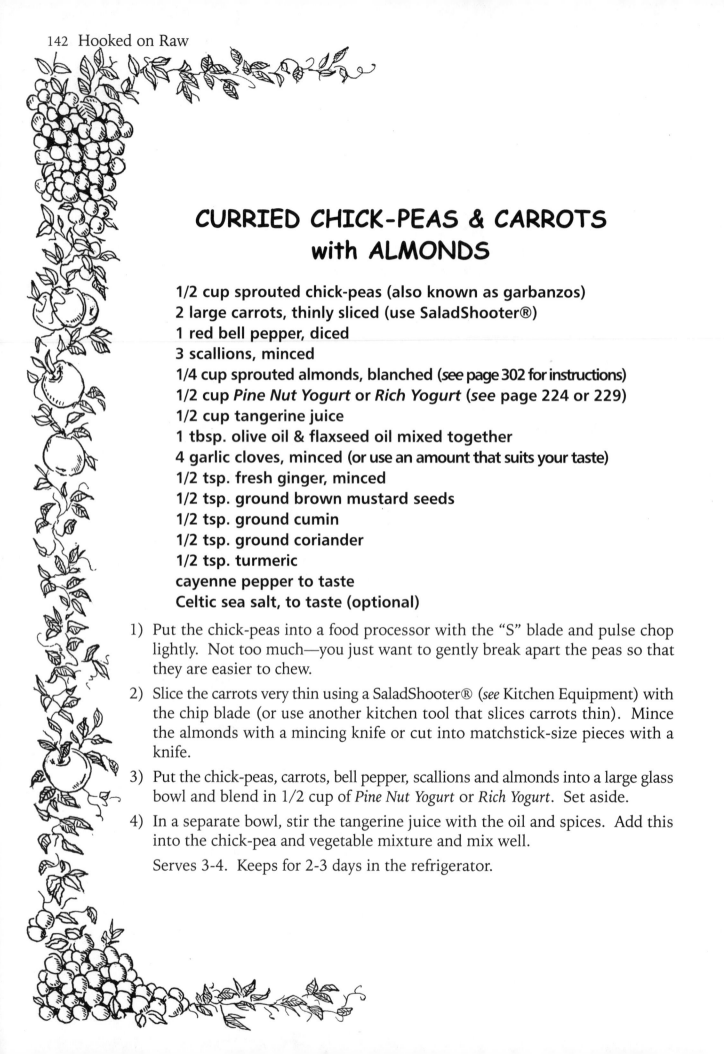

CURRIED CHICK-PEAS & CARROTS
with ALMONDS

1/2 cup sprouted chick-peas (also known as garbanzos)
2 large carrots, thinly sliced (use SaladShooter®)
1 red bell pepper, diced
3 scallions, minced
1/4 cup sprouted almonds, blanched (*see* page 302 for instructions)
1/2 cup *Pine Nut Yogurt* or *Rich Yogurt* (*see* page 224 or 229)
1/2 cup tangerine juice
1 tbsp. olive oil & flaxseed oil mixed together
4 garlic cloves, minced (or use an amount that suits your taste)
1/2 tsp. fresh ginger, minced
1/2 tsp. ground brown mustard seeds
1/2 tsp. ground cumin
1/2 tsp. ground coriander
1/2 tsp. turmeric
cayenne pepper to taste
Celtic sea salt, to taste (optional)

1) Put the chick-peas into a food processor with the "S" blade and pulse chop lightly. Not too much—you just want to gently break apart the peas so that they are easier to chew.

2) Slice the carrots very thin using a SaladShooter® (*see* Kitchen Equipment) with the chip blade (or use another kitchen tool that slices carrots thin). Mince the almonds with a mincing knife or cut into matchstick-size pieces with a knife.

3) Put the chick-peas, carrots, bell pepper, scallions and almonds into a large glass bowl and blend in 1/2 cup of *Pine Nut Yogurt* or *Rich Yogurt*. Set aside.

4) In a separate bowl, stir the tangerine juice with the oil and spices. Add this into the chick-pea and vegetable mixture and mix well.

Serves 3-4. Keeps for 2-3 days in the refrigerator.

COLLARD ROLLS

1 recipe of *Veggie Seed Paté* (*see* page 158)
1/2 bunch collard greens
clover, alfalfa or mixed sprouts
cucumber, julienne
tomato, julienne

OPTIONAL MARINADE: flaxseed or olive oil
lemon
Nama Shoyu and/or Celtic sea salt

1) Wash the collard leaves and shake off the water. **Marinating the leaves is optional.*** If you choose to do it, baste the inside of the leaves with the marinade, and place the leaves into a large bowl, one on top of another, as follows—one leaf with the marinated side facing up, next leaf with the marinated side facing down, and continue until you have done about half a bunch of leaves. Put a piece of parchment paper on top of the leaves and then put a heavy weight on top of the parchment paper. Cover with a clean dishtowel and let marinate in the refrigerator overnight. (For the heavy weight, use a half-gallon glass or plastic jug filled with water.)

2) When ready to prepare the *Collard Rolls*, drain out the marinade (save for another use, such as adding to salad dressings or sauces).

3) Cut the middle stalk out of the collard leaf (this can be saved for juicing). This leaves two sides of the large leaf which can then be cut into pieces for stuffing. These can be cut any size you want. Approx. 3" X 3" is good. Put a tablespoon of *Veggie Seed Paté* on one end of the leaf, add some sprouts, cucumber and tomato julienne, and roll the collard leaf tightly. Make as many as you want.

Keeps for a few days in the refrigerator.

*NOTE: The reason for marinating is to soften up the leaves enough so that you will enjoy eating them raw. If you already enjoy eating raw collards and don't find the leaves too tough, then eliminate this step. I usually do. You could also make the rolls with chard leaves, which are a little softer and easier to chew.

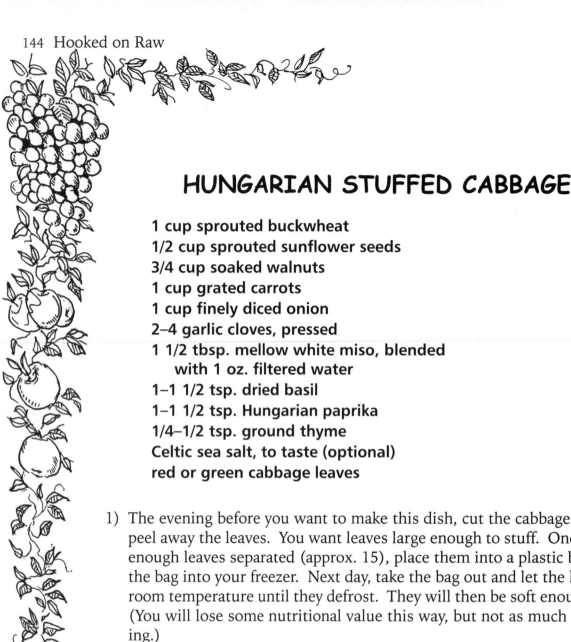

HUNGARIAN STUFFED CABBAGE

1 cup sprouted buckwheat
1/2 cup sprouted sunflower seeds
3/4 cup soaked walnuts
1 cup grated carrots
1 cup finely diced onion
2–4 garlic cloves, pressed
1 1/2 tbsp. mellow white miso, blended
    with 1 oz. filtered water
1–1 1/2 tsp. dried basil
1–1 1/2 tsp. Hungarian paprika
1/4–1/2 tsp. ground thyme
Celtic sea salt, to taste (optional)
red or green cabbage leaves

1) The evening before you want to make this dish, cut the cabbage in half and peel away the leaves. You want leaves large enough to stuff. Once you have enough leaves separated (approx. 15), place them into a plastic bag and put the bag into your freezer. Next day, take the bag out and let the leaves sit at room temperature until they defrost. They will then be soft enough to stuff. (You will lose some nutritional value this way, but not as much as by cooking.)

2) Briefly process the first three ingredients in a food processor with the "S" blade. Put into a large bowl and mix with the remaining ingredients. Start with less of the spices and add more to your own taste.

3) Stuff the cabbage leaves by putting a heaping tbsp. or more of the mixture onto a cabbage leaf and then roll the leaf, tucking in the ends as you go. Once you have rolled it, you can cut the rest of the cabbage leaf away with a sharp knife.

Makes approx. 15 cabbage rolls, 3-4 to a serving. Keeps for 3 days in the refrigerator.

SERVE PLAIN OR WITH:

- *Dill Sauce* (*see* page 215).
- *Italian Tomato Sauce* (*see* page 212).

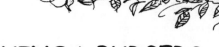

BUCKWHEAT-QUINOA BURGERS

1 recipe *Hungarian Stuffed Cabbage* (make stuffing only—
** *see* opposite page)**
1/2 cup sprouted quinoa
1 cup soaked walnuts

1) Follow step #2 only of the *Hungarian Stuffed Cabbage* recipe. Set aside.

2) Put the soaked walnuts through the Champion or Green Power juicer with the blank (homogenizer) in place. Scrape the paste out of the juicer housing. (With this small amount, a lot of it will be stuck in there.) Or you could put the walnuts into a food processor and using the "S" blade, blend to a paste, adding a little water if necessary.

3) Add the sprouted quinoa and the walnut paste to the Hungarian stuffing and mix well together with your hands. The walnut paste helps to hold the burger ingredients together. Form into burger-shaped patties and serve as is, or dehydrate as follows:

> For rare: dehydrate at 95° F for 4 hours.
>
> For medium: dehydrate at 95° for 10 hours.
>
> For well done: dehydrate at 95° for 24-36 hours.

Makes 9 Burgers. You'll probably want to double or triple the recipe. Keeps for up to a week in a sealed container in the refrigerator.

SERVING SUGGESTION: Serve on *Jamie & Kim's Flax Crackers* (page 265) with *Almond Mayonnaise* (page 185), mustard (opt.), tomato and onion.

SPINACH ROLLS

1 recipe *Creamed Spinach*   **1 1/2 cups tomato julienne**
1 1/4 cups cucumber julienne   **3/4 cup grated zucchini**
3/4 cup alfalfa or clover sprouts   **1/3 cup desalted olives (*see* Glossary)**

1) Make *Creamed Spinach* (*see* page 207). Pour the *Creamed Spinach* onto Teflex-lined dehydrator trays in the form of circles. This amount of *Creamed Spinach* should make approx. 6 to 7 circles. Dehydrate at 95° F for approx. 24 hours or until dry, but flexible.

2) Stuff with the julienned vegetables and serve immediately. Does not keep well.

Serves 3–6.

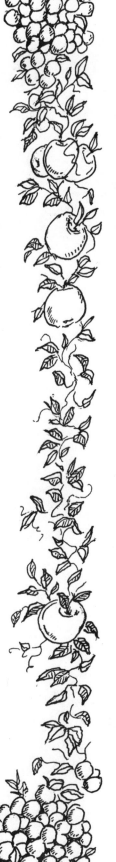

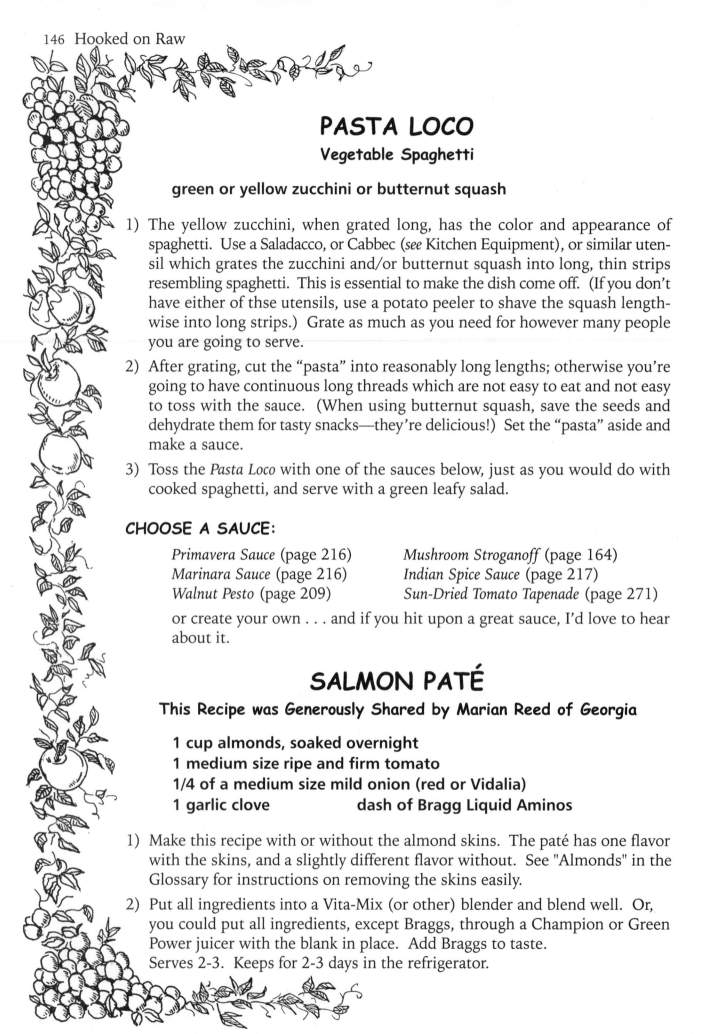

PASTA LOCO
Vegetable Spaghetti

green or yellow zucchini or butternut squash

1) The yellow zucchini, when grated long, has the color and appearance of spaghetti. Use a Saladacco, or Cabbec (*see* Kitchen Equipment), or similar utensil which grates the zucchini and/or butternut squash into long, thin strips resembling spaghetti. This is essential to make the dish come off. (If you don't have either of thse utensils, use a potato peeler to shave the squash lengthwise into long strips.) Grate as much as you need for however many people you are going to serve.

2) After grating, cut the "pasta" into reasonably long lengths; otherwise you're going to have continuous long threads which are not easy to eat and not easy to toss with the sauce. (When using butternut squash, save the seeds and dehydrate them for tasty snacks—they're delicious!) Set the "pasta" aside and make a sauce.

3) Toss the *Pasta Loco* with one of the sauces below, just as you would do with cooked spaghetti, and serve with a green leafy salad.

CHOOSE A SAUCE:

Primavera Sauce (page 216)   *Mushroom Stroganoff* (page 164)
Marinara Sauce (page 216)   *Indian Spice Sauce* (page 217)
Walnut Pesto (page 209)   *Sun-Dried Tomato Tapenade* (page 271)

or create your own . . . and if you hit upon a great sauce, I'd love to hear about it.

SALMON PATÉ
This Recipe was Generously Shared by Marian Reed of Georgia

1 cup almonds, soaked overnight
1 medium size ripe and firm tomato
1/4 of a medium size mild onion (red or Vidalia)
1 garlic clove   dash of Bragg Liquid Aminos

1) Make this recipe with or without the almond skins. The paté has one flavor with the skins, and a slightly different flavor without. See "Almonds" in the Glossary for instructions on removing the skins easily.

2) Put all ingredients into a Vita-Mix (or other) blender and blend well. Or, you could put all ingredients, except Braggs, through a Champion or Green Power juicer with the blank in place. Add Braggs to taste.
Serves 2-3. Keeps for 2-3 days in the refrigerator.

NOTE: This recipe is so simple and so delicious. If the paté comes out too loose, you could add more almonds to firm it up.

VARIATION: For a stronger salmon-like flavor, cover the paté with a cotton cloth and let sit out at room temperature overnight. In the morning, refrigerate.

SQUAGHETTI WITH GARLIC & OIL

> **1 medium butternut squash**
> **4 oz. olive oil (extra-virgin)**
> **4 cloves garlic (pressed)**
> **1/2–3/4 cup *Pine Nut Parmezan or Three Nut Parmezan* (see**
>   **page 226 or 231)**
> **Celtic sea salt, to taste**
> **garnish: minced parsley**

1) Grate the butternut squash into spaghetti-like threads with a Saladacco (*see* Kitchen Equipment). Cut the threads a little so that they will be easier to eat.

2) In a small bowl, mix the oil, garlic and Celtic sea salt.

3) Toss the Squaghetti with the garlic and oil until well coated. Add the *Pine Nut Parmezan* and toss again. Sprinkle with a little minced parsley.

   Serves 4.

VARIATION: Add one or a combination of diced tomatoes, mushrooms, bell peppers and finely chopped basil.

STUFFED SEA LEAVES

> **1/2 package of Alaria (Wild Atlantic Wakame, sold by the**
> **Maine Coast Sea Vegetable Co., works well in this recipe)**

STUFFING: Use one of the following:

Pecan Wild Rice Loaf (page 161)   *Toona* (page 135)
Neat Loaf (page 137)   *Hungarian Stuffed Cabbage stuffing* (page 144)
Veggie Seed Paté (page 158)   *Walnut Curry Paté* (page 162)

1) Soak Alaria for an hour in filtered water. Drain and pat dry with a clean cotton tea towel or paper towels.

2) Unfold the Alaria and lay flat on counter. Put approx. 1 tsp. of stuffing in middle and then roll into a packet, tucking in the sides as you go.

   Makes approx. 28 packets. Keeps for 2 days in the refrigerator.

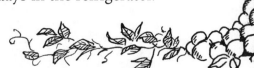

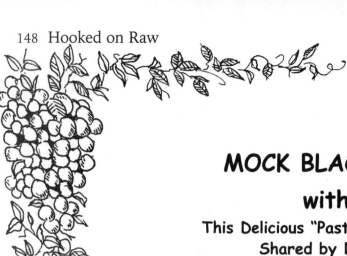

MOCK BLACK INK PASTA
with PESTO

This Delicious "Pasta" Recipe was Generously Shared by Doris Djolit Beigel

**1 package hiziki
filtered water
3 tomatoes,* diced**

1) Soak the hiziki in filtered water, enough to cover, for 30 minutes. Rinse 3 times and drain well.

2) Dice the tomatoes and set aside.

PINE NUT PESTO:

**1 cup pine nuts, soaked and rinsed (soak a few extra to
    sprinkle on top)
4 1/2 cups fresh basil, gently packed (remove stems and
    discolored leaves)
1/2 cup fresh mint leaves, gently packed
3 medium to large garlic cloves, finely chopped
4 1/2 tbsp. olive oil (extra-virgin)
1/2 of a slightly rounded tsp. Celtic sea salt
1 1/2 tsp. Nama Shoyu
approx. 3 tbsp. filtered water**

3) While the hiziki is soaking, make the *Pine Nut Pesto*. Start by putting the garlic into the food processor with the "S" blade running. Then add in the pine nuts, followed by basil and mint, Celtic sea salt and Nama Shoyu. Add in the oil and water last. Process until smooth.

4) Set aside 1 cup of hiziki and 1/2 cup of pesto for garnishing. Toss the remainder of the hiziki "pasta" with the remaining *Pine Nut Pesto*. When serving, put the tossed "pasta" in the center of the plate and surround it with the reserved plain hiziki.   Add extra dollops of pesto on top. Sprinkle with diced tomatoes, extra olive oil and extra soaked pine nuts. Garnish with mint and basil leaves.

Serves 4. Keeps for 2 days in the refrigerator.

*You could skin the tomatoes, but it is optional.

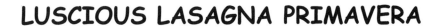

LUSCIOUS LASAGNA PRIMAVERA

(Without Noodles)

1) Make one recipe of *Almond Ricotta* without Veggie Chips (see page 225)

2) Make one recipe of *Italian Tomato Sauce (see page 212)*

PRIMAVERA FILLING:

1 large zucchini
1/2 med. red onion
1/2 red bell pepper
1 tomato
2 each of shiitake, crimini and regular mushrooms
1/4 cup fresh basil, minced
1/2 lemon, juiced
1 oz. olive oil (extra-virgin)
3 garlic cloves, pressed
1/2 tsp. oregano
Celtic sea salt, to taste
1/2 cup pumpkin seeds
1/4 cup pine nuts (optional)

3) With a mandoline or similar utensil, slice the zucchini, onion, red bell pepper, tomato and mushrooms very thin. Set aside in a large bowl.

4) Make a marinade by mixing the lemon, basil, oil, garlic, oregano and Celtic sea salt and toss gently with the vegetables. Make sure the vegetables are coated. You might have to separate the pieces of zucchini. Marinate at room temperature for half an hour.

5) Grind the pumpkin seeds and the pine nuts in a SaladShooter® or nut mill and set aside. (This is your "Parmezan" cheese.)

TO ASSEMBLE THE LASAGNA:

6) In a large casserole, spoon a layer of tomato sauce, then a layer of marinated vegetables, then a layer of *Almond Ricotta*, and continue alternating the layers until you are out of ingredients. Sprinkle "Parmezan" on the top.

Serves 6. Keeps for 2-3 days in the refrigerator.

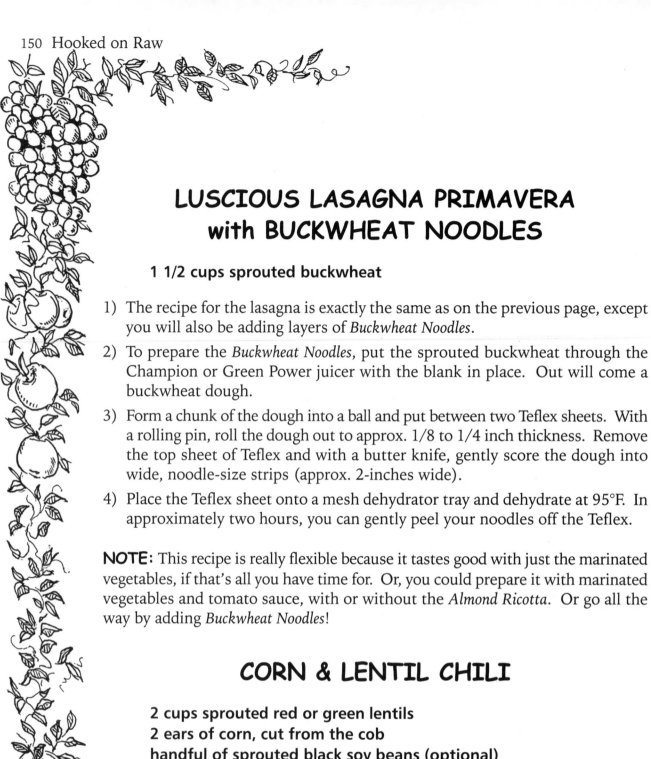

LUSCIOUS LASAGNA PRIMAVERA
with BUCKWHEAT NOODLES

1 1/2 cups sprouted buckwheat

1) The recipe for the lasagna is exactly the same as on the previous page, except you will also be adding layers of *Buckwheat Noodles*.

2) To prepare the *Buckwheat Noodles*, put the sprouted buckwheat through the Champion or Green Power juicer with the blank in place. Out will come a buckwheat dough.

3) Form a chunk of the dough into a ball and put between two Teflex sheets. With a rolling pin, roll the dough out to approx. 1/8 to 1/4 inch thickness. Remove the top sheet of Teflex and with a butter knife, gently score the dough into wide, noodle-size strips (approx. 2-inches wide).

4) Place the Teflex sheet onto a mesh dehydrator tray and dehydrate at 95°F. In approximately two hours, you can gently peel your noodles off the Teflex.

NOTE: This recipe is really flexible because it tastes good with just the marinated vegetables, if that's all you have time for. Or, you could prepare it with marinated vegetables and tomato sauce, with or without the *Almond Ricotta*. Or go all the way by adding *Buckwheat Noodles*!

CORN & LENTIL CHILI

2 cups sprouted red or green lentils
2 ears of corn, cut from the cob
handful of sprouted black soy beans (optional)
1 recipe *Sun-Dried Tomato Tapenade* (see page 271)

1) In a bowl mix the lentils, soy beans and corn. (Try to get the freshest corn possible, otherwise it will be too starchy and its flavor will not be satisfying.)

2) Add in some *Sun-Dried Tomato Tapenade* (how much to add in depends on your own taste) and mix well.

Serves 2-3. Keeps 2 days in the refrigerator.

HOT TAMALE PIE

8 oz. dried sweet corn*
1 1/4 cup cucumber and celery juices (any combination)
1–2 garlic cloves, pressed
1/4 tsp. Celtic sea salt
1 recipe *Chedda Sauce* (*see* page 210)
2 mushrooms, sliced thin
1 fresh ear of corn, cut from the cob
1/4 red bell pepper, finely diced
1/4 red onion, finely diced
1/4–1/2 jalapeño pepper, seeded, and finely diced

1) Use only "dried sweet corn." Other kinds of dried corn do not work for this recipe. Put the dried sweet corn into a seed/nut grinder and grind fine. Set aside.

2) Prepare the cucumber and celery juices.** Add pressed garlic and Celtic sea salt and stir.

3) Pour the juices over the ground sweet corn and mix well with a large spoon. Let sit for 1/2 to 1 hour. This is your tamale "masa."

4) Between two layers of parchment paper, put a chunk of the tamale masa and roll it out with a rolling pin. In 2 individual casserole dishes, spread a layer of the tamale masa. (If the masa doesn't readily peel off the parchment paper, use a spatula to scoop it up in sections.) Over the masa, spread a layer of *Chedda Sauce*. Then sprinkle most of the vegetables on top of the *Chedda Sauce*, saving a little to garnish the top.

5) Roll out another thin layer of masa, and place it over the vegetables. The masa doesn't have to completely cover the whole casserole. Over the masa, spoon on some more *Chedda Sauce* and sprinkle the top with the remaining vegetables.

6) Serve as is, or put into the dehydrator for 2 hours.

Serves 2-4. Keeps for two days in the refrigerator.

NOTE: Goes well with a *Gorgeous Greens Salad* (*see* page 178), or try *Watercress and Red Bell Pepper Salad* (*see* page 171).

* If your health food store does not carry Neshaminy Valley Natural Foods brand of "dried sweet corn," you can order it from the Organic Provisions mail order catalog (*see* Source Index).

** You could use any combination of cucumber, celery or even tomato juice (freshly made, of course).

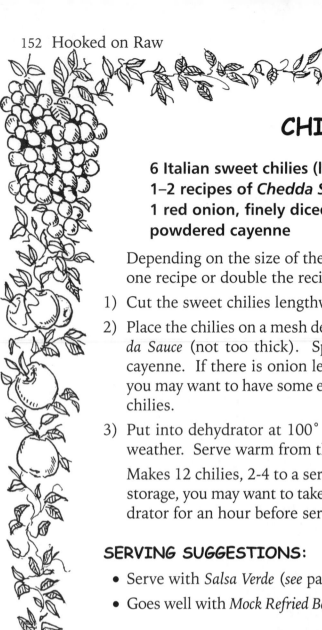

CHILI RELLENO

6 Italian sweet chilies (like Cubanelles or Anaheims)
1–2 recipes of *Chedda Sauce* (*see* page 210)
1 red onion, finely diced
powdered cayenne

Depending on the size of the sweet chilies, you will need either to make one recipe or double the recipe for *Chedda Sauce*.

1) Cut the sweet chilies lengthwise and take out the seeds.

2) Place the chilies on a mesh dehydrator tray and fill the cavities with the *Chedda Sauce* (not too thick). Sprinkle with finely diced onion and powdered cayenne. If there is onion left over, put it onto the dehydrator tray also, as you may want to have some extra semi-dehydrated onion to sprinkle over the chilies.

3) Put into dehydrator at 100˚ F for 10 to 15 hours; try 5-7 hours in warmer weather. Serve warm from the dehydrator.

Makes 12 chilies, 2-4 to a serving. Keeps for 2 days in the refrigerator. After storage, you may want to take the chill off by putting them back into the dehydrator for an hour before serving.

SERVING SUGGESTIONS:

- Serve with *Salsa Verde* (*see* page 212) and a large green salad.
- Goes well with *Mock Refried Bean Stuffing & Salsa Verde*. (*see* pages 154 and 212)

CHILI NON-CARNE

1 cup sprouted barley
1 cup soaked walnuts
1 cup corn, cut from the cob
1 bell pepper, any color, diced small
2 carrots, diced small
1/2 cup diced zucchini
1 cup diced tomato
1/2 cup diced onion
1/2 cup Greek black olives, pitted, chopped & desalted
** (*see* Glossary)**
1/2 tsp. homemade *Italian Seasoning* (*see* page 292) or use
** store bought**
1/4 tsp. chili powder
1 1/2–2 cups *Italian Tomato Sauce* (*see* page 212);

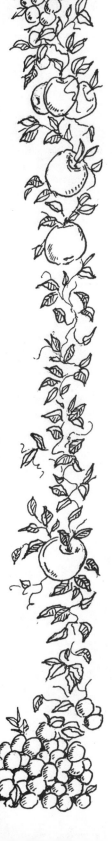

use ONLY 1 large fig when making it)

1) Lightly pulse chop the barley and walnuts in a food processor with the "S" blade. It should be small and chunky, not pasty. Transfer to a large bowl.

2) Add in the corn, diced vegetables, olives, *Italian Tomato Sauce,* and spices, and mix well. Taste and adjust flavors.

   Serves 4-6. Keeps for 2 days in the refrigerator.

VARIATIONS:

- Form little balls from the *Veggie Seed Paté* (*see* page 158) with your hands, and dehydrate at 95° F for 4 hours. Add into the Chili before serving.

- Or add in some *Almond-Beet Nut Roll* (*see* page 160), shaped into little balls.

SPROUTED SWEET BROWN RICE

"Sweet Brown Rice" is a variety of brown rice. It looks kind of like short grain brown rice, but it is a little different. It is used a lot for making rice pudding.

1) Soak any amount you need of sweet brown rice in filtered water for 24-36 hours, at room temperature, changing the water once (twice in humid weather, as you don't want the rice to ferment).

2) Drain, rinse and drain again, then set out to sprout. Rinse and drain the rice twice a day for approx. 2 days, by which time you should see the tiny sprouts appear. Sometimes rice has to be put into a warm spot to encourage it to sprout.

   Store in filtered water in the refrigerator. Keeps for 2-3 days; after that it gets bitter.

SERVING SUGGESTIONS:

- It's good spooned on top of the *Green Power Soup* (*see* page 193).
- Use it in place of, or in addition to, wild rice in recipes.
- Use it in the *Sweet Brown Rice Pudding* recipe (*see* page 287).

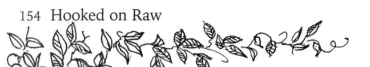

TACOS IN THE RAW

MOCK REFRIED BEAN STUFFING:

 2 cups sprouted aduki beans
 1 cup walnuts, soaked overnight
 2 avocados, mashed
 2–4 lemons, juiced (add to taste)
 1 garlic clove, pressed
 2–4 tsp. ground cumin
 1/2–1 tsp. ground coriander (optional)
 1/2 tsp. cayenne (or to taste—start with LESS)
 Celtic sea salt, to taste

1) Put sprouted aduki beans through the Champion juicer with the juicer screen in place. You read it right. Don't use the juicer blank. This is because if you use the blank, you will get a paste that is too hard. If you juice it, you get a paste (as a pulp residue) and some juice also, which you then mix together to obtain the right consistency. Set aside in a bowl.

2) Drain the walnuts and process in a food processor using the "S" blade.

3) Add the walnut mixture to the aduki paste. Add all the rest of the above ingredients and mix well.

GAZPACHO SAUCE:

2 tomatoes	3/4 cup cilantro
1 red bell pepper	1–2 lemons, juiced
1 green bell pepper	1 tsp. dried oregano
1 onion	

4) Mince all the sauce ingredients with a mincing knife or pulse chop in a food processor with the "S" blade. Add lemon juice and oregano and toss. Put 1/3 of the sauce into a blender and blend well. Add the blended sauce back in with the rest of the sauce.

ASSEMBLING THE TACOS:

5) For taco shells, use cabbage leaves or romaine leaves or any vegetable that forms a little cup that you can put the bean stuffing into, top with the *Gazpacho Sauce* and ENJOY!

Serves 6. Keeps 2-3 days in the refrigerator.

VARIATION: For a "meatier" flavor, add some *Neat Loaf* (*see* page 137) when assembling the tacos

BURRITO FIESTA

1) As a Burrito wrap, use either a sturdy purple cabbage leaf that forms a cup shape or a firm romaine lettuce leaf. You could also take large green cabbage leaves, put them into the dehydrator for 5-10 minutes to soften them up and use them to stuff your burrito ingredients in the form of cabbage rolls.

2) Choose your wrap and then stuff with any combination below.

THERE'S NO BEEF BURRITO:

1 recipe *Neat Loaf* (page 137)
avocado, cubed
tomato, julienne
red bell pepper, julienne

CALIFORNIA BURRITO:

1 recipe *Mock Refried
    Bean Stuffing* (page 154)
1 recipe *Mango Salsa con Clase* (page 214)
drizzle with *Lynn's Honey
    Mustard Dressing* (page 188)

CHILI BURRITO:

1 recipe *Chili Non-Carne* (page 152)
avocado, cubed
clover or alfalfa sprouts

GUACAMOLE BURRITO:

1 recipe *Guacamole* (page 174)
very fresh corn, cut from
    the cob
any salsa recipe

SPICY JAMAICAN "JERK" VEGGIES

4 cups asparagus, julienne
4 cups chopped mushrooms
2 cups snow peas, julienne
2 cups string beans, destring and julienne
1 red bell pepper, julienne
1 onion, diced
2 garlic cloves, pressed
4 tbsp. olive oil
2 oz. filtered water
1 tbsp. *Jamaican Jerk Seasoning* (see page 289)
Celtic sea salt or Nama Shoyu, to taste

1) Combine all vegetables in a large bowl. Set aside.

2) In a small bowl, blend olive oil, water and seasoning to make a sauce. **Don't forget to add a tsp. of honey to the *Jerk Seasoning*.**

3) Pour the sauce over the vegetables and toss until well coated. Serve as is or put into the dehydrator, set at 95° F, for 1–2 hours.

Serves 4. Keeps for 2-3 days in the refrigerator.

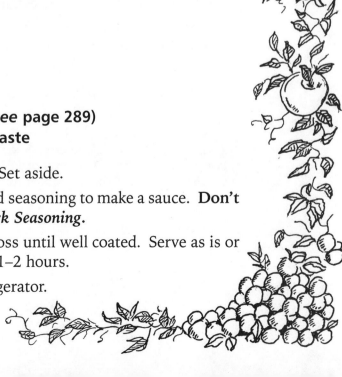

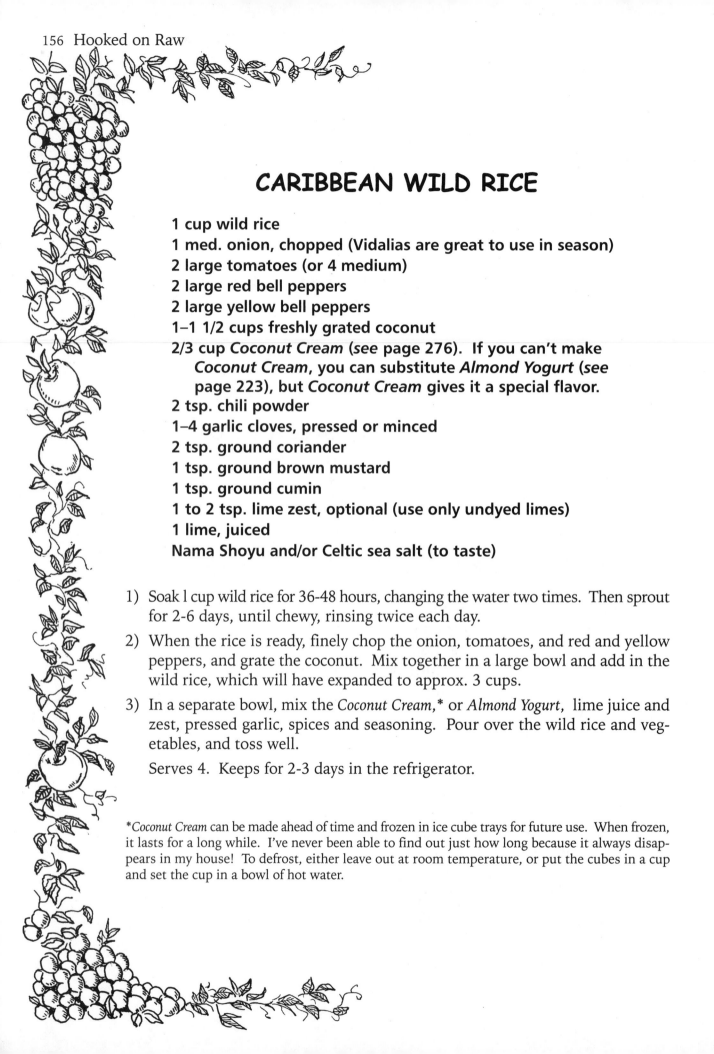

CARIBBEAN WILD RICE

1 cup wild rice

1 med. onion, chopped (Vidalias are great to use in season)

2 large tomatoes (or 4 medium)

2 large red bell peppers

2 large yellow bell peppers

1–1 1/2 cups freshly grated coconut

2/3 cup *Coconut Cream* (*see* page 276). If you can't make *Coconut Cream*, you can substitute *Almond Yogurt* (*see* page 223), but *Coconut Cream* gives it a special flavor.

2 tsp. chili powder

1–4 garlic cloves, pressed or minced

2 tsp. ground coriander

1 tsp. ground brown mustard

1 tsp. ground cumin

1 to 2 tsp. lime zest, optional (use only undyed limes)

1 lime, juiced

Nama Shoyu and/or Celtic sea salt (to taste)

1) Soak l cup wild rice for 36-48 hours, changing the water two times. Then sprout for 2-6 days, until chewy, rinsing twice each day.

2) When the rice is ready, finely chop the onion, tomatoes, and red and yellow peppers, and grate the coconut. Mix together in a large bowl and add in the wild rice, which will have expanded to approx. 3 cups.

3) In a separate bowl, mix the *Coconut Cream*,* or *Almond Yogurt*, lime juice and zest, pressed garlic, spices and seasoning. Pour over the wild rice and vegetables, and toss well.

Serves 4. Keeps for 2-3 days in the refrigerator.

Coconut Cream can be made ahead of time and frozen in ice cube trays for future use. When frozen, it lasts for a long while. I've never been able to find out just how long because it always disappears in my house! To defrost, either leave out at room temperature, or put the cubes in a cup and set the cup in a bowl of hot water.

COCONUT RICE

1 1/2 cups sprouted Manitok wild rice (or any wild rice,
  sprouted) OR a combination of 3/4 cup sprouted wild
  rice and 3/4 cup Sprouted *Sweet Brown Rice* (*see* page 153)
1 cup shredded carrots
1 cup fresh shredded coconut (light brown shell)
1/4 cup unhulled sesame seed (soaked overnight)
1/4 cup raisins or currants
1 1/2 tbsp. of combination olive oil and flaxseed oil
1 tsp. cinnamon
1/2 tsp. ground cumin
1/2 tsp. ground black mustard
pinch of powdered cloves (optional)
pinch of fresh ground white pepper (optional)
Celtic sea salt, to taste

1) Mix the first five ingredients together in a bowl. Set aside.

2) In a small bowl, stir oil and spices together. Pour onto the coconut/rice
 mixture and toss well. Taste and adjust the seasonings.

 Serves 2. Keeps for 2-3 days in the refrigerator.

VARIATION: For a savory version of this recipe, eliminate the raisins and cinnamon, and add pressed garlic.

UNBAKED BEANS

2 cups soybean sprouts
3/4 cup *Sun-Dried Tomato Tapenade* (*see* page 271)
chili powder, to taste
cayenne, to taste

1) Don't use store bought soybean sprouts because they are allowed to grow too
 long, and don't deliver the flavor you want in this dish. You need to sprout
 the soybeans just until the sprouts are about 1/4 inch or less. The idea is that
 you want them to look like beans, not sprouts.

2) Put the soybean sprouts into some hot water for a few minutes to warm them
 up (make sure you can put your finger into the water without burning it). Drain
 well, put the sprouts into a bowl and mix with the *Sun-Dried Tomato Tapenade*
 and spices. Enjoy!

 Serves 2–4. Keeps 2 days or longer in the refrigerator.

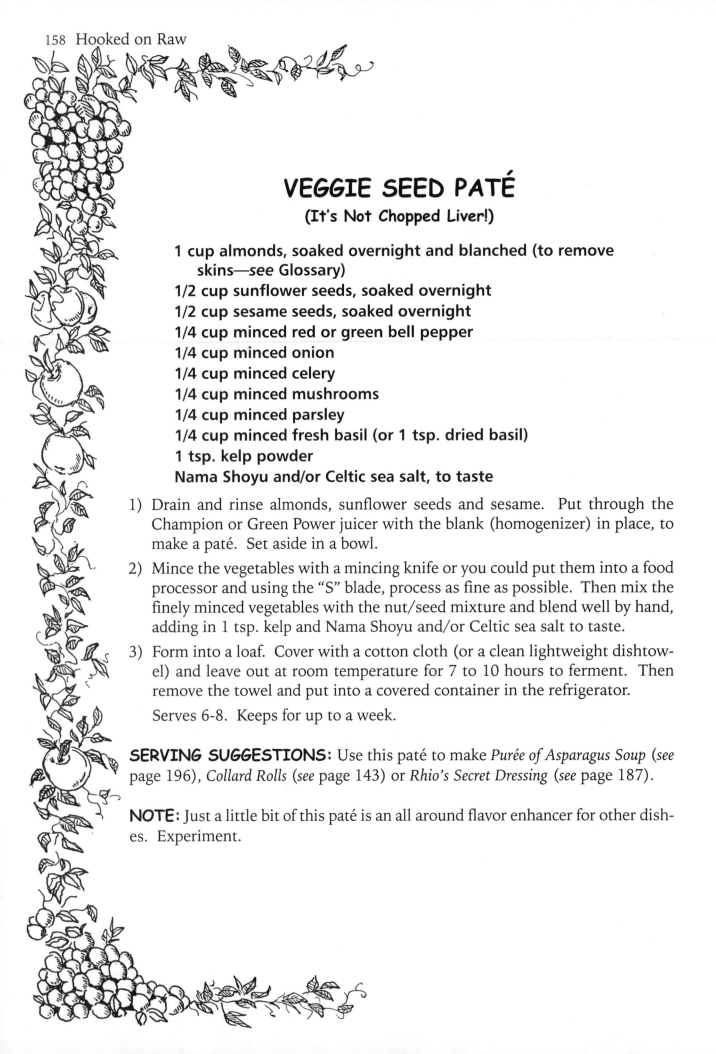

VEGGIE SEED PATÉ
(It's Not Chopped Liver!)

1 cup almonds, soaked overnight and blanched (to remove skins—*see* Glossary)
1/2 cup sunflower seeds, soaked overnight
1/2 cup sesame seeds, soaked overnight
1/4 cup minced red or green bell pepper
1/4 cup minced onion
1/4 cup minced celery
1/4 cup minced mushrooms
1/4 cup minced parsley
1/4 cup minced fresh basil (or 1 tsp. dried basil)
1 tsp. kelp powder
Nama Shoyu and/or Celtic sea salt, to taste

1) Drain and rinse almonds, sunflower seeds and sesame. Put through the Champion or Green Power juicer with the blank (homogenizer) in place, to make a paté. Set aside in a bowl.

2) Mince the vegetables with a mincing knife or you could put them into a food processor and using the "S" blade, process as fine as possible. Then mix the finely minced vegetables with the nut/seed mixture and blend well by hand, adding in 1 tsp. kelp and Nama Shoyu and/or Celtic sea salt to taste.

3) Form into a loaf. Cover with a cotton cloth (or a clean lightweight dishtowel) and leave out at room temperature for 7 to 10 hours to ferment. Then remove the towel and put into a covered container in the refrigerator.

Serves 6-8. Keeps for up to a week.

SERVING SUGGESTIONS: Use this paté to make *Purée of Asparagus Soup* (*see* page 196), *Collard Rolls* (*see* page 143) or *Rhio's Secret Dressing* (*see* page 187).

NOTE: Just a little bit of this paté is an all around flavor enhancer for other dishes. Experiment.

MEDITERRANEAN LOAF
with Kalamata Olives & Sun-Dried Tomato Topping

NUT AND VEGETABLE BASE:

> **2 cups sprouted almonds, blanched**
> **1 1/2 cups sprouted sunflower seeds**
> **1 cup celery (slice the celery into 1/2" pieces to cut the threads)**
> **1/2 cup carrot**
> **1/2 onion**
> **2 garlic cloves**
> **1/8–1/4 cup Kalamata olives, desalted***
> **1 handful basil**
> **Celtic sea salt, to taste**

1) First, put the sun-dried tomatoes to soak so they will be ready by the time you get to the topping.

2) Next, put all the ingredients above, except the Celtic sea salt, through a Champion or Green Power juicer with the blank (homogenizer) in place. Season, blend well and set aside.

SUN-DRIED TOMATO TOPPING:

> **1 1/2 cups sun-dried tomatoes, soaked 1-2 hours in 1 cup of celery juice. You could also soak the sun-dried tomatoes in filtered water.**
> **2 tbsp. olive oil (extra-virgin)**
> **1 garlic clove**
> **a few leaves of basil**
> **handful of Kalamata olives**
> **for garnish: Kalamata olives and parsley**

3) Blend the topping ingredients in a food processor with the "S" blade, adding just enough water to make a thick paste-like sauce.

4) On a large flat plate spread out the nut and vegetable base about 1/2 inch thick. Frost the top with the *Sun-Dried Tomato Topping* and garnish artistically with the minced Kalamata olives, and finely chopped parsley.

Serves 4-6. Keeps for 3 days in the refrigerator.

*See "Olives" in Glossary for how to remove salt.

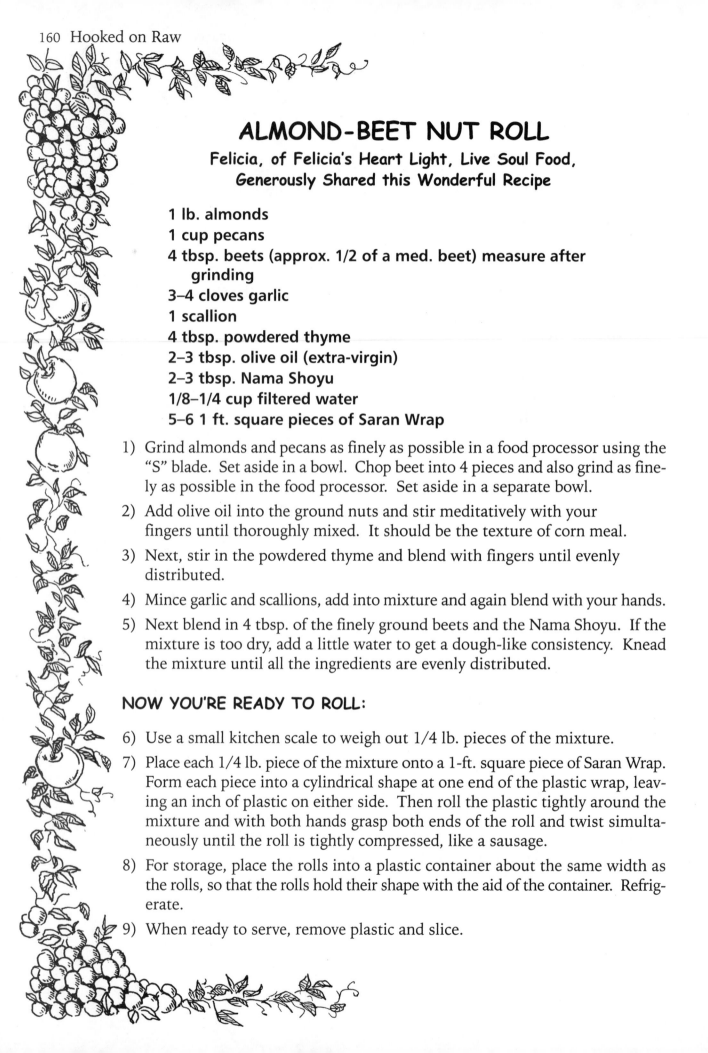

ALMOND-BEET NUT ROLL

Felicia, of Felicia's Heart Light, Live Soul Food, Generously Shared this Wonderful Recipe

1 lb. almonds
1 cup pecans
4 tbsp. beets (approx. 1/2 of a med. beet) measure after
    grinding
3–4 cloves garlic
1 scallion
4 tbsp. powdered thyme
2–3 tbsp. olive oil (extra-virgin)
2–3 tbsp. Nama Shoyu
1/8–1/4 cup filtered water
5–6 1 ft. square pieces of Saran Wrap

1) Grind almonds and pecans as finely as possible in a food processor using the "S" blade. Set aside in a bowl. Chop beet into 4 pieces and also grind as finely as possible in the food processor. Set aside in a separate bowl.

2) Add olive oil into the ground nuts and stir meditatively with your fingers until thoroughly mixed. It should be the texture of corn meal.

3) Next, stir in the powdered thyme and blend with fingers until evenly distributed.

4) Mince garlic and scallions, add into mixture and again blend with your hands.

5) Next blend in 4 tbsp. of the finely ground beets and the Nama Shoyu. If the mixture is too dry, add a little water to get a dough-like consistency. Knead the mixture until all the ingredients are evenly distributed.

NOW YOU'RE READY TO ROLL:

6) Use a small kitchen scale to weigh out 1/4 lb. pieces of the mixture.

7) Place each 1/4 lb. piece of the mixture onto a 1-ft. square piece of Saran Wrap. Form each piece into a cylindrical shape at one end of the plastic wrap, leaving an inch of plastic on either side. Then roll the plastic tightly around the mixture and with both hands grasp both ends of the roll and twist simultaneously until the roll is tightly compressed, like a sausage.

8) For storage, place the rolls into a plastic container about the same width as the rolls, so that the rolls hold their shape with the aid of the container. Refrigerate.

9) When ready to serve, remove plastic and slice.

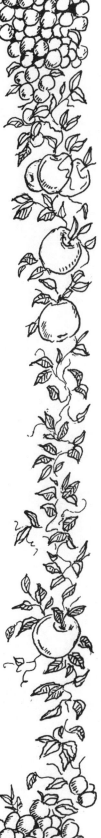

Yield: 5–6 1/4 lb. rolls. Keeps for up to 2 weeks in the refrigerator. This is highly concentrated, so eat moderate portions (a serving is approx. 2 oz.). Serve with a large leafy green salad.

VARIATIONS:

- Form into round patties or balls. These can be used as is or dehydrated for 4 hours at 95° F.
- Make an *Almond-Beet Nut Loaf* by pressing mixture into a loaf pan.

NOTE: For those who enjoy the flavor of sausage, this does the trick. A more biogenic version of the foregoing recipe can be made by using soaked, sprouted, and peeled almonds, and soaked pecans. This version will keep for 6 days in the refrigerator.

PECAN-WILD RICE LOAF

3 cups pecans, soaked 3 hours
2 cups carrots (cut into chunks to measure)
1 red bell pepper
1/2 cup chopped shallot or onion
1/2 cup chopped fresh basil
1/2 cup chopped fresh cilantro
1 cup sprouted mung beans
1 cup sprouted wild rice
2 1/2 lemons, juiced
2 tsp. curry powder
1 tsp. coriander powder
1/4 tsp. cayenne (or to taste)
Nama Shoyu and/or Celtic sea salt, to taste

1) Put pecans and carrots through the Champion or Green Power juicer with the blank in place. It comes out like a paté. Set aside in a large bowl.

2) Put the red bell pepper, shallots or onion, basil and cilantro into a food processor & blend well using the "S" blade. Add this mixture into the paté.

3) Then, add in the sprouted mung beans and wild rice, lemon juice and spices. Mix very well by hand. Taste and adjust flavors. Shape into a loaf and transfer to a serving platter. Garnish with pecan halves and red bell pepper rings in a pleasing design.

Serves 6. Keeps 2-3 days in refrigerator. Goes well with *Apple-Cranberry Relish* (*see* page 269).

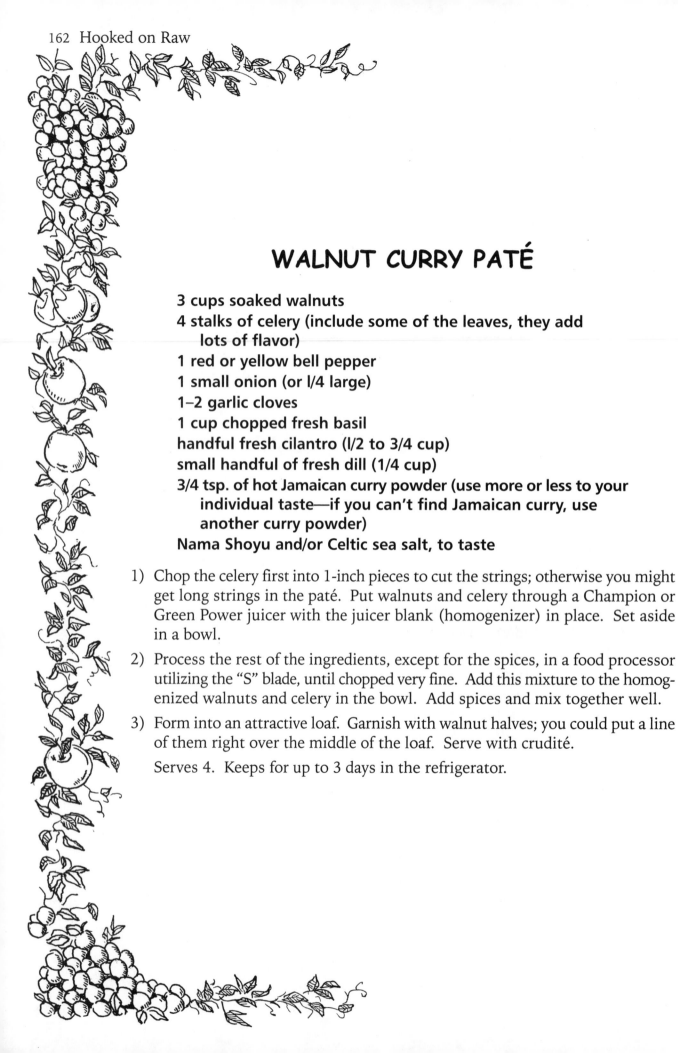

WALNUT CURRY PATÉ

3 cups soaked walnuts
4 stalks of celery (include some of the leaves, they add
lots of flavor)
1 red or yellow bell pepper
1 small onion (or l/4 large)
1–2 garlic cloves
1 cup chopped fresh basil
handful fresh cilantro (l/2 to 3/4 cup)
small handful of fresh dill (1/4 cup)
3/4 tsp. of hot Jamaican curry powder (use more or less to your
individual taste—if you can't find Jamaican curry, use
another curry powder)
Nama Shoyu and/or Celtic sea salt, to taste

1) Chop the celery first into 1-inch pieces to cut the strings; otherwise you might get long strings in the paté. Put walnuts and celery through a Champion or Green Power juicer with the juicer blank (homogenizer) in place. Set aside in a bowl.

2) Process the rest of the ingredients, except for the spices, in a food processor utilizing the "S" blade, until chopped very fine. Add this mixture to the homogenized walnuts and celery in the bowl. Add spices and mix together well.

3) Form into an attractive loaf. Garnish with walnut halves; you could put a line of them right over the middle of the loaf. Serve with crudité.

Serves 4. Keeps for up to 3 days in the refrigerator.

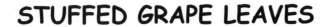

STUFFED GRAPE LEAVES

20 fresh grape leaves
2 oz. olive oil (extra-virgin)
dash of Nama Shoyu and Celtic sea salt

2 lemons, juiced
2 garlic cloves, pressed

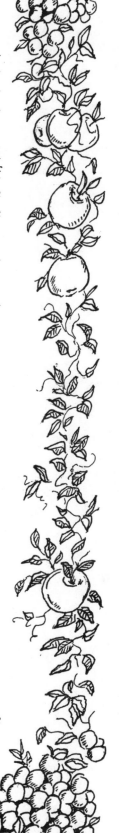

1) In a bowl, combine all the ingredients (except the grape leaves) to create a marinade. Coat each grape leaf thoroughly by dipping both sides into the marinade. Put the grape leaves into a plastic container, pour on any remaining marinade and let sit at room temperature for an hour. Then put the covered container into the freezer overnight.

2) When you're ready to stuff the grape leaves, take them out of the freezer and let them sit at room temperature until defrosted. Drain and pat top side of leaf dry with a cotton cloth or paper towel. (These leaves are not soft like the store bought ones that have been cooked and/or pasteurized. You will have to chew them a bit.)

3) Stuff the grape leaves with either the *Neat Loaf* (*see* page 137) or *Hungarian Stuffed Cabbage* mix (*see* page 144).

Keeps for 3 days in the refrigerator. Serve with sliced tomatoes or with *Armenian* or *Tabbouleh Salad* (*see* page 182 or 172).

BROCCOLI & MUSHROOMS
with Sweet & Sour Sauce

1/4 lb. shiitake mushrooms, chopped small
4 cups broccoli florets, chopped small
1 red bell pepper, chopped small
1 cup sprouted sunflower seeds
1 cup sprouted wild rice or sprouted barley

1) Put the vegetables, seeds and grains into a large bowl and set aside.

SWEET & SOUR SAUCE:

2 tbsp. grated ginger (peel the ginger first, before grating)
1 red hot chili pepper, seeded and minced
1/4 cup olive oil (extra-virgin)
1 recipe *Prune Paste* (*see* page 270)
Nama Shoyu to taste

2) In a small bowl, combine the grated ginger, hot chili pepper, olive oil and *Prune Paste*. Stir well.

3) Toss the vegetables and grains with the *Sweet & Sour Sauce*.

Serves 4-6. Keeps for 1 day in the refrigerator.

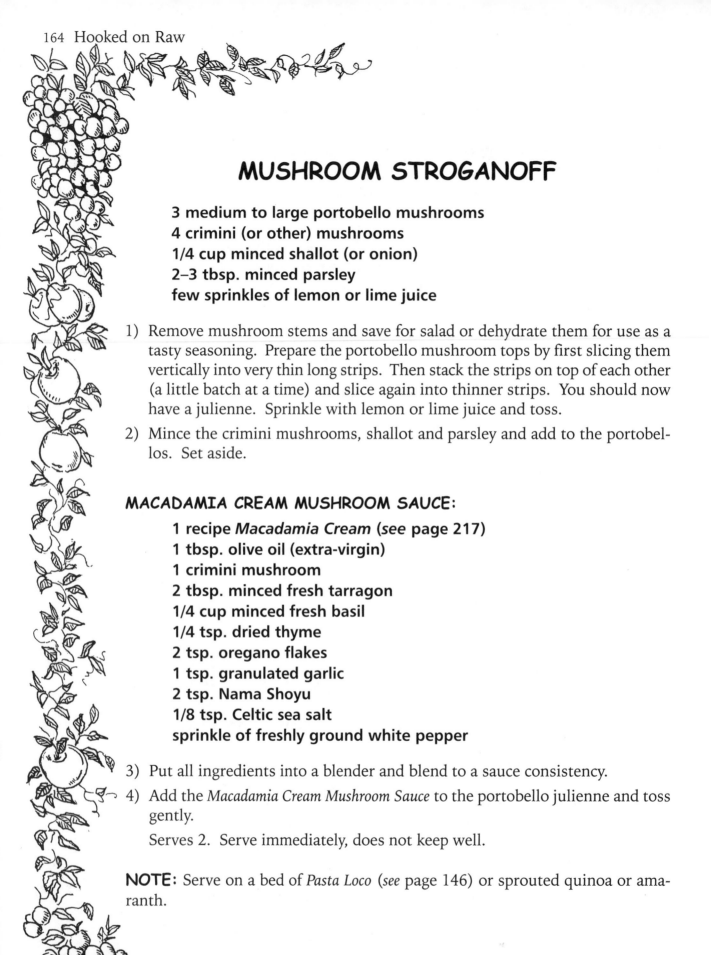

MUSHROOM STROGANOFF

3 medium to large portobello mushrooms
4 crimini (or other) mushrooms
1/4 cup minced shallot (or onion)
2–3 tbsp. minced parsley
few sprinkles of lemon or lime juice

1) Remove mushroom stems and save for salad or dehydrate them for use as a tasty seasoning. Prepare the portobello mushroom tops by first slicing them vertically into very thin long strips. Then stack the strips on top of each other (a little batch at a time) and slice again into thinner strips. You should now have a julienne. Sprinkle with lemon or lime juice and toss.

2) Mince the crimini mushrooms, shallot and parsley and add to the portobellos. Set aside.

MACADAMIA CREAM MUSHROOM SAUCE:

1 recipe *Macadamia Cream* (*see* page 217)
1 tbsp. olive oil (extra-virgin)
1 crimini mushroom
2 tbsp. minced fresh tarragon
1/4 cup minced fresh basil
1/4 tsp. dried thyme
2 tsp. oregano flakes
1 tsp. granulated garlic
2 tsp. Nama Shoyu
1/8 tsp. Celtic sea salt
sprinkle of freshly ground white pepper

3) Put all ingredients into a blender and blend to a sauce consistency.
4) Add the *Macadamia Cream Mushroom Sauce* to the portobello julienne and toss gently.

Serves 2. Serve immediately, does not keep well.

NOTE: Serve on a bed of *Pasta Loco* (*see* page 146) or sprouted quinoa or amaranth.

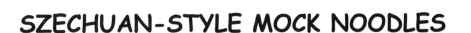

SZECHUAN-STYLE MOCK NOODLES

2 cups each of zucchini and butternut squash, grated into
    long spaghetti-like strips (measure after grating)
1 cup daikon radish, grated into long spaghetti-like strips
1 red or yellow bell pepper, julienne
1/2 cup arame, soaked 10 minutes and drained
1 cup mung bean sprouts
2 scallions, thinly sliced on the diagonal
1/4 cup grated, raw Valencia peanuts
1/4 cup freshly grated coconut

1) Using a Saladacco or a similar utensil that grates vegetables into long, thin strips resembling spaghetti, grate the zucchini, butternut squash and daikon radish until you have 5 cups of "vegetable spaghetti." Cut the threads into reasonably long bite-size pieces. (The threads come out of the Saladacco as multiple continuous strings.) Put into a bowl and set aside.

2) Prepare the rest of the ingredients above and toss with the vegetable spaghetti.

SZECHUAN SAUCE:

2 tbsp. sesame oil (Flora Oils—*see* Source Index)
2–4 garlic cloves, pressed
2 tsp. grated or pressed ginger
3 tbsp. raw sesame tahini
1 tbsp. Nama Shoyu
1/2 tsp. anise powder (or freshly ground fennel seed)
sprinkle of cayenne
enough filtered water to thin to a sauce consistency
garnish: soaked black sesame seeds

3) In a small bowl blend all the sauce ingredients, except the sesame seeds.

4) Pour the sauce over the "spaghetti" and vegetables and toss very well to coat. Garnish with black sesame seeds.

Serves 2-3. Keeps for 2 days in the refrigerator.

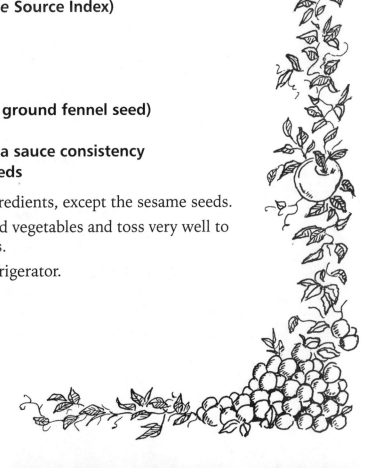

QUICK NORI ROLLS

5 nori sheets (use black nori; if it looks green,
   it has been toasted)
4 cups grated Jerusalem artichokes* (or use carrots)
1 avocado, mashed
1 lemon, juiced
1 garlic clove, pressed (optional)
Nama Shoyu or Celtic sea salt, to taste

1) Scrub the Jerusalem artichokes with a vegetable brush. Do not peel. You may however, need to break off some of the knobs when rinsing because sometimes soil gets trapped in there and you want to be sure and clean it out. Grate the Jerusalem artichokes and sprinkle with lemon juice to prevent oxidation (otherwise they will turn dark).

2) Mash avocado to a cream with a fork and mix into the grated artichokes. Add in Nama Shoyu and/or Celtic sea salt and garlic to taste. Mix well.

3) Put 3 heaping tbsp. onto one side of a nori sheet, and roll. To seal the roll, run half a cut lemon over the edge of the nori and press together. Serve immediately. Does not keep for long because the moisture of the filling makes the nori sheet soggy after a while. If you want the rolls to last a while longer; before stuffing, line the entire nori sheet with clover sprouts or romaine lettuce leaves. (Cut the rib out of the romaine using only the soft leafy sections.)

Makes 5 rolls. Each roll can be cut into 4 pieces, so you have either 20 small or 5 large rolls.

*Jerusalem Artichoke aka Sunchokes (see Glossary).

VEGGIE SUSHI ROLLS

As Inspired by Dafna Mordecai of the
"Accent on Wellness" Show (NYC)

There are many flavorful combinations that you can stuff into nori to create *Veggie Sushi Rolls* . . . following are just a few. After getting the hang of it, go on to create your own.

GENERAL INSTRUCTIONS: Take a piece of nori (get the black, untoasted kind), place it on a sushi mat, then layer the ingredients on top of the nori to about 1 1/2 inches from the edge. Then roll the mat over tightly, lift the top of the mat off and continue rolling the nori. Once rolled, seal the edges with a little lemon juice or water.

HERE ARE SOME DELICIOUS COMBINATIONS FOR THE FILLING:

#1   Avocado, mashed or sliced
     Sprouted almonds, sliced
     Tomato, sliced or diced
     Carrot, grated
     Squeeze of lemon

#2   Avocado, mashed or sliced
     Cucumber, cut into long slivers
     Basil or dill, minced
     Squeeze of lemon

#3   Avocado, mashed or sliced
     Pistachios, soaked for 1 hour
       and then mashed
     Tomato, sliced or diced
     Carrots, finely grated
     Squeeze of lemon

#4   Avocado, mashed or sliced
     Pear, sliced
     Red bell pepper, julienne
     Dill, minced
     Raisins or currants, soaked
     Squeeze of lemon

DIPPING SAUCES FOR SUSHI ROLLS

CUCUMBER-TAHINI SAUCE:

Sesame tahini
Lemon juice
Cucumber and celery juice
Fresh dill, minced
Celtic sea salt, to taste (optional)

Put all ingredients, except the minced dill, into the blender and blend well. Transfer to a bowl and stir in the minced dill.

DATE-CUCUMBER SAUCE:

Cucumber & celery juice
Nori
Dates
Soak water from dates
Lime juice
Celtic sea salt, to taste (optional)

Blend all ingredients in a blender.

SUGGESTION: Serve with *Wasabi Mousse* (*see* page 269) on the side.

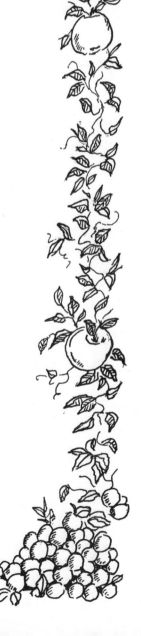

SEA LEIGH SPECIAL

1/2 package sea palms (a sea vegetable)
2 fresh ears of corn, cut from the cob
1/2 red bell pepper, julienne

DRESSING:

1 tomato
1/2 cup sun-dried tomato, soaked 2 hours in either freshly
   made tomato juice or in a blended whole tomato (use 1
   extra tomato for this and blend with a little water)*
1/2 stalk celery
1 tsp. dark unpasteurized miso
8 basil leaves
1/2 tsp. powdered dill
1/4 tsp. Mexican blend powder
1 tbsp. olive oil (extra-virgin)
sprinkle of Celtic sea salt

1) Put the sea palms into a bowl and cover with filtered water. Let sit until soft and pliable; approx. 1/2 to 1 hour.

2) Put all the dressing ingredients into a blender and blend well.

3) Cut the sea palms into bite-size pieces. Mix in a bowl with the corn and bell pepper. Add dressing and toss well.

   Serves 2. Keeps for two days in the refrigerator.

*If you're pinched for time, soak the dried tomatoes in filtered water

SAVORY EGGPLANT STEW
with Tomatoes

1 eggplant, sliced very thin
2 lemons, juiced
2 tbsp. sesame oil (or extra-virgin olive oil)
1 tbsp. Nama Shoyu
1/2 onion, sliced thin
1 cup sprouted hulled barley
1 cup soaked walnuts, drained (soak overnight or at least
   1 hour)
1 large tomato, cut into bite-size chunks
1–2 cloves garlic, pressed
1/2 tsp. poultry seasoning
Nama Shoyu or Celtic sea salt, to taste

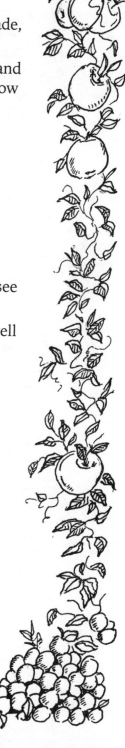

1) Slice the eggplant very thin using a mandoline or similar type equipment. Stack the slices on top of each other and cut in half the long way. Set aside.

2) Make a marinade out of the lemon juice, oil and Nama Shoyu. Pour the marinade over the eggplant and toss so that all the eggplant is coated.

3) Put the barley and walnuts into the food processor and using the "S" blade, process for 15 seconds. Add this to the eggplant mixture.

4) Add in onions, chunked tomatoes, pressed garlic, poultry seasoning and Nama Shoyu or Celtic sea salt, to taste. Toss to mix everything well. Allow to sit for one hour before serving.

Serves 4. Best when eaten freshly made.

MIDDLE EASTERN EGGPLANT STEW
with Dried Fruit

1) Prepare as per steps 1 through 3 in previous *Savory Eggplant Stew* recipe (see opposite page).

2) Instead of the ingredients in step 4 above, add in the following and toss well to mix.

> **1 cup dried prunes (soak 2-3 hours, drain and chop)**
> **1 cup dried apricots (soak 2-3 hours, drain and chop)**
> **1 tsp. cinnamon**
> **1/2 tsp. freshly grated nutmeg**
> **1/2 tsp. turmeric**
> **pinch of Celtic sea salt**

3) Allow to sit for one hour before serving.

Serves 4. Keeps for 2 days in the refrigerator.

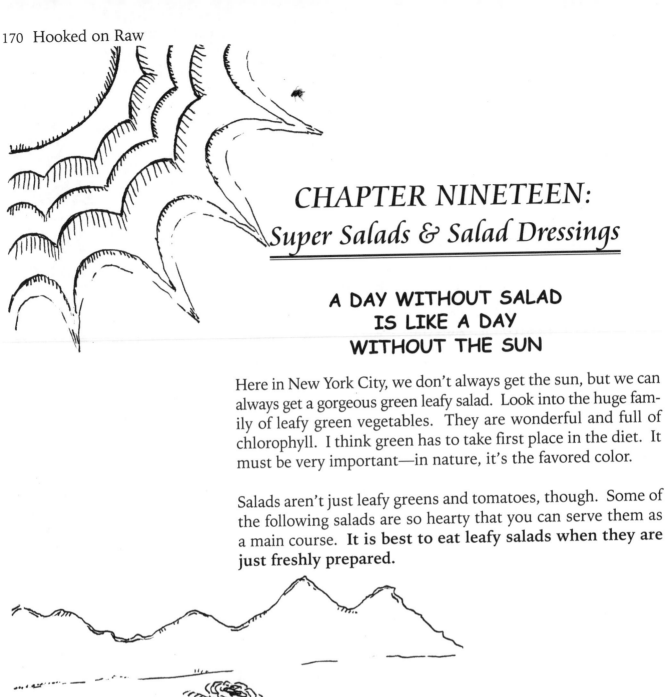

CHAPTER NINETEEN:
Super Salads & Salad Dressings

A DAY WITHOUT SALAD
IS LIKE A DAY
WITHOUT THE SUN

Here in New York City, we don't always get the sun, but we can always get a gorgeous green leafy salad. Look into the huge family of leafy green vegetables. They are wonderful and full of chlorophyll. I think green has to take first place in the diet. It must be very important—in nature, it's the favored color.

Salads aren't just leafy greens and tomatoes, though. Some of the following salads are so hearty that you can serve them as a main course. **It is best to eat leafy salads when they are just freshly prepared.**

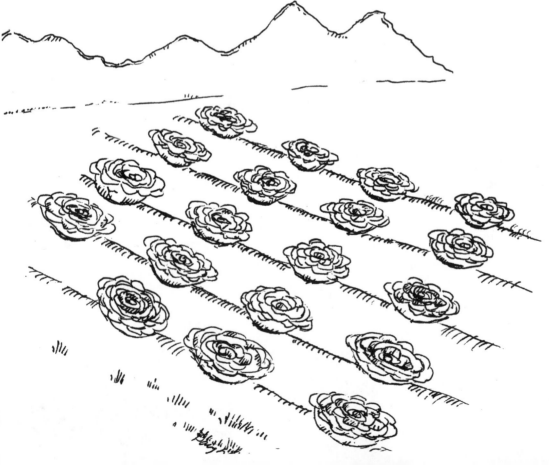

WATERCRESS & RED BELL PEPPER SALAD

2 bunches watercress, chopped
3 red bell peppers, julienne
1/2 cup pumpkin seeds, ground
3 tbsp. dehydrated onion, flaked or powdered (or use fresh
    minced onion, to taste)
1–2 garlic cloves, pressed
small piece of fresh ginger, pressed (use garlic press)
1/2 lemon, juiced
1 tbsp. flaxseed oil (or use 1 tbsp. of half flaxseed oil and
    half sesame oil)
Nama Shoyu or Celtic sea salt, to taste (optional)
for garnish: clover or alfalfa sprouts

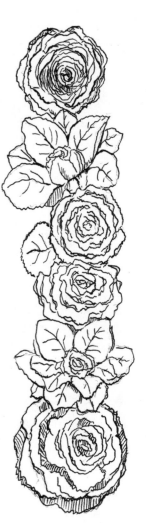

1) Mix the first four ingredients together in a large bowl. Set aside.

2) In a small bowl, blend the oil, lemon juice and seasonings, to taste. Pour over the salad and toss well. Transfer to serving bowls and garnish with clover or alfalfa sprouts all around the edge.

Serves 2-4, depending on how hungry you are. Keeps 1 day in the refrigerator.

LEIGH'S LENTIL SALAD

1 cup lentil sprouts
2 tomatoes, diced
1/2 onion, diced
1 medium cucumber, diced
1 cup clover or alfalfa sprouts

Try *Some Like it Hot Marinade* (cilantro & cayenne,
    optional) as a dressing (*see* page 270) or use
    a dressing of your choice.

1) Mix all ingredients together in a bowl and toss with the dressing.

Serves 2. Keeps 1-2 days in the refrigerator.

TABBOULEH SALAD

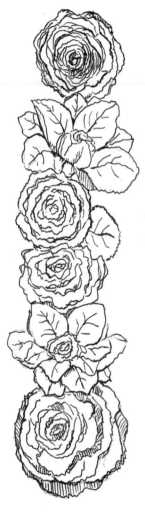

3 cups sprouted hulled buckwheat*
7 oz. carrot juice
2 1/2 large tomatoes, diced
1 1/2 cups finely chopped parsley
3/4 cup finely chopped scallions
2 tbsp. lemon juice
2 tbsp. olive oil (extra-virgin)
1 tsp. of flaxseed oil (optional)
1 tsp. dried mint or 2 tsp. fresh, minced
dash of Nama Shoyu or Celtic sea salt

1) Mix all ingredients together in a large bowl. Taste and adjust flavors.

   Serves 3-4. Keeps 2 days in the refrigerator.

*I use hulled, sprouted buckwheat in the *Tabbouleh Salad* instead of the traditional bulghur wheat. Bulghur wheat is a pre-cooked product when you buy it. Sprouted buckwheat makes a tasty substitute.

BEET-HIZIKI SALAD

1 medium beet, grated
1 tbsp. dry hiziki
l/2 cup sprouted sunflower seeds
olive oil (extra-virgin)
lemon juice
1 garlic clove, pressed (optional)
dash of Nama Shoyu or Celtic sea salt

1) Rinse hiziki. Soak it in filtered water until it swells up (about an hour).

2) The dry hiziki will have swelled to 1/2 cup. Drain, rinse and chop it a little. In a bowl, mix the hiziki with the grated beet and sunflower seeds, adding a little olive oil, lemon juice, l clove of pressed garlic (optional) and a dash of Nama Shoyu or Celtic sea salt. Mmm . . . delicious!

   Serves 1-2. Keeps for 2 days in the refrigerator.

FENNEL SALAD
with Cranberry Vinaigrette

1/2 fennel, sliced thin
3 oranges, cut into small chunks (with seeds removed)
1/2 cup Greek, black, sun-dried olives, desalted and minced
   (see "Olives" in Glossary for instructions on how to get
   the salt out)
1/3 cup dried cranberries, soaked 1 hour and drained

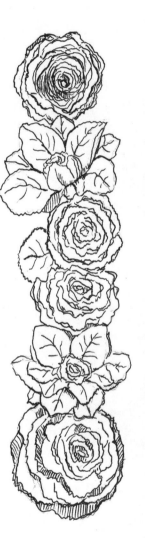

1) In a large bowl, mix the fennel, oranges, olives and cranberries and set aside.

CRANBERRY VINAIGRETTE:

   1/2–3/4 cup dried cranberries, soaked 1 hour
   juice of one orange
   3 tbsp. minced shallots
   1 tsp. olive oil (extra-virgin)
   raw honey (optional)
   Trocomare (optional)

2) Make a cranberry purée by putting the rehydrated cranberries through the Champion or Green Power juicer with the juice screen installed. You'll get purée instead of juice because the cranberries are dried, not fresh. You need to come out with 2 tbsp. of cranberry purée.

3) In a small bowl, mix the cranberry purée with orange juice, shallots and olive oil. If it's not sweet enough, add a little honey.

4) Pour onto the salad and toss gently. Add a sprinkle of Trocomare to taste.

   Serves 2. Keeps 2 days in the refrigerator.

FENNEL SLAW
with Pomegranate

1 fennel bulb, including some of the feathery top
1/3 of a pomegranate
handful of raw pistachio nuts
3 tbsp. *Pine Nut Yogurt* (see page 224) or any seed or
   nut yogurt
Celtic sea salt (optional)

1) Slice the fennel very thin on a mandoline or V-Slicer (see Kitchen Equipment). Put into a bowl and add in the *Pine Nut Yogurt*, pomegranate seeds and pistachio nuts, and toss well. Add Celtic sea salt, to taste.

   Serves 2. Keeps for 2 days in the refrigerator.

INDIAN COLE SLAW

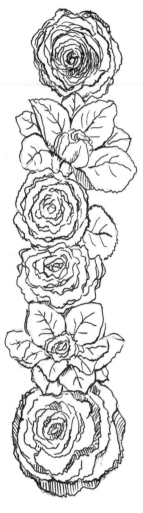

3 cups finely chopped green cabbage
3 cups chopped tomatoes
1 cup fresh grated coconut
1/2 cup peanuts,* ground (make sure they're raw, not
　　roasted)
1 large date, soaked, pitted and mashed
2 tbsp. lemon juice
2 tbsp. peanut oil (Flora Oils) or use olive oil
1/2 tsp. ground brown mustard seed
1/2 tsp. ground cumin seed
1/4 tsp. turmeric
pinch asafoetida (*see* Glossary)
1 tbsp. minced jalapeño, or to taste (optional)
Nama Shoyu and/or Celtic sea salt, to taste

1) Mix first 4 ingredients together in a large bowl and set aside.

2) In a small bowl, mash the soaked date, add in the balance of the ingredients, and blend to a smooth dressing.

3) Pour the dressing into the cabbage and tomato mixture and mix well.

　　Serves 4. This salad keeps well for 2-3 days in the refrigerator.

*Sunorganic Farm sells raw, organic, Valencia peanuts (*see* Source Index).

GUACAMOLE

2 medium avocados
1/3 cup chopped onion
1 small tomato, diced
1/2 cup diced cucumber
1/3 cup diced red bell pepper
1/2 lemon, juiced
1 tbsp. red bell pepper powder (optional)
1/8 tsp. Celtic sea salt

1) Mash or cube the avocados and mix with the vegetables and spices.

　　Serves 2. Best eaten when freshly made, but keeps for 2 days in the refrigerator. When storing, leave the avocado pits in the *Guacamole* to help maintain freshness. Serve on a bed of leafy greens.

SERVING SUGGESTIONS:

- Goes well with the *Tex-Mex Salad* (*see* page 177).
- Delicious with *Tacos in the Raw* (*see* page 154).

RAINBOW SUPER SLAW

1 green cabbage, grated or sliced very thin
1/3 red cabbage, grated or sliced very thin
2 tomatoes, chopped
1/2 carrot, grated
1 red bell pepper, julienne
large handful of arame*
Pine Nut Yogurt or any yogurt recipe (*see* page 224)
lime or lemon juice to taste
Nama Shoyu or Celtic sea salt, to taste

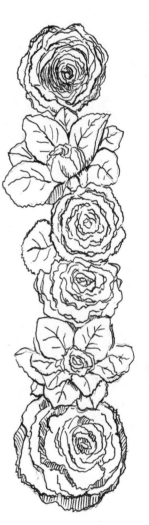

1) Soak the arame in filtered water for 5-10 minutes, then drain.

2) In a large bowl, mix all the vegetables with the *Pine Nut Yogurt* (which substitutes for mayonnaise), lemon or lime juice, and seasoning, to taste.

   Serves 4. Keeps for 3 days in the refrigerator.

ALTERNATIVE: Use *Almond Mayonnaise* instead of yogurt (*see* page 185).

*A mild-flavored sea vegetable (seaweed), the inclusion of which doesn't change the flavor of the slaw.

SEA VEGETABLE SALAD

1 package Ohsawa
   "Sea Vegetable Salad"
1 tomato, chopped
1 cucumber, chopped
1/2 cup grated daikon radish
3 shiitake mushrooms, sliced

1/2 cup sprouted
   sunflower seeds
1 tbsp. sesame oil
   (Flora Oils)
2 tbsp. lemon juice
1 garlic clove, pressed

1) Put the dried "Sea Vegetable Salad" into a bowl and cover with filtered water. Let sit for an hour, then drain the water. Transfer to another bowl, add in the other vegetables and set aside.

2) Make a dressing with the oil, lemon and garlic. Pour over the vegetables and toss well.

   Serves 2. Keeps for 2 days in the refrigerator.

SPINACH CAESAR SALAD

1 large bunch spinach
1/2 cup pumpkin seeds, ground
1–2 garlic cloves, pressed
1/2 lemon, juiced
1/2–1 tsp. prepared Dijon mustard (*see* Glossary)
2 tbsp. olive oil (extra-virgin)
dash of Celtic sea salt
sprinkle of freshly ground white pepper

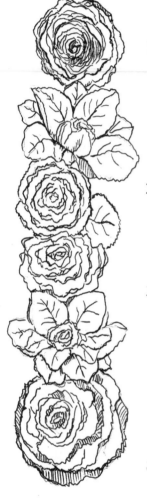

1) Rinse the spinach very well under running water, one leaf at a time. Make sure there is no soil or sand in the bottom part near the roots. Sand in your salad is not tasty! Another way to wash spinach is to put the leaves into a large bowl and fill it with water. Then shake the leaves in the water and the soil should fall to the bottom of the bowl. Once clean, spin the spinach leaves dry in a salad spinner and put into a large bowl. Tear or cut leaves into bite-size pieces.

2) Grind the pumpkin seeds. I like to use a kitchen utensil called a Salad-Shooter® (*see* Kitchen Equipment), or you can use a coffee or nut grinder. Add the ground seeds to the spinach and toss well. (The pumpkin seeds are a substitute for the Parmesan cheese used in conventional Caesar salad recipes).

3) In a small bowl, blend 1 or 2 pressed cloves of garlic, lemon juice, Dijon mustard, olive oil, a sprinkle of white pepper and Celtic sea salt. Pour over the spinach and toss well.

Serves 2-4. Keeps for 1 day in the refrigerator.

CAESAR SALAD

Substitute 1 large head of romaine lettuce for the spinach in the above recipe.

FAST & TASTY

tomatoes, chopped
buckwheat lettuce or pea greens, chopped
chives, scallions or shallots, minced
flaxseed oil

1) Make as much as you need for the number of people being served. Generally use 1/2 to 1 tbsp. of oil per person. Toss well. Best eaten when freshly made.

TEX-MEX SALAD

1 1/2 cups sprouted red lentils
1 1/2 cups fresh corn kernels, cut from the cob
1 1/2 cups diced red bell pepper
1 cup diced celery
1/2 cup minced Spanish onion

1) Mix above ingredients together in a large bowl and set aside.

HOT SAUCE:

1/4 cup lime juice
1 tbsp. olive oil (extra-virgin)
1 tbsp. flaxseed oil
2–3 cloves garlic, minced or pressed
1/2 jalapeño pepper, finely minced (optional)
2 tsp. chili powder
1/8 tsp. dry yellow mustard powder (optional)
dash of cayenne
dash of Nama Shoyu or Celtic sea salt
1/4 cup pine nuts
2 oz. filtered water
cilantro and/or scallions, minced
clover sprouts for garnish

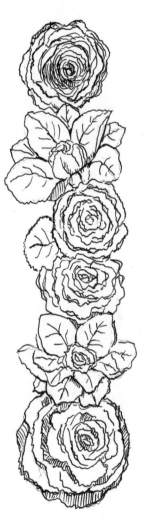

2) In a small bowl, mix together the lime juice, oil and spices (except for the cilantro). Stir well. Pour over the salad and toss.

3) In a blender, put 1/4 cup pine nuts, 2 oz. water and about 1/2 cup of the salad and blend to a cream. Add cream into salad and toss again. Garnish with clover sprouts all around the edge of the bowl and sprinkle minced cilantro and scallions on top.

Serves 3-4. Keeps for 2 days in the refrigerator. Goes well with *Guacamole* (*see* page 174).

CAULIFLOWER & MUNG

1 medium cauliflower, chopped
2–3 cups mung bean sprouts
1 recipe *Lynn's Honey-Mustard Dressing* (*see* page 188)

1) Mix the cauliflower and mung beans in a bowl. Add dressing and toss.

Serves 2-4. Keeps for 3 days in the refrigerator.

SPINACH SALAD—INDIAN STYLE

4 cups spinach, finely chopped
4 tbsp. freshly grated coconut
2 tbsp. ground, raw Valencia peanuts

1) Mix the finely chopped spinach with the coconut and ground peanuts in a large bowl and set aside.

INDIAN SPICE DRESSING:

1 tbsp. olive and flaxseed oils, mixed
1 tbsp. lemon juice
1 date, soaked and mashed
1/2 tsp. ground cumin
sprinkle of asafoetida
dash of Nama Shoyu or Celtic sea salt

2) Mash the date with a fork and combine with the other dressing ingredients. Pour the dressing over the salad and toss well.

Serves 2. Keeps for 2 days in the refrigerator.

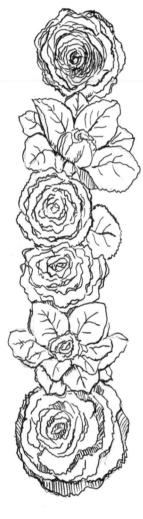

GORGEOUS GREENS

It is recommended that you have a gorgeous green salad every single day. In Italy, they say that a day without salad is like a day without the sun.

Gorgeous Greens is a salad made with a variety of leafy greens such as:

- **succulent leaf lettuces: bibb, red leaf, romaine, etc.**
- **spicy greens: arugula, watercress, nasturtium leaves, etc.**
- **bitter greens: chicory, escarole, dandelion, radicchio, etc.**
- **wild herbs, if you can get them: lamb's quarters, chickweed, purslane, etc., and**
- **edible flowers: squash blossoms, nasturtiums, red clover, marigolds, chrysanthemums, etc.**

Put together a selection from the different categories, keeping the first category predominant. Wash and spin dry in a salad spinner. Toss with your favorite dressing. Best when eaten freshly made.

HOOKED ON ROOTS SALAD

1 cup grated sweet potato
1 cup grated daikon radish
1 cup grated rutabaga
1 cup grated Jerusalem artichoke
1 cup grated beet
1/2 cup pumpkin seeds, grated
1 1/2 large avocados
1–2 garlic cloves, pressed
1–2 tbsp. lemon juice
Celtic sea salt, to taste (optional)

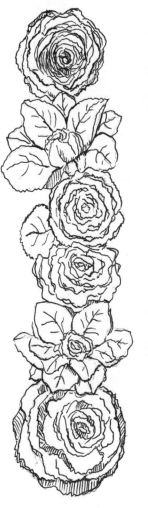

1) Wash the roots with a vegetable brush but don't peel, unless you see a part that looks bad. Cut all blemished parts out. Make sure the roots are not waxed. I've seen rutabagas heavily waxed, and in that case it is wise to peel.

2) Grate all the roots and put into a bowl. A handy tool for this job is a Salad-Shooter® (*see* Kitchen Equipment). Add mashed avocado, grated or ground pumpkin seeds (the SaladShooter® works for seeds also), pressed garlic, a squeeze of lemon juice and a dash of Celtic sea salt and blend well.

Serves 4-6. Keeps for 2 days in the refrigerator.

NOTE: This is a delicious way to introduce raw roots to people who say they "just can't eat raw roots." (Experiment with other combinations of roots.)

EASY-CHEEZY SLAW

cabbage, grated
Chedda Sauce (*see* page 210)
lemon juice
raisins or currants
Nama Shoyu and/or Celtic sea salt, to taste
garnish: tomatoes and cucumbers

1) Grate enough green cabbage for the number of people being served. Mix with some *Chedda Sauce*, and add lemon juice, raisins, Nama Shoyu and/or Celtic sea salt to taste. Garnish with slices of tomatoes and cucumbers.

Keeps for 2 days in the refrigerator.

CARLYN'S SALAD
Inspired by a Lovely Evening Spent at Carlyn's House

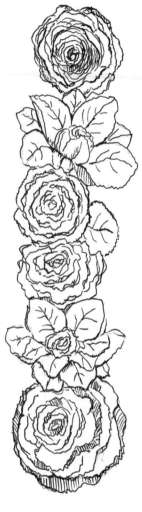

1 bunch arugula
1 large avocado, cubed
1 large red bell pepper, diced
1 large tomato, diced
1/2 medium white onion, minced
1 handful cilantro, cut up fine

1) Put all the salad ingredients into a large bowl and set aside.

SIMPLE DRESSING:

1 1/2 tbsp. olive oil (extra-virgin)
1/2 lemon, juiced
1 garlic clove, pressed
Spike
Herbamare
oregano
white pepper, freshly ground

2) In a small bowl stir the dressing ingredients, adding the spices according to your own taste.

3) Pour the dressing over the salad and toss.

Serves 2. Best when eaten freshly made.

HUNGARIAN SAUERKRAUT SALAD

1 cup *Hungarian Sauerkraut* (*see* page 228)
1 red bell pepper, diced
1 large tomato, diced
1 cucumber, diced
1/2 onion, diced
1 tbsp. olive oil (extra-virgin)
handful of raisins (optional)
dash of Nama Shoyu or Celtic sea salt

1) Put all the ingredients into a bowl and toss gently.

Serves 2. Keeps for 2 days in the refrigerator.

VARIATIONS: Instead of oil, try using:

- 1/4 cup of soaked pine nuts, blended in a blender with a little water.
- 1/4 cup of any nut yogurt recipe.

URAD DAL SPROUT SALAD

2 cups sprouted urad dal*
1/2 avocado
1/2 small lemon, juiced
1/3 cup minced shallot
Nama Shoyu or Celtic sea salt, to taste
for garnish: clover or alfalfa sprouts and chunks of
    tomatoes

1) Sprout the urad dal as you would any other bean. When sprouted, put into a bowl with the minced shallot.

2) In another small bowl mash the avocado with a fork and mix with the lemon juice. Then mix the mashed avocado with the urad dal sprouts and blend well by hand. Add a dash of Nama Shoyu or Celtic salt. Garnish with clover or alfalfa sprouts and chunks of tomato.

Serves 2. Keeps for 2 days in the refrigerator.

*Urad Dal is a small bean from India. It has a grayish black exterior and the kernel is cream colored. It is extremely easy to sprout. Make sure you purchase whole beans, not split ones. They are available in stores that sell products from India.

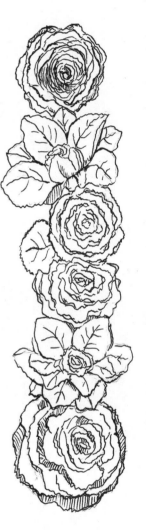

SUN-DRENCHED NITUKE

1 1/2 cups carrots, cut into matchstick-style pieces
1 1/2 cups beets, cut into matchstick-style pieces
1 cup Chinese snow peas, julienne
1/2 cup onion, diced small
1/4 cup sesame seeds, soaked overnight or for at least
    3 hours
1–2 tbsp. sesame oil
1/2 lime, juiced
1 garlic clove, pressed
Nama Shoyu, to taste

1) Yes, it takes a little patience to cut the vegetables into matchstick-size pieces but it makes all the difference in the success of this dish.

2) Mix all ingredients, except the onions and oil, together in a bowl and toss well. Cover with a screen and place in the hot sun for 4 hours. When ready to serve, add in the onions and oil and toss again.

If no sun is available, then add in the onions and oil, toss, and marinate in the refrigerator overnight before serving.

Serves 2. Keeps for 2-3 days in the refrigerator.

CUCUMBERS & CREAM SALAD

cucumber
Pine Nut or *Almond Yogurt* (*see* **page 224 or 223**)
lemon or lime juice
Celtic sea salt to taste

1) Take any amount of cucumber, enough for the amount of people you will be serving, and slice very thin. A mandoline is good for this. Toss with the yogurt, lemon or lime juice and a sprinkle of Celtic sea salt.

NOTE: Try to buy unwaxed, organic cucumbers from a farmer's market or get the Kirby cucumbers. Kirby cucumbers are generally not covered with wax because they are used to make pickles.

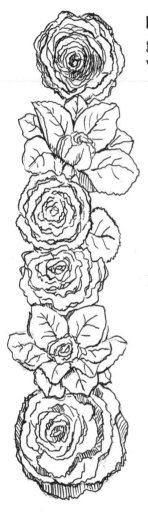

AVOCADO QUICKIE

1 avocado, cubed
2 tomatoes, chopped
1 cucumber, chopped
clover or alfalfa sprouts

1) Mix the avocado, tomatoes and cucumber and toss together in a bowl, then serve over a bed of clover or alfalfa sprouts.

Serves 1. Best when eaten freshly made.

ARMENIAN SALAD

1 large cucumber, diced
1 cup chopped celery
1/2 cup finely diced radishes
1/2 cup Kalamata olives or Greek, black olives
1/2 cup walnuts, soaked overnight (or at least 2 hours)
1 tbsp. olive and flaxseed oil, combined
1 tbsp. lemon juice

1) Soak the pitted olives in distilled water overnight to get rid of most of the salt. Next day—drain, rinse and chop the olives. (Desalted olives can be stored in the refrigerator for up to 3 weeks.) Drain, rinse and chop the walnuts also.

2) Combine all the ingredients in a salad bowl and toss.

Serves 2. Keeps for 2 days in the refrigerator.

RED CABBAGE SLAW WITH ARAME

3 cups grated red cabbage
1 medium carrot, grated
1/2 red bell pepper, julienne
2–3 heaping tbsp. dry arame (a sea vegetable)
1/2 lemon, juiced
3 oz. yogurt (use any of the seed or nut yogurt recipes)
1 tsp. cold-pressed sesame oil (*see Source Index*
     under Flora, Inc.)
Celtic sea salt, to taste

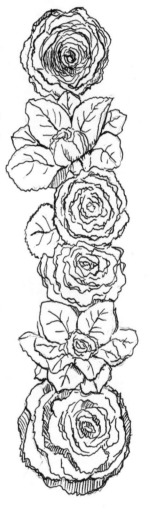

1) Soak the arame in filtered water for 5 minutes, then drain, rinse, and chop.

2) Combine the first four ingredients together in a large bowl. Add in the yogurt, oil and lemon juice. Toss well and season with a sprinkle of Celtic sea salt.

   Serves 2. Keeps for 2-3 days in the refrigerator.

GERMAN POTATO SALAD

5 cups grated red potatoes (a SaladShooter® works well)
filtered water to cover
1 cup diced red bell pepper
1 carrot, diced
3 tbsp. dehydrated onion flakes
2 tsp. Dijon mustard
1 recipe *Almond Mayonnaise*
Celtic sea salt, to taste
1/4 cup fresh minced dill
dash of paprika & cayenne
garnish: 2–3 tbsp minced chives,
1–2 tbsp. minced parsley

1) Scrub the potatoes but don't peel. Finely grate the red potatoes and put into a large bowl. Cover with filtered water and refrigerate overnight.

2) Next day, drain and rinse the potatoes. Squeeze as much liquid out of them as possible. Put into a large bowl, add bell pepper, carrots and dehydrated onion flakes. Set aside.

3) Add dill, mustard, and spices to the *Almond Mayonnaise*.

4) Mix the *Almond Mayonnaise* with the potatoes and vegetables. Toss well.

5) Garnish salad with minced chives and parsley.

   Serves 4. Serve immediately. Best when eaten freshly made.

Salad Dressings

Freshly harvested organic and wild vegetables are delicious on their own, but oh, with a little dressing, they become divine! Some of the sauces in the "Sauces, Dips & Spreads" section also make tasty salad dressings.

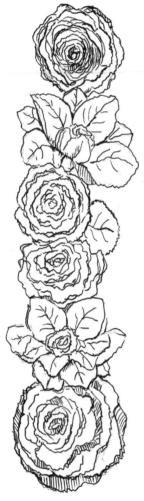

CAESAR DRESSING
This Dressing is Wonderful on Leafy Greens

2 tbsp. olive oil (extra-virgin)
1/2 lemon, juiced
1–2 garlic cloves, pressed
1/2–1 tsp. prepared Dijon mustard
dash of freshly ground white pepper
Celtic sea salt, to taste
1/2 cup pumpkin seeds, ground
1–2 tbsp. pine nuts, ground (optional)

1) Mix first six ingredients together in a small bowl.

2) When assembling a salad, first spin the leafy greens in a salad spinner. Transfer the greens to a bowl and toss the salad first with the ground pumpkin seeds and pine nuts, then add in the dressing and toss again.

Yield: enough for a large leafy salad for 2-4. Make fresh each time.

CREAMY FRENCH AVOCADO DRESSING

1 cup carrot juice
1/2 avocado
1 garlic clove
1/2 medium lemon, juiced (or to taste)
1 tsp. fresh dill
1/8–1/4 tsp. Celtic sea salt

1) In a juicer, prepare carrot juice.

2) Transfer the carrot juice to a blender, add in the rest of the ingredients and blend to a creamy consistency.

Yield: approx. 1 cup. Prepare and serve. Do not store.

ALMOND MAYONNAISE

1/2 cup sprouted almonds, blanched (*see* Glossary)
1 tbsp. soaked pine nuts (*optional*)
1 heaping tbsp. agar-agar flakes
1/2 clove garlic
1/2–3/4 cup filtered water (put 2 ice cubes in the water)
1 cup organic, unrefined oil (a good combination is 1/2
  extra-virgin olive & 1/2 sesame or sunflower oil* with
  1 tbsp. of flaxseed oil)
3 tbsp. lemon juice
1/2 tsp. unpasteurized apple cider vinegar
1/2 tsp. raw honey
1/4–1/2 tsp. Celtic sea salt
1/8 tsp. yellow mustard powder or 1/2 tsp. prepared
  stone-ground mustard
1/8 tsp. white pepper (grind fresh in a peppermill)

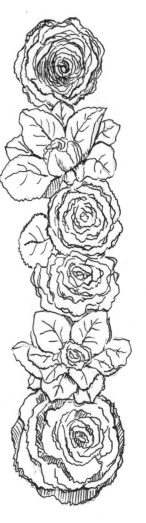

1) Place a small glass bowl and a wire whisk into the freezer for later use.

2) Put the almonds, pine nuts, agar-agar flakes, garlic and 1/2 cup of the water into the blender and blend very well, adding more water if necessary. (The ice cubes are in the water to keep it cold, which helps to solidify the mayonnaise when you add the oil.)

3) When the almonds are broken down to a fine cream, start adding in the oil very slowly. Have the blender running on medium or high (depending on your blender). The mayonnaise will start to thicken. If it gets thin, add in an ice cube or two, which will thicken it up again.

4) When all the oil is absorbed into the almond mixture, transfer the mayonnaise to the small chilled bowl and add in the lemon, vinegar and honey slowly, beating constantly with the wire whisk. Then, add in the Celtic sea salt and spices. Taste and adjust the flavors. Store in a glass jar in the refrigerator.

Makes almost 2 cups. Keeps for up to 3 weeks in the refrigerator.

NOTE: If the mayonnaise separates (and gets thin) when you add in the lemon juice and spices, it is usually because you added them in too fast and didn't whisk all the while. Should this happen, put the whole thing back into the blender, add in another 1/2 tbsp. agar-agar flakes and 2 to 3 ice cubes, and blend again. It should thicken up. If it still doesn't, put the mayonnaise into the refrigerator, and after a while it will thicken from the cold.

*Flora Oils makes **genuinely** cold-pressed sesame or sunflower oil—*see* Source Index.

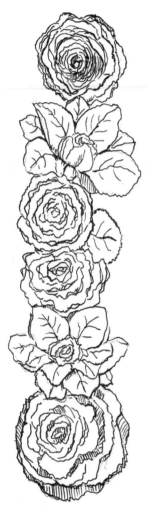

GOLDEN DOUBLE T DRESSING

2 heaping tbsp. raw sesame tahini
1 medium lime, juiced
1 tsp. turmeric
1/2–3/4 tsp. curry powder
1/2 tsp. dillweed
1/4–1/2 tsp. prepared Dijon mustard
1/4 tsp. Celtic sea salt
filtered water

1) Put all ingredients into a small bowl and with a spoon, blend well. Add enough water to thin to pancake batter consistency.

Enough for one huge salad. Keeps for up to a week in the refrigerator.

CHEEZY TOFU DRESSING

1 recipe *Creamy Tofu* (*see* page 230)
1/4 cup raw sesame tahini
1 tsp. prepared Dijon mustard
1 cup filtered water
1 tsp. basil flakes
1 tsp. dillweed
1/4 tsp. cayenne (or to taste)
1 tsp. dehydrated garlic granules
1 tbsp. finely cut fresh chives
Celtic sea salt, to taste

1) Put all ingredients into a bowl and blend together by hand.

Yield: 2 cups. Keeps for 2 days in the refrigerator, but is better the 1st day.

PAPAYA FRENCH DRESSING

2 cups papaya
1/2 cup orange juice
1/4 cup olive oil (extra-virgin)
1–2 small garlic cloves
1 tsp. agar-agar flakes
1 tsp. ground thyme
dash of Celtic sea salt

1) Put all ingredients into a blender and blend well.

Yield: approx. 1 1/2 cups. Best used the same day, but keeps for 2 days (you may have to reblend).

RHIO'S SECRET DRESSING

1–2 tbsp. *Veggie Seed Paté* (*see* page 158)
1–2 garlic cloves, pressed
1/4 lemon or lime, juiced
1 tbsp. cold-pressed sesame or olive oil
1 tbsp. any nut or seed yogurt
whey* or filtered water (use enough to thin out the
    dressing)
Celtic sea salt, to taste

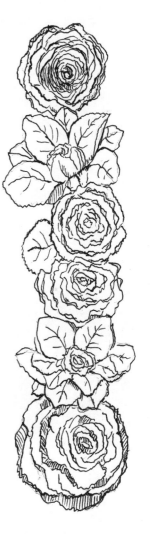

1) Blend all ingredients together in a small bowl.

Yield: enough for a very large leafy green salad. If you want to make more dressing to have on hand, double or triple the recipe. Keeps for 3 days in the refrigerator.

*This is a liquid that is produced when making nut or seed yogurts. It separates from the soft curd and goes to the bottom of the jar.

QUICK & BASIC

2 tbsp. olive oil (extra-virgin)
2 tbsp. fresh lemon juice or 1 tbsp. apple cider vinegar
1 garlic clove, pressed
Celtic sea salt to taste

1) Blend all ingredients together in a small bowl. Adjust flavor to your taste.

Enough for 1 large salad. Serve immediately.

TAHINI-LIME DRESSING

3 rounded tbsp. raw sesame tahini
4 tbsp. olive oil (extra-virgin)
3 limes, juiced
6–12 garlic cloves
1 tsp. prepared Dijon mustard
1/2 tsp. Celtic sea salt
1/4 cup filtered water

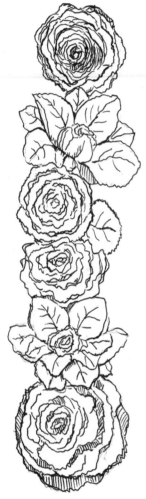

1) Using a mortar and pestle, mash the garlic cloves and Celtic sea salt until the garlic breaks down to a paste.

2) Transfer to a small bowl, add in the other ingredients and blend well.

Enough for 3 large salads. Keeps for up to a week in the refrigerator.

SUSIE'S SASSY LEMON DRESSING

Graciously Shared by my Sister Susie
So Simple and yet So Good!

1 cup lemon juice
1/2 cup olive oil (extra-virgin)
6 large garlic cloves
Celtic sea salt, to taste

1) Put all ingredients into a blender and blend very well.

Yield: 1 2/3 cups. Keeps for 2 weeks or more in the refrigerator, as the lemon preserves it. After storing, shake well before using.

LYNN'S HONEY-MUSTARD DRESSING

Inspired by a Lovely Farm Lady in Puerto Rico

6 oz. olive oil (extra-virgin)
2 tbsp. apple cider vinegar
2 tbsp. prepared Dijon mustard
2 oz. raw honey
2 tbsp. garlic powder
1/4 tsp. Celtic sea salt

1) Put all ingredients into a blender and blend to a creamy consistency.

Yield: 1 cup. Keeps for 2 weeks or more in the refrigerator.

CREAMY MINT DRESSING
with a Lemon Tang

1/2 cup sprouted sunflower seeds
1/3 cup olive oil
1/2 cup filtered water (or whey)
1/4 cup lime juice
2 garlic cloves
fresh mint leaves to taste, minced (use dried mint, if
    fresh is not available)
1 tsp. onion powder
1/4 tsp. Celtic sea salt

1) Put all ingredients into a blender and blend to a creamy consistency.
    Yield: 1 cup. Keeps for 4 days in the refrigerator.

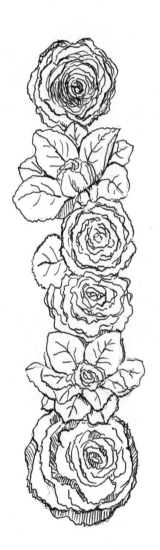

THOUSAND ISLAND DRESSING

1 recipe *Almond Mayonnaise* (*see* page 185)
2 rounded tbsp. *Sun Dried Tomato Tapenade* (*see* page 271)
2 tbsp. finely diced dill sour pickles or fresh cucumbers
1 tbsp. minced fresh dill
1 tsp. Dijon mustard
1/2 tsp. paprika

1) Put all ingredients into a bowl and blend well with a wire whisk.
Yield: approx. 1 pint. Keeps for 3 days in the refrigerator.

AVOCADO DRESSING

1 medium avocado
1 cup almonds, blanched
2 tbsp. soaked pine nuts
1 cup filtered water
1–2 lemons, juiced

1 tbsp. olive oil (extra-virgin)
1 tsp. Dijon mustard
2 tbsp. finely chopped dill
1 tbsp. finely chopped chives
Celtic sea salt, to taste

1) Put avocado, nuts and water into a blender and blend to a sauce consistency. Transfer to a bowl and mix in the other ingredients with a wire whisk.
Yield: 1 1/2 cups. Serve immediately.

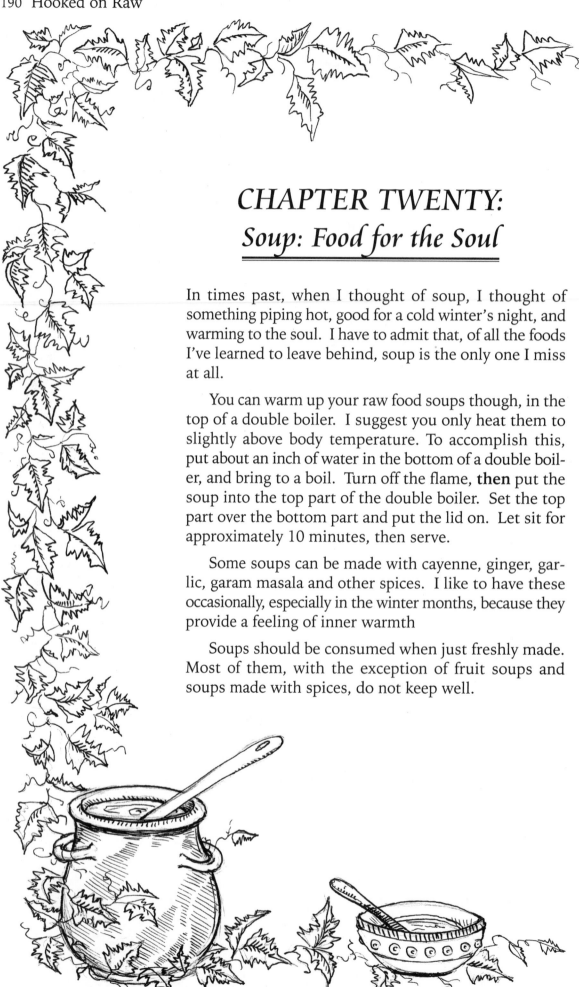

CHAPTER TWENTY:
Soup: Food for the Soul

In times past, when I thought of soup, I thought of something piping hot, good for a cold winter's night, and warming to the soul. I have to admit that, of all the foods I've learned to leave behind, soup is the only one I miss at all.

You can warm up your raw food soups though, in the top of a double boiler. I suggest you only heat them to slightly above body temperature. To accomplish this, put about an inch of water in the bottom of a double boiler, and bring to a boil. Turn off the flame, **then** put the soup into the top part of the double boiler. Set the top part over the bottom part and put the lid on. Let sit for approximately 10 minutes, then serve.

Some soups can be made with cayenne, ginger, garlic, garam masala and other spices. I like to have these occasionally, especially in the winter months, because they provide a feeling of inner warmth

Soups should be consumed when just freshly made. Most of them, with the exception of fruit soups and soups made with spices, do not keep well.

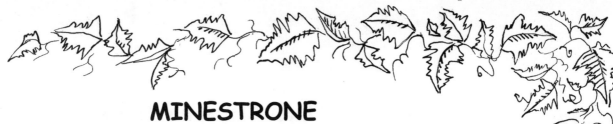

MINESTRONE

4–6 chard leaves (save stems for another use)
1/2 cup sprouted chick peas or 1 fresh corn,
    cut from the cob
1 large tomato, diced
1/2 red bell pepper, diced
1 1/2 cups sprouted wild rice
1 cup dried sweet corn (*see* Source Index)
3/4 cup filtered water
1–2 tbsp. olive oil (extra-virgin)
1 tbsp. *Vegetable Seasoning & Broth* AND
    2–3 tbsp. *"Organic Vegetable Mix"* (*see* page 291)
1 tbsp. mellow white miso (opt.)
Celtic sea salt and/or Nama Shoyu, to taste
3 cups filtered water, heated (don't boil)

1) Cover the dried sweet corn with 3/4 cup water and set aside.

2) Put the chick-peas into a food processor and using the "S" blade pulse chop lightly. Transfer to a large soup tureen.

3) Put the chard leaves into the food processor and using the "S" blade process as finely as possible. Transfer to the soup tureen.

4) Put all the other ingredients, including the dried sweet corn, into the soup tureen and stir well. If using miso, blend by hand with a little water first. Taste and adjust flavors.

    Yield: approx. 2 quarts. Keeps for 2 days in the refrigerator.

REFRESHING FRUIT SOUP

1/3 of a pineapple
1 bunch grapes
1 apple
1 tomato
1/2 lemon or lime

TOPPING: Any nut or seed yogurt—or try *Macadamia Cream* (*see* page 217)

1) Put all of the fruit through a juicer. Serve with or without a dollop of nut or seed yogurt.

    Serves 2. Keeps for 2 days in the refrigerator.

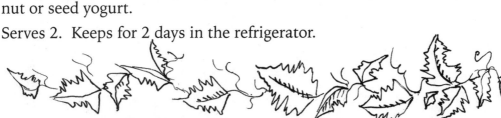

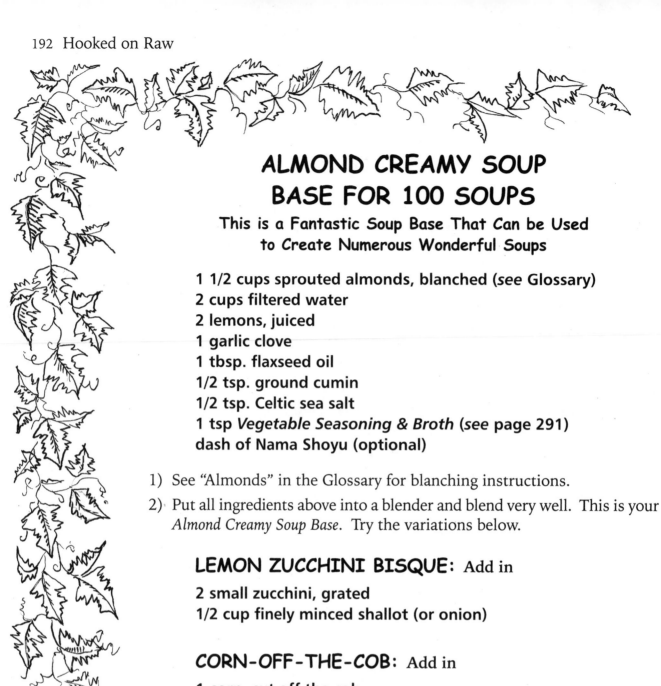

ALMOND CREAMY SOUP BASE FOR 100 SOUPS

This is a Fantastic Soup Base That Can be Used to Create Numerous Wonderful Soups

1 1/2 cups sprouted almonds, blanched (*see Glossary*)
2 cups filtered water
2 lemons, juiced
1 garlic clove
1 tbsp. flaxseed oil
1/2 tsp. ground cumin
1/2 tsp. Celtic sea salt
1 tsp *Vegetable Seasoning & Broth* (*see page 291*)
dash of Nama Shoyu (optional)

1) See "Almonds" in the Glossary for blanching instructions.

2) Put all ingredients above into a blender and blend very well. This is your *Almond Creamy Soup Base*. Try the variations below.

LEMON ZUCCHINI BISQUE: Add in

2 small zucchini, grated
1/2 cup finely minced shallot (or onion)

CORN-OFF-THE-COB: Add in

1 corn, cut off the cob
1/4 cup finely minced shallot
1/4 red bell pepper, finely chopped
2 mushrooms, finely chopped

ALMOND-BEET BORSCHT: Add in

1/2 beet, grated
1/2 cup chopped cucumber
1/4 cup finely minced chives
sprinkle of chopped dill

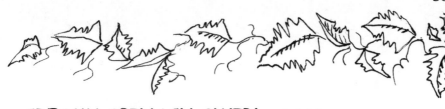

CREAMY SPINACH SWIRL: Add in

1/2 bunch spinach
1/2 tsp. garam masala

Divide the soup base in half. Put one half back into the blender with spinach and garam masala and blend well. Pour the white soup base into 2 or 4 soup bowls, then pour the green spinach blend into each bowl. With a spoon stir gently. It will swirl out and look like the colors in a Matisse painting. Beautiful and delicious!

Serves 2-4. Because of the spices, this soup will keep for 2 days in the refrigerator.

GREEN POWER SOUP

2 cups cucumber juice
2 1/2 cups *Marinated Collard Ribbons* (see page 206)
1/4–1/2 avocado (If you're on a reducing diet, use only 1
    or 2 tbsp. to cream it up a bit)
1/4–1/2 lemon, juiced
1 garlic clove
1–2 tsp. mellow white miso (optional)

1) Prepare the cucumber juice in a juicer, then put it into a blender with all the rest of the ingredients and blend to a creamy consistency.

2) Any sprouts which you have on hand, such as lentils, wild rice, mung beans, etc. can be spooned on top of the soup before serving,

Serves 1 or 2. Best when eaten freshly made.

VARIATION: Instead of the cucumber juice, you could use a combination of celery and zucchini juice or you could use chard stem or collard stem juice. Chard and collard stems are the thick stalk or rib in the middle of the leaf.

NOTE: If you're using the soup as part of a body cleansing process, eliminate the miso.

*This also works with marinated kale, red and green chard ribbons, and beet tops (separately or combined). It is not absolutely necessary to marinate the leaves in order to make the soup. I usually use the leaves as they come, but marinating is suggested here because most people are not accustomed yet to the raw taste.

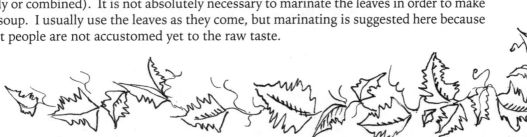

BORSCHT

1 medium beet
5 large carrots
1 lemon, peeled—leave the white pith on
1/2 large cucumber, minced
1–2 shallots, minced
1 scallion, minced
2 heaping tbsp. red lentil sprouts (optional)
2 heaping tbsp. any yogurt or plain seed cheese
   (*see* Chapter 23)

1) In a juicer, prepare beet, carrot and lemon juices. Stir them together and pour into two bowls.

2) Top each bowl with some minced cucumber, shallot or scallion, and a dollop of yogurt or seed cheese. If available, the red lentil sprouts are a delicious addition.

Serves 2. Best when eaten freshly made.

"HOT" CREAM OF CAULIFLOWER SOUP

1/2 cup carrot juice
1/2 cup *Almond Milk* (*see* page 249)
2 one-inch slices of ginger, juiced (or to taste)
1 small cauliflower, chopped (approx. 2-3 cups)
1/2 avocado
2 oz. hot filtered water (optional)
1 tsp. garam masala
1 tsp. curry powder
1 tsp. red bell pepper powder

1) In a juicer, make the carrot and ginger juice.

2) Put the juices into the blender with the *Almond Milk* and all the other ingredients, except the hot water, and blend well. After the soup is well blended, add in the hot water, blend briefly and serve "hot." The addition of the hot water makes this into a warm soup.

Serves 2. Serve with *Macaroon Chews* (*see* page 256) and you'll think you're in exotic India!

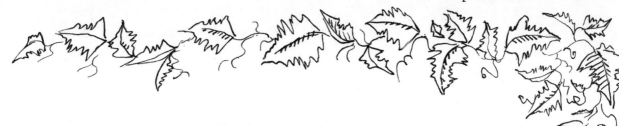

TOMATO SURPRISE SOUP

1 cup winter squash juice (spaghetti squash or butternut
are good—juice the rind, and the seeds—put everything
through, except the stem)
1 cup Jerusalem artichoke* juice
1 medium red bell pepper
1 medium lemon
1 large tomato
1 slice onion
1 tsp. unpasteurized mellow white miso
sprinkle of cayenne (optional)

1) Scrub the squash and Jerusalem artichokes with a vegetable brush, but do not peel. If there are any blemished areas, cut them out. Using a juicer, prepare one cup of squash juice and one cup of Jerusalem artichoke juice. Pour these juices into the blender jar.

2) Peel the lemon, being careful to leave the white pith** on, cut in half, then put through the juicer with the red bell pepper. Add these juices to the blender jar.

3) Add the tomato, onion and miso and blend well. Sprinkle with cayenne if desired.

Makes 2 servings. Best when eaten freshly made.

NOTE: This soup came as a complete surprise to me one day when I didn't have much in the refrigerator and I didn't feel like going shopping. (It was a New York deep-freeze winter.) I started by making the juices (an unlikely combination I probably never would have tried, except that was all there was). I then added the miso, onion and tomato. Surprise! It was delicious and satisfying! I tried it out on (who else?) Leigh, who previously wouldn't eat raw winter squash for nothin' . . . he didn't even know the squash was in there, and now he enjoys it!

*Also known as sunchokes.

**Pith: This is the white part, just under the peel of all citrus fruits. It is very rich in rutin, a bioflavonoid. When you use the pith in juice, you get a more nutritionally complete juice, plus the juice is thicker.   And, when used in juice or soup, the pith does not taste bitter, as it might when eaten alone.

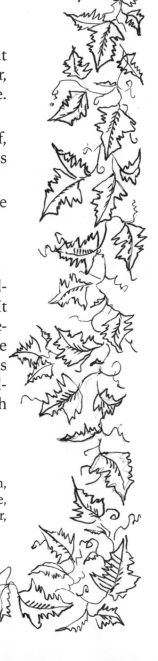

SPICY INDIAN SPINACH SOUP

1 large bunch spinach
1 cup cucumber juice
1/4–1/2 cup *Pine Nut Yogurt* (see **page 224**)
1 tsp. garam masala
1/2 tsp. ground coriander
1/4 tsp. turmeric
1/4 tsp. fresh ground white pepper
1/8 tsp. asafoetida
pinch of nutmeg
dash of cayenne
2 tsp. Nama Shoyu

1) Wash the spinach very well—you don't want sand in your soup.
2) Blend all ingredients in a blender.

Serves 2. Keeps for 2 days in the refrigerator because the spices preserve it. After storage, shake well before serving.

ALTERNATE SUGGESTION:

• **INDIAN SPICE FLAKY BREAD:** Pour soup onto dehydrator trays lined with Teflex and dehydrate at 95° F for approx. 24 hours or until crisp, then peel off. One recipe makes 4 to 5 spice bread slices. These are very thin, kind of flaky and they melt in your mouth. A good accompaniment to Indian-style menus.

PURÉE OF ASPARAGUS SOUP

2 cups chopped asparagus
1 cup water or Rejuvelac
1 tbsp. *Veggie Seed Paté* (see **page 158**)
1 shiitake (or other mushroom)
1 small garlic clove
dash of Celtic sea salt

1) Put all ingredients into a blender and blend well. Serve immediately.

Serves 1 or 2. Best when eaten freshly made.

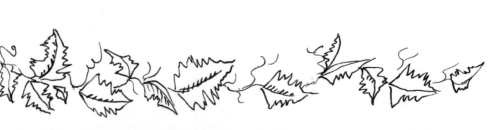

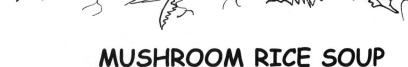

MUSHROOM RICE SOUP

2 cups rough chopped mushrooms
filtered water, enough to cover the mushrooms
1 tbsp. Nama Shoyu
1/2 tsp. Celtic sea salt
1/4–1/2 avocado
1 garlic clove
1 cup warm filtered water
1/2 cup *Sprouted Sweet Brown Rice* (*see* page 153)

1) In a medium size bowl, mix the water, Nama Shoyu and Celtic sea salt. Toss the mushrooms with this mixture and put them into the refrigerator overnight. When ready to prepare the soup, drain the liquid out and discard.

2) Put the mushrooms in a blender with 1 cup warm filtered water, the avocado, and garlic. Blend to a cream (or leave chunky, if you like).

Serve in bowls and ladle in some *Sprouted Sweet Brown Rice*.

Serves 2. Serve immediately.

CREAM OF CELERY ROOT SOUP

8 oz. cucumber juice
1 1/2 cups chopped celery root (*see* Glossary)
1/2 tomato
2 oz. lemon juice
4 heap. tbsp. sprouted sunflower seed
4 heap. tbsp. sprouted pine nuts or 1/4 avocado
1–2 garlic cloves
1 heap. tbsp. red bell pepper powder
dash of Nama Shoyu or Celtic sea salt

1) Make sure to wash the celery root very well, as soil can become trapped in the gnarls.

2) Prepare the cucumber juice in a juicer. Transfer the juice to a blender, add in chopped celery root and the balance of the ingredients. Blend well

Serves 2. Serve immediately.

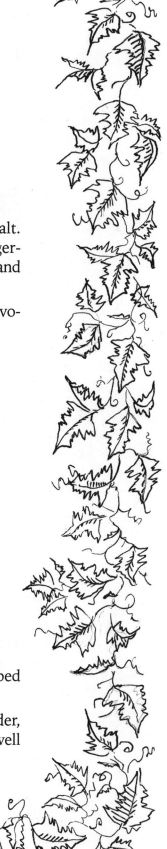

DR. ANN'S ENERGY SOUP

Dr. Ann Wigmore, one of the pioneers of the modern day living foods movement, innovated Energy Soups as a form of light, easy to digest nourishment. She actually developed them for herself because, as a busy woman, she wanted to obtain the optimum nutrition in the shortest possible time. (Eating a salad and chewing it thoroughly takes 30-45 minutes.) Dr. Ann developed Energy Soups as the ultimate food for energy. They are easy-to-digest nourishment; the perfect daily food for cleansing and balancing the body at a slow and natural pace and, most assuredly, a good food for people with digestive system problems. I recommend all of Ann Wigmore's books. She was an advanced, spiritual woman, clearly ahead of her time. *Dr. Ann's Energy Soup* has many, many variations. Following are two basic recipes.

ENERGY SOUP #1

1 large or 2 small apples
1 cup *Rejuvelac* (*see* page 227) or use filtered water
1/2 cup dulse leaves*
1 tbsp. sprouted lentils or peas
1–5 cups of green leaves, such as buckwheat lettuce,
    sunflower greens, parsley, etc. (see more extensive
    list on the following page)
1/2–1 avocado

1) Blend apple, *Rejuvelac* (or water), dulse and sprouted lentils or peas in a blender, then add the avocado and as much leafy greens as you want, from 1–5 cups, and blend again. (I like it heavy on the greens but you might have to work up to it.)

Serves 2. Best when eaten freshly made

NOTE: If made with *Rejuvelac* it will keep all day because the *Rejuvelac* keeps the soup from oxidizing. If made with water, serve immediately.

*Dulse is a dark purple sea vegetable.

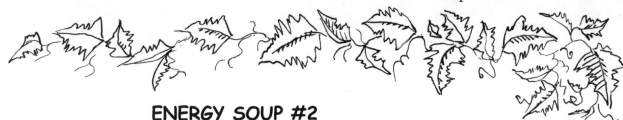

ENERGY SOUP #2

1 tbsp. sprouted lentils
1 tbsp. sprouted whole peas
1 small piece of carrot
1 small piece of sweet potato, squash or Jerusalem
artichoke
1 cup *Rejuvelac* (*see* page 227) or use filtered water
1 large apple (or 2 small)
1/2 cup dulse leaves*
1–5 cups of buckwheat lettuce, sunflower greens and/or
any other greens (see list below)
1/2–1 avocado
handful of fresh cilantro or basil for flavor (optional)

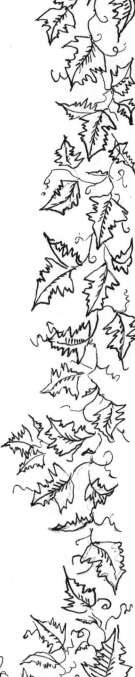

1) Put the first four ingredients into the blender with *Rejuvelac* or water. (Cut up the carrot and sweet potato a little so they blend easier.) Start the blender and liquefy. Add all the other ingredients and blend well.

Serves 2–3. Best when eaten freshly made.

VARIATIONS: Replace the apple and avocado with either:

- 1/2–1 papaya
- 1/2–1 large mango
- 1/3–1/2 cup seed cheese
- 1 ripe plantain (you'll know it's ripe because the peel will be halfway to almost black but the fruit will not be mushy)

PARTIAL LIST OF GREEN LEAF IDEAS

ROTATE THE GREENS (use one or a combination)

buckwheat lettuce	**parsley**
sunflower greens	**spinach**
pea greens	**carrot tops**
leaf lettuce	**beet tops**
alfalfa & clover sprouts	**kale**

collard leaves (cut stalk out and save for juice)
chard leaves (cut stalk out and save for juice)
cactus pads
edible weeds, such as: purslane, plantain, malva, filaree, chick-
weed, lamb's-quarters, comfrey, goutweed, young dande-
lion, leaf amaranth, etc.

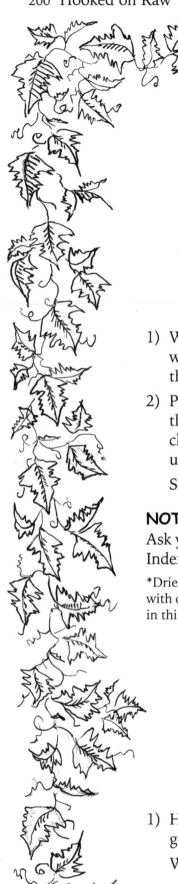

CORN CHOWDER

2 ears of corn
2 cups of *Almond Milk* (*see* page 249)
1 tbsp. soaked pine nuts (optional)
2 shallots, minced
1/2 cup dried sweet corn*
1/2 cup sprouted red lentils
1/2–1 tsp. ground cumin
dash of Nama Shoyu or Celtic sea salt

1) With a sharp knife cut the corn off the cobs. Put the kernels into a blender with the *Almond Milk* and the pine nuts. Blend very well, then strain through a muslin cloth. Squeeze out all the liquid. Discard the pulp.

2) Put the liquid into a soup tureen, add the rest of the ingredients and adjust the flavors to suit your taste. The dried sweet corn will be too tough to chew at first, so let the soup sit at room temperature for about 30 minutes. This softens the dried corn enough to make it chewable.

Serves 2-3. Best when eaten freshly made.

NOTE: Neshaminy Valley Natural Foods distributes "Dried Sweet Corn." Ask your health food store to carry it. (*See* "Organic Provisions" in the Source Index.)

*Dried sweet corn is a variety of fresh corn which has been dehydrated. Don't confuse it with other dried corn meant for corn bread or tortillas. Those types of corn will not work in this recipe.

VEGETABLE BROTH

1 heaping tbsp. *Vegetable Seasoning & Broth*
    (*see* page 291)
1 tbsp. Greek, sun-dried black olives, desalted* and minced
1 cup filtered water
1/2 tsp. olive or flaxseed oil (optional)
dash of Celtic sea salt

1) Heat the filtered water to hot, but not so hot that you can't put your finger in.

When ready, stir in the ingredients. Enjoy!

*For instructions on desalting the olives, *see* "Olives" in the Glossary.

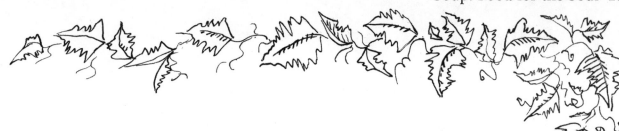

QUICK BLENDER SOUP
in Five Minutes Flat

This is a formula for making *Quick Blender Soup*:

1) Start off with 1 or 2 large tomatoes. Roughly chop them and put into the blender. Add in any raw vegetables, leafy green vegetables or sprouts. Use mostly vegetables that grow above the ground. If you want to use a root vegetable, put in only 1 or 2 small chunks.

SUGGESTED COMBINATIONS:

Quick Soup 1	Quick Soup 2	Quick Soup 3
tomatoes	tomatoes	cucumber
celery leaves	asparagus	tomato
spinach	spinach	spinach
sprouts	shiitake mushroom	buckwheat lettuce
onion	avocado	sunflower greens
garlic		chives or dill
lemon		
avocado (optional)		

These soups are a little bland, so to make them more interesting, you can add some other ingredients on top of the soup before serving. Try one or a combination of the following:

> chopped chives
> chopped scallions
> diced cucumbers and/or tomatoes
> sprouted sunflower seeds
> chopped olives, desalted (*see* Glossary)
> *Vegetable Seasoning & Broth* (*see* page 291)

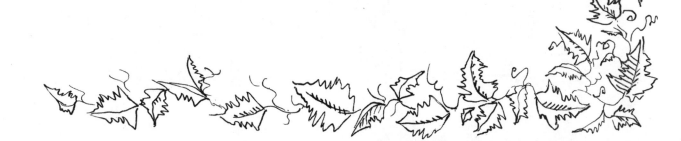

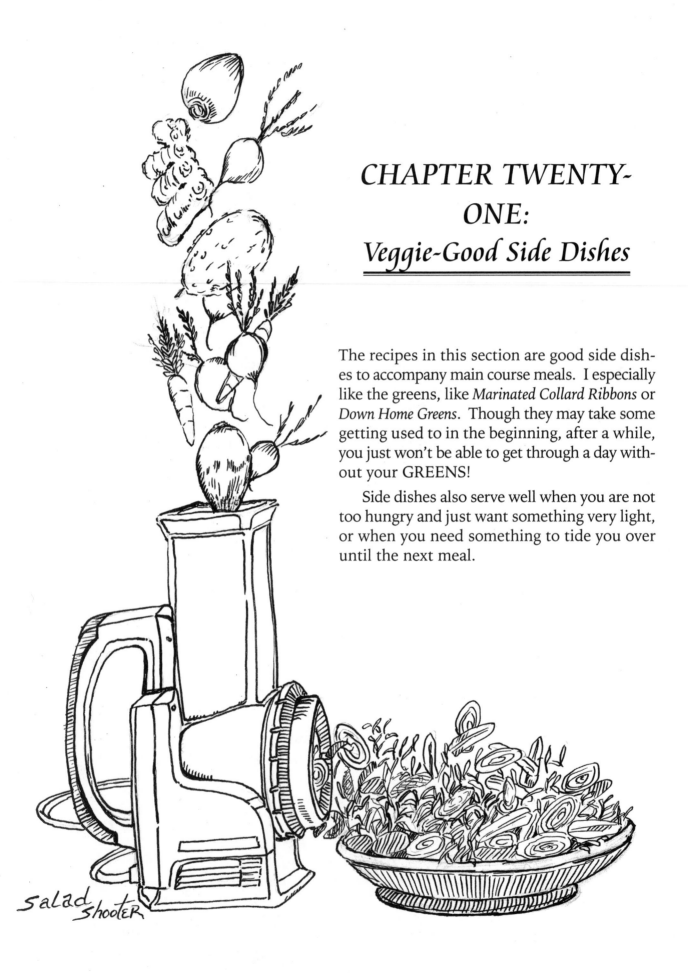

CHAPTER TWENTY-ONE:
Veggie-Good Side Dishes

The recipes in this section are good side dishes to accompany main course meals. I especially like the greens, like *Marinated Collard Ribbons* or *Down Home Greens*. Though they may take some getting used to in the beginning, after a while, you just won't be able to get through a day without your GREENS!

Side dishes also serve well when you are not too hungry and just want something very light, or when you need something to tide you over until the next meal.

salad
shooter

GREEN BEANS JULIENNE
with Raisins & Walnuts

3 cups green beans, julienne
2 oz. raisins, soaked 1 hour in just enough water
    to cover
4 oz. walnuts, soaked 1 hour (try black walnuts for
    an unusually tasty treat)
1 lime, juiced
1 sweet orange, juiced
dash of Nama Shoyu or Celtic sea salt
pinch of freshly ground white pepper

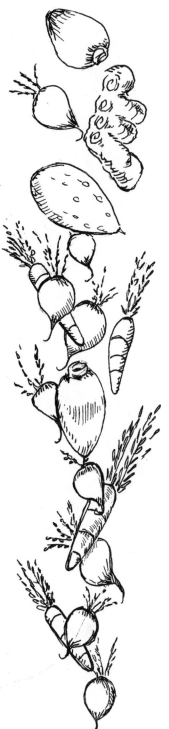

1) Drain the water out of the raisins and save for another use. Drain and rinse the walnuts. Toss all the ingredients together in a bowl.

Serves 4. Keeps for 2 days in the refrigerator.

CACTUS JULIENNE

2 cactus pads, julienne*
1/2 cup fresh grated coconut
1/4 cup fresh-ground, raw peanuts
1 1/2 tbsp. combination olive oil and flaxseed oil
1 date, pitted, soaked and mashed
1/8 tsp. asafoetida
1/2 tsp. ground brown mustard seeds
1/2 tsp. or more of fresh green chili, seeded
    and minced
dash of Nama Shoyu or Celtic sea salt

1) Wash the cactus pads and make sure to remove the thorns. Cut each pad in half and then in half again. Using a V-Slicer or similar piece of kitchen equipment, prepare a cactus pad julienne.

2) Transfer to a bowl and grate in the coconut and peanuts. Mix together the rest of the ingredients to make a dressing. Pour onto the cactus and toss gently.

Serves 1 or 2. Serve immediately. Doesn't keep well.

*NOTE: Once cut, cactus pads ooze a thick gel-like liquid. If you find that this does not appeal to your taste, then before preparing the recipe, put the cactus julienne into the dehydrator at 95° F for a couple of hours to dry up the liquid somewhat. This makes it more pleasant to eat, for some people.

DOWN HOME GREENS

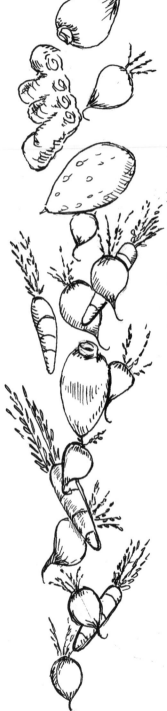

1 bunch collard greens
1 bunch kale or swiss chard
2 tbsp. flaxseed oil
1/4 lemon, juiced
3 tbsp. unpasteurized apple cider vinegar
1 1/2 tbsp. unheated honey
1–2 garlic cloves, pressed
1 tsp. ground cumin
1/2 scant tsp. Celtic sea salt

1) Wash the greens and cut out the rib going almost all the way down the middle of the leaf (save for juicing).

2) Lay the greens one on top of the other and then fold in half and roll the whole bunch into a tight roll. (You'll probably have to do this twice to use all the greens.) Starting at one end of the roll, cut into very thin slivers. Put the slivers into a large bowl and set aside.

3) In a small bowl, mix the rest of the ingredients and blend well into a dressing.

4) Toss the greens with the dressing until they are well coated. Cover and let marinate in the refrigerator overnight. They could also be served just freshly prepared, but you may need time to get used to the flavor.

Serves 2-4. Keeps for 2-3 days in the refrigerator.

SESAME TURNIPS

2 cups small diced turnips
1 recipe *Simple Marinade* (*see* page 206)
1 cup red bell pepper, julienne
1/2 cup scallions or leeks, sliced very thin
1 garlic clove, pressed
1/2 lemon, juiced
1/4 cup raw sesame tahini
sprinkle of sesame seeds

1) Toss the turnips with the *Simple Marinade* to coat well. Let marinate overnight in the refrigerator.

2) The next day add the rest of the ingredients to the turnips and mix well.

Makes approx. 3 1/2 cups. Keeps for 3-4 days in the refrigerator.

CURRIED SUGAR SNAP PEAS

3 cups sugar snap peas, Chinese snow peas or any
    edible podded peas, julienne
3 tbsp. freshly grated coconut

1) De-string the peas and prepare julienne.

2) Mix peas with the freshly grated coconut and set aside in a bowl.

CURRY DRESSING:

1 tbsp. olive oil (extra-virgin)
1/2 medium lemon, juiced
1 date, pitted, soaked and mashed
1/2 tsp. ground brown mustard seeds
1/2 tsp. ground cumin seeds
1/2 tsp. garam masala
1/4 tsp. turmeric powder
pinch asafoetida
Nama Shoyu to taste or sprinkle of Celtic sea salt
garnish: 2 tbsp. freshly chopped cilantro

3) Mix the oil, lemon juice, mashed date, spices and seasoning. Pour
this dressing onto the peas and toss well. Sprinkle with chopped
cilantro.

Serves 2-4. Keeps in the refrigerator for 2-3 days.

SIMPLY FENNEL

1 fennel
1 tbsp. olive oil (extra-virgin)
1/4 cup pumpkin seeds, grated
sprinkle of Celtic sea salt or Nama Shoyu

1) Slice the fennel bulb very thin with a V-Slicer, mandoline or similar
piece of kitchen equipment. Put into a bowl. Mince a small amount
of the fennel leaves (about 3/4 cup) and add to the bowl.

2) Grate the pumpkin seeds with the SaladShooter® or a nut grinder
(*see* Kitchen Equipment). Add the grated pumpkin seeds, oil and seasoning to the fennel and toss well.

Serves 2. Keeps for 2 days in the refrigerator.

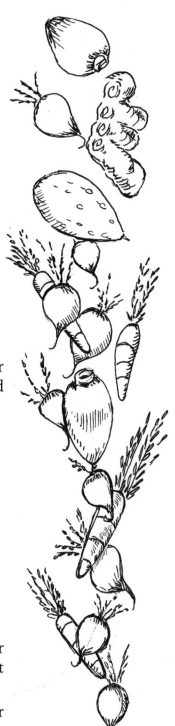

PURSLANE

1 large bunch purslane (a wild vegetable)
1 recipe *Tahini/Miso Dip* (see page 213)

1) Cut the purslane into bite-size pieces and toss with *Tahini/Miso Dip*, which has been blended with a little water. Serves 2-4.

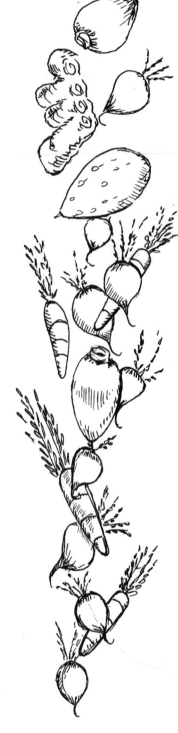

MARINATED COLLARD RIBBONS

1 bunch collard greens

SIMPLE MARINADE:

1–1 1/2 tbsp. olive oil and flaxseed oil mixed
1/2–1 lemon or lime, juiced
1 tbsp. Nama Shoyu or a sprinkle of Celtic sea salt

1) Wash the collard greens and cut out the stems or ribs which go almost all the way down the middle of the leaf (save for juicing).

2) Lay the collard leaves one on top of the other and then fold in half and roll the whole bunch into a tight roll. Starting at one end of the roll, cut into very thin slivers. Put the resulting ribbons into a large bowl. Add the marinade and toss until all the ribbons are well coated. Cover the greens and let marinate in the refrigerator overnight.

Serves 2. Keeps for 2-3 days in the refrigerator.

ALTERNATIVE: You could weigh down the greens by covering them first with some parchment paper and then putting a heavy weight on top of them, such as a half gallon plastic or glass water jug filled with water. The weight helps the marinade penetrate into the leaves to soften them up. Marinate overnight.

SERVING SUGGESTIONS:

- Add sprouted, blanched, dehydrated almonds, red bell pepper julienne, and diced onions, shallots or scallions. Toss.
- Add mellow white miso mixed with a little water and pressed garlic. Toss.
- Use in *Green Power Soup* recipe (*see* page 193)

NOTE: This is one of my favorite recipes, I could eat a ton of it and do! It's a good way to get greens into your diet. Check out the *Down Home Greens* recipe also (*see* page 204)

*This recipe also works well with red and green chard leaves, kale and beet tops. Wild leafy plants, such as leaf amaranth (callaloo) and lamb's-quarter, etc. can be chopped and mixed with the marinade for a delicious alternative to cultivated vegetables.

MASHED BUTTERNUT SQUASH

1 small to medium butternut squash
1-2 tbsp. olive oil (extra-virgin) and flaxseed oil mixed
1 lemon or lime, juiced
Nama Shoyu, to taste, or a sprinkle of Celtic sea salt

1) Wash the squash but do not peel. Cut off the stem and only take out the seeds if they are very large. Sometimes the squash has small immature seeds which can be left in for this dish. Slice the butternut squash very thin using a V-Slicer, SaladShooter® or similar piece of kitchen equipment.

2) Put into a bowl and toss with a marinade made of oil, lemon or lime juice and Nama Shoyu or Celtic sea salt. Toss well so that all the squash is coated. Cover and let marinate in the refrigerator overnight.

3) Next day, put the squash through the Champion or Green Power juicer with the blank (homogenizer) in place. If you want it smoother, put it through twice.

Serves 3-4. Keeps for 2-3 days in the refrigerator.

BEETS IN ORANGE VINAIGRETTE

3 cups grated beets
juice of 3-4 oranges
1 tsp. olive oil
1 tsp. thyme
dash of Celtic sea salt and freshly ground white
  pepper

1) Mix all ingredients together in a bowl.

Serves 4-6. Keeps for 3 days in the refrigerator.

CREAMED SPINACH

1 bunch spinach, chopped (approx. 4-5 cups)

1 medium tomato, quartered	**1 avocado**
1/2 cup shallot	**1 cup sprouted pine nuts**
(or 1/2 med. onion)	**1/2 lime, juiced**
1/4 cup fresh dill	**1 tbsp. Nama Shoyu**
(or 1 tsp. dried)	

1) Put all ingredients into a food processor and, using the "S" blade, process until smooth.

Serves 4. Keeps for 2 days in the refrigerator.

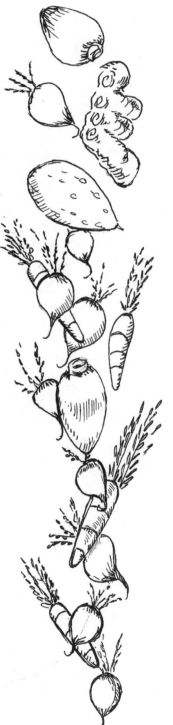

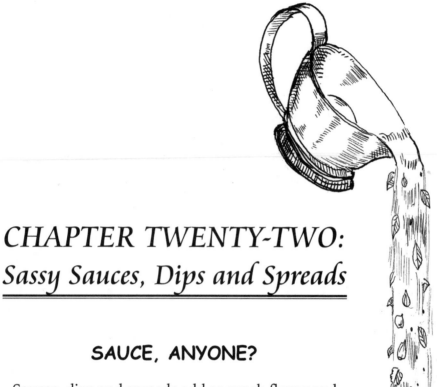

CHAPTER TWENTY-TWO:
Sassy Sauces, Dips and Spreads

SAUCE, ANYONE?

Sauces, dips and spreads add so much flavor and variety into your menus. You can never get bored. My *Honey of a Pistachio Spread* is divine on celery sticks.

Try a large plate of colorful, crunchy crudité with a tempting dip . . . Mmm good!

Or how about zucchini pasta with a freshly made pesto or marinara sauce?

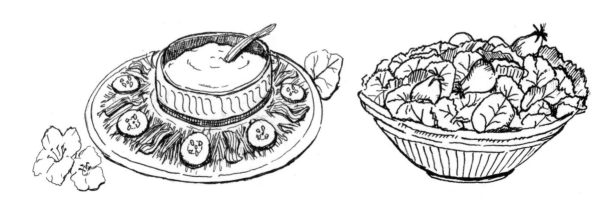

FRENCH LENTIL TAPENADE

1/2 cup sprouted French lentils
1/2 cup Nicoise or Kalamata olives (take the pits out
    and soak in distilled water overnight to remove
    most of the salt)
1 tbsp. capers (soak overnight in distilled water)
1 garlic clove
1/4 cup fresh parsley
1/2 lemon or lime, juiced
3 tbsp. olive oil (extra-virgin)

1) Drain the water out of the olives and capers and rinse well.

2) Put all the ingredients into a food processor and, using the "S"
    blade, process as fine as possible.

Makes about 1 cup. Keeps for 1 week.

NOTE: Good as a topping for raw crackers.

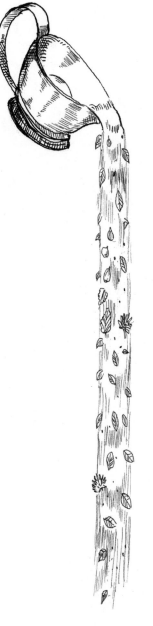

WALNUT PESTO

1/2 cup walnuts, soaked overnight (or for at least
    1 hour)
1 tbsp. pine nuts, soaked overnight (or for at least
    1 hour)
1 1/2 cups fresh basil leaves
1/2 cup spinach leaves
2 medium cloves garlic
1/4 cup olive oil (extra-virgin)
Celtic sea salt or Nama Shoyu, to taste
freshly ground white pepper, to taste

1) Place everything, except the oil and seasoning, in a food processor,
    and using the "S" blade, blend well. Then slowly add the oil through
    the food tube of the processor. Add Celtic sea salt (or Nama Shoyu)
    and white pepper to taste.

Yield: 1 cup. Keeps for up to 5 days in the refrigerator.

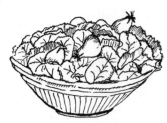

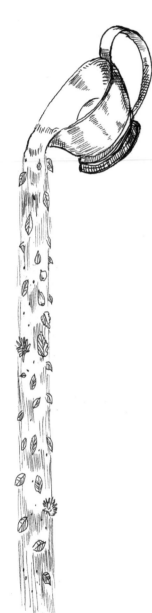

CHEDDA SAUCE

3/4 cup soaked pine nuts
1/2 cup soaked sunflower seeds
1 large red bell pepper, seeded
1/2 lemon, juiced
1 1/2 tbsp. nutritional yeast flakes (*see Glossary*)
1 small clove garlic, optional
2 tsp. Nama Shoyu

1) Soak the pine nuts overnight (or for at least 2 hours) in filtered water. Do the same with the sunflower seeds. (Or use sprouted nuts and seeds.)

2) Cut the red bell pepper into small pieces and put into the blender first. The bell pepper releases liquid so you won't have to add any water to the recipe. Rinse the soaked pine nuts and sunflower seeds and add to blender. Then add the other ingredients and blend well. If the red bell pepper doesn't liquefy readily, add a little water (not too much).

Yield: 1 1/4 cups. Keeps for 2-3 days in the refrigerator.

ALTERNATIVE: For those who don't appreciate the flavor of pine nuts, you can make the recipe with 1 cup of sprouted, blanched almonds, and reduce the sunflower seeds to 1/4 cup. Add in 1–2 tbsp. of soaked macadamia nuts, which makes the sauce creamier (optional). The rest of the ingredients remain the same.

SERVING SUGGESTIONS:

- Good as a sauce on finely chopped broccoli or Brussels sprouts (*see* page 137 for *Broccoli with Chedda Sauce*).

- Use as the filling for the *Chili Relleno* recipe (*see* page 152).

- **CHEDDA CHEEZ:**
  This sauce can also be made into a cheddar-type cheese by dehydrating it. Spread the sauce out 1/4" thick on a Teflex-lined dehydrator tray and dehydrate at 95° F for one to two days. The resulting sheet can then be cut into pieces or crumbled up with your hands and used like grated cheese. It will keep for more than 2 weeks in the refrigerator, but don't crumble yet—just break the sheets so you can fit them into a container for storage and cut or crumble them as needed.

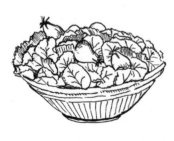

HUMMUS

2 cups sprouted chick-peas (garbanzos)
1/2 cup unhulled sesame seeds, soaked overnight
1 cup raw sesame tahini
2–3 lemons, juiced
2–3 garlic cloves
1 tbsp. olive oil (extra-virgin)
handful of parsley, minced
half a handful of mint, minced
dash of freshly ground white pepper (use a peppermill)
Nama Shoyu or Celtic sea salt, to taste

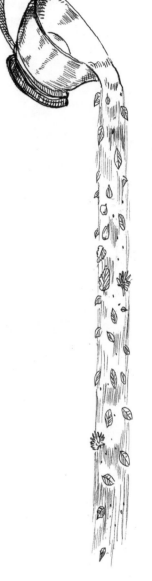

1) The success of this recipe depends upon the chick-peas being slightly fermented. So when you sprout them, let the process continue until the peas have a slightly fermented taste. This changes the flavor of the raw chick-peas to be more pleasing. It takes the edge off. (Sometimes the chick-peas will go bad before they ferment, so to avoid losing your chick-peas after they are sprouted, go to #2 below and note the **Exception**.)

2) Put the sprouted chick-peas into the food processor with the "S" blade and process about 15 seconds to break up the peas. Transfer the peas to a bowl and put in 1 tbsp. of olive oil, juice of 1 lemon and Nama Shoyu or Celtic sea salt. Toss well and let marinate in the refrigerator overnight. The marinade "cold cooks"* the chick-peas, further enhancing the flavor of your final dish.

   EXCEPTION: If the sprouted chick peas didn't taste like they were slightly fermented to you, then marinate by leaving them at room temperature for an additional 5-8 hours.

3) Next, put the drained sesame seeds, sesame tahini, garlic and the marinated chick-peas through the Champion or Green Power juicer** with the blank in place. For a smoother *Hummus*, put them through two times. Mix the resulting paté with the remaining lemon juice, and spices. Blend well by hand, adding a little water if necessary, to get the consistency you want.

   Yield: almost 3 cups. Keeps for 3-4 days in the refrigerator. Serve as a dip with crudité.

NOTE: If you like *Hummus* with a red bell pepper flavor, add up to 5 tbsp. *Red Bell Pepper Powder* (*see* page 290).

*No enzymes are lost and all the nutrients are enhanced by fermenting.

**If you don't have a Champion or Green Power juicer, you can make *Hummus* in a food processor by using the "S" blade, and adding a little water to blend as smooth as possible.

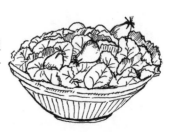

ITALIAN TOMATO SAUCE

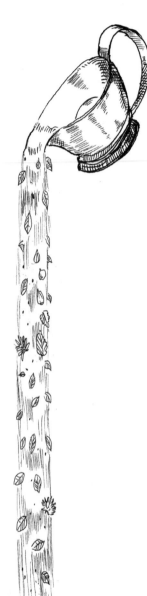

1 large tomato
1/2 onion
1–2 dried figs or dates, soaked 1 hour
1 additional tomato, blended (to soak sun-dried tomatoes)
1 cup sun-dried tomatoes, soaked 2 hours in the liquid from one blended tomato
3/4 cup basil
1/4–1/2 jalapeño pepper (or to taste), seeded
1 heaping tbsp. pine nuts (optional)
1 garlic clove
1/4 tsp. *Italian Seasoning*, (see page 292) or use store bought
dash olive oil (extra-virgin)
Celtic sea salt, to taste

1) After letting the sun-dried tomatoes soak for 2 hours, put all ingredients into a blender and blend well. (You could also soak the sun-dried tomatoes in filtered water instead of soaking them in blended fresh tomato. Drain the water first, before making the sauce.)

Makes a little over 8 oz. Keeps for 2 days in the refrigerator. After storage, stir well before using.

SERVING SUGGESTIONS: Use over *Pasta Loco* (*see* page 146), in *Chili non-Carne* (*see* page 152), or in *Luscious Lasagna Primavera* (*see* page 149).

SALSA VERDE

6 large tomatillos,* minced or diced small
1 med. green bell pepper, minced or diced small
1/2 cup minced onion
1 avocado, diced small
1–2 garlic cloves, minced or pressed
1 cup minced cilantro
Celtic sea salt, to taste

1) Prepare all the vegetables. Put into a bowl and toss together with a dash of Celtic sea salt.

Yield: 4 cups. Keeps for 2 days in the refrigerator.

*Tomatillos are the tomatoes commonly used in Mexico. They are small and green with a papery husk around them (*see* Glossary).

APRICOT BUTTER

1 1/2 cups dried apricots, soaked overnight
1/2 cup macadamia nuts, soaked overnight

1) In a food processor using the "S" blade, process the apricots and macadamias to a smooth butter.

Yield: 1 1/2 cups. Keeps for up to 1 week in the refrigerator.

SERVING SUGGESTIONS: Great as a topping for sliced apples, pears, jicama and chayote.

BUTTAH

1 cup olive oil (extra-virgin)
1/8–1/4 tsp. Celtic sea salt
1 tbsp. agar-agar flakes

1) Put ingredients into a blender and blend very well.
2) Pour the mixture into an ice cube tray, filling each cube only halfway, and freeze.
3) Every time you need a butter substitute, take out a cube and let it sit for a couple of minutes before serving.

SERVING SUGGESTION: Serve with *Essene Bread* (*see* page 257).

TAHINI/MISO DIP

1 orange, juiced
6 tbsp. raw sesame tahini
2 tsp. red miso
1 scallion, finely chopped

1) Put first three ingredients into a food processor, using the "S" blade. Transfer to a bowl and blend in the chopped scallion.

Makes 1 cup. Keeps for a week or more in the refrigerator.

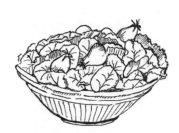

HONEY OF A PISTACHIO SPREAD

1 cup raw pistachios
1 tbsp. unheated honey
sprinkle of Celtic sea salt
squeeze of lemon (some people like it with lemon
and some without)

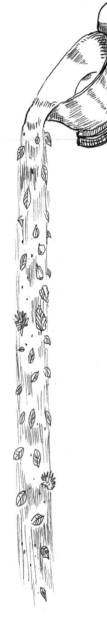

1) Put ingredients into a food processor & process using the "S" blade.
   Yield: 1 cup. Keeps for up to a week.

SERVING SUGGESTION: Spread on celery sticks and serve them as an appetizer. Mmmm good!

FILBERT SUN SAUCE

1/2 cup sprouted filberts
1/2 cup sprouted sunflower seeds
1 cup filtered water
1 lemon, juiced
2 soaked dates (soak in water until soft)
2 tsp. mellow white miso

1) Put all ingredients into a blender and blend until smooth.
   Yield: 2 1/4 cups.   Keeps for 2-3 days in the refrigerator.

MANGO SALSA CON CLASE

1 cup diced mango
1 large lemon or lime, juiced
1 small jalapeno, seeded and minced
2 tbsp. minced chives or scallions
1/8 tsp. Celtic sea salt
a pinch of habanero pepper powder or cayenne

1) Mix all ingredients together in a bowl.
   Yield: 1 cup. Keeps for 2 days in the refrigerator.

HERBED TOFU DIP

1 recipe *Creamy Tofu* (*see* page 230)
2 tbsp. olive oil (extra-virgin)
1/2 medium onion, chopped
1 garlic clove, pressed
2 tbsp. sesame tahini

1/4 cup finely cut cilantro
4–5 basil leaves, finely cut
1 tsp. Nama Shoyu

1) Put the *Creamy Tofu* into a bowl with all the other ingredients and, with a spoon, blend until smooth.

Yield: 2 cups. Keeps for 4-5 days in the refrigerator.

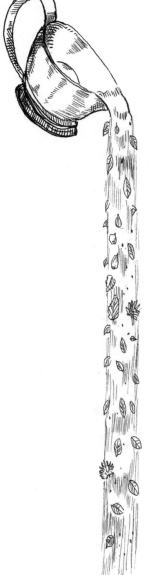

SUNFLOWER DIP

2 cups sprouted or soaked sunflower seeds
2–3 celery stalks, including leaves, chopped
1 tbsp. sesame tahini mixed with 1 oz. filtered water
3 garlic cloves
1 1/2 lemons, juiced
1 tsp. Dijon mustard
1 tbsp. chopped chives
1 diced tomato
1/2 tsp. *Vegetable Seasoning & Broth* (*see* page 291)
Nama Shoyu & Celtic sea salt, to taste

1) Blend all the ingredients, except the chives and tomato, very well in a food processor, utilizing the "S" blade.

2) Transfer to a bowl, add in the tomatoes and chives, mix and serve.

Yield: 2 cups. Keeps for 2 days, but best when freshly made.

DILL SAUCE

1 cup sprouted almonds, blanched (*see* Glossary)
2 tbsp. soaked or sprouted pine nuts
1/2 cup, or more, of filtered water
1 tbsp. olive oil (extra-virgin)
1 tbsp. finely chopped dill
1 tbsp. finely chopped chives
Celtic sea salt, to taste

1) Put almonds, pine nuts and water into a blender and blend until the nuts have a sauce consistency. Transfer to a bowl.

2) Add other ingredients, and mix with a wire whisk until blended.

Yield: 3/4 cup. Keeps for 3 days in the refrigerator.

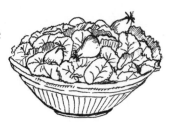

MARINARA SAUCE

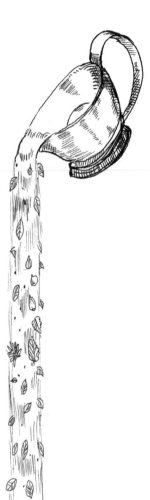

2 tomatoes, chopped
1 tsp. fresh oregano
1/4 cup soaked, sun-dried tomatoes
1/4 cup fresh basil
2 tsp. jalapeño pepper
1/2 cup soaked prunes, pitted
2 tsp. Nama Shoyu
1 cup diced mushrooms
2 tbsp. currants
1 tbsp. olive oil (extra-virgin)
2 tbsp. minced shallots
2–3 tbsp. apple cider vinegar
2 garlic cloves
1 tsp. slippery elm powder (look for it in an
   herb shop)

1) In a food processor, using the "S" blade, process all the ingredients, except mushrooms and shallots, to a creamy sauce.

2) Transfer to a bowl. Add in the mushrooms and shallots and stir. Serve over *Pasta Loco* (*see* page 146).

Yield: 2–3 cups. Keeps for 3 days in the refrigerator.

PRIMAVERA SAUCE

1 red bell pepper, diced small
1 green bell pepper, diced small
1 tomato, diced small
1/2 cup finely cut fresh basil
2 tbsp. dehydrated garlic granules
1/4 tsp. dried oregano
1/2 cup Kalamata or Greek black olives, desalted &
   finely cut (*see* Glossary for instructions on
   desalting)
1/2 cup olive oil, extra-virgin
dash of Celtic sea salt (opt.)

1) Mix all ingredients together in a bowl and mash a bit with a wire whisk.

Yield: 3 cups. Keeps for approximately 3 days in the refrigerator.

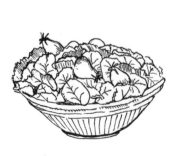

MACADAMIA CREAM

**2 cups macadamias,* soaked in filtered water for
  4 hours**
2 cups filtered water
1 tbsp. agar-agar flakes

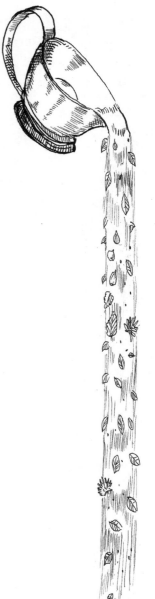

1) Drain and rinse the nuts. Blend the nuts with 2 cups of filtered water in a Vita-Mix—*see* Kitchen Equipment. (In a regular blender you can do it in two batches. You may have to blend longer, so the nuts break down to a fine cream.)

2) Take the blended cream and strain through a muslin cloth or bag. You should have approx. 20 oz. of liquid. Put the liquid back into the blender, add the agar-agar flakes and blend well. Pour into a wide-mouth glass jar and put into the refrigerator. In a few hours, the cream will have thickened and risen to the top of the jar. When ready to serve, spoon the cream off the top, as needed.

Yield: 12 oz. Keeps for 3 days in the refrigerator.

*Shelled macadamias go rancid very quickly. Sometimes they are already rancid when you buy them. Sunorganic Farm (*see* Source Index) sells fresh, organic macadamias which are excellent.

INDIAN SPICE SAUCE

1 cup mashed avocado
1 cup *Macadamia Cream* (see recipe above)
1/2 cup olive oil, extra-virgin
1 one-inch slice of ginger (or to taste)
1/2 jalapeño, minced
1 garlic clove, pressed
1 1/2 tbsp. *Indian Spice Seasoning* (see page 291)
1 tsp. ground cumin
Celtic sea salt and Nama Shoyu, to taste

1) Put all ingredients into a bowl, and with a wire whisk, mash and blend until a smooth sauce is produced.

Yield: 2 cups. Keeps for 2 days in the refrigerator.

SERVING SUGGESTIONS: Toss with *Pasta Loco* (*see* page 146) or mix into sprouted quinoa or amaranth.

CHAPTER TWENTY-THREE:
The Ancient Art of Culturing Foods

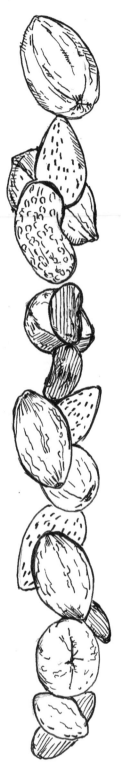

Cultured food is as old as the earliest civilizations, perhaps even older. In modern as well as ancient times, wine, beer, cheese and yogurt have been examples of cultured products. These days, however, our "modern" methods of producing these products have rendered them less than excellent for our health. The making of most wine and beer now involves chemicals to "speed" the fermentation process, and our yogurts and cheeses have been pasteurized, rendering them unsuitable for human consumption. Most cheese now is being made with genetically engineered enzymes,[1] such as Chymosin, Aspartic proteinase enzyme from R. miehei and others.

NUT AND SEED CHEESES, YOGURTS, NUT MILK, CREAM, KEFIR, ETC.

There are several categories of dairy-like products which can be made from nuts and seeds such as:

1) Yogurt

2) Yogurt Cheese (This is rich, like sour cream)

3) Seed (and Nut) Cheese

4) Nut and Seed Milks and Creams

5) Kefirs and Lassis

6) Mock Cheddars

7) Grated Parmesan Type Cheese

Following is a broad overview of preparation methods.

YOGURT

The yogurt you get from nuts and seeds is softer in texture than dairy yogurt. If you want it firmer, you must go a step further and make yogurt cheese. Basically, to make a yogurt: Put a combination of soaked and sprouted nuts and/or seeds that is pleasing in flavor in the blender with water or Rejuvelac (see page 227) and blend to a fine cream. Then strain the resulting liquid through an undyed cotton or muslin cloth (*see* "Clothcrafters, Inc." in the Source Index) to separate the pulp from the milk. The discarded pulp can be used to

---

[1]Genetic Engineering of foods aka Biotechnology (see Chapter 9).

make cookies. (Cheesecloth won't work for straining the liquid because the holes are too big, but I have seen occasionally, in the kitchen supply stores, a very tightly woven cheesecloth which would work.) Put the milk into a glass jar, cover with a dry cotton or muslin cloth or a clean lightweight kitchen towel and let sit at room temperature for approximately 8-12 hours. At the end of this time, the solids will have separated from the liquid whey, which will stay on the bottom of the jar. Put the yogurt into the refrigerator to solidify more. Serve by scooping out carefully from the top. Don't agitate the jar or you will mix the yogurt back in with the whey.

YOGURT CHEESE

Yogurt cheese is more like dairy yogurt in texture. You can make yogurt cheese from any of the yogurt recipes. Once the yogurt is made, separate the yogurt from the whey by making a hole at the top edge of the yogurt and gently pour out the whey. Then get a strainer with feet (supports) and set the strainer inside a glass bowl. Line the strainer with muslin cloth and pour the yogurt into the cloth. Fold the cloth closed over the yogurt and set the whole thing in the refrigerator overnight. This extra step drains more whey out of the yogurt. By the next day, you will have a rich, creamy yogurt cheese.

SEED (AND NUT) CHEESE

The first step in preparing seed (and nut) cheese and yogurt is the same; you blend soaked and sprouted nuts and/or seeds in the blender with water or *Rejuvelac*. It's what you do next that determines whether you produce a yogurt or a cheese. For cheese: Pour the blended liquid into a Cheese Bag (*see* Kitchen Equipment) and squeeze out a little of the liquid (the liquid you squeeze out is nut cream, which is delicious), then hang the bag over the sink or over a bowl and leave at room temperature for 8 to 12 hours. Additional liquid will drip out of the bag.

After the cheese is done, take it out of the bag and store it in a glass jar in the refrigerator. Seed cheeses have a unique flavor of their own, depending upon what combination of nuts and/or seeds you've used. And they can also be seasoned with minced vegetables and herbs.

The above is one method of preparing seed cheese. You can also make seed cheese in bowls and bottles.

NUT AND SEED MILKS

To make a nut and/or seed milk: Blend soaked and sprouted nuts and/or seeds with water or *Rejuvelac*, usually 3 1/2 to 6 cups of water per cup of nuts and 2 1/2 to 4 cups of water per cup of seeds, or anywhere in between for a combination of nuts and seeds. How much water you use is all a matter of personal taste. Once the nuts and seeds are blended well, strain them through a muslin or cotton cloth to separate the milk from the pulp.

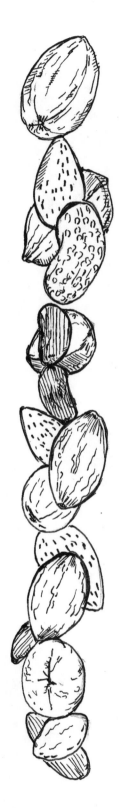

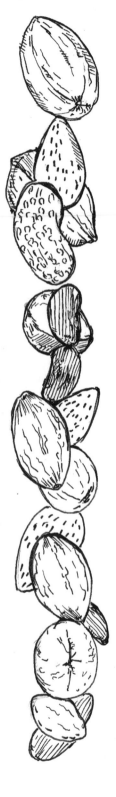

NUT AND SEED CREAMS

To make a nut and/or seed cream: Follow the same instructions used for the nut and seed milks, but use much less water, so you come out with a thick cream. Pine nuts, almonds or macadamias produce the best tasting creams.

KEFIR (usually pronounced Kee-fur)

Kefir is a fermented beverage made from either cow or goat milk using kefir grains as a starter. Its use dates back to ancient times and it is said to have originated in the Caucasus Mountains of the former Soviet Union. No one knows how the original kefir grains appeared, but back then kefir was fermented naturally in bags made of animal hides.

Kefir grains contain a complex mixture of both bacteria and yeasts. By mixing milk with active kefir cultures and allowing the milk to sit at room temperature, a delicious, naturally fermented drink is obtained. Originally it was made with raw milk. Unfortunately, today it is made from pasteurized milk. Scientists studying the live organisms found in kefir have reported the following potential benefits:

- It inhibits putrefactive and pathogenic microorganisms because of its huge quantity of lactic bacteria

- It is highly digestible, and its acidity and enzymes stimulate the digestion of other foods.

- It normalizes bowel function, restores the intestinal flora, assists in controlling harmful yeast overgrowth, and stimulates peristalsis and the production of digestive juices in the intestinal tract.

- It provides the body with easily assimilated proteins, minerals, vitamins, enzymes, beneficial live microorganisms and natural antibiotic-like substances

I called Lifeway Foods to find out if I could use the kefir culture (that they sell) with almond and other nut milks, instead of dairy milk, and was told that it was possible. So I started experimenting. I found that the procedure is very similar to that used in the making of nut and seed yogurts. The kefir product has a slightly more tart flavor. (*see Almond Kefir* recipe-page 222. Also, for a source of kefir grains, *see* "Kefir Culture" in the Source Index.)

LASSI

Traditionally, Lassi is a product made with soured milk. My recipe for *Lassi* (*see* page 246) consists of a beverage blended from a nut and/or seed yogurt with the whey added back in, and then flavored with fruits and spices.

MOCK CHEDDAR SAUCE AND CHEESE

This is an unfermented seed sauce blended with vegetables and nutritional yeast powder, which gives it a cheddar-like flavor. (*see* page 210 for *Chedda Sauce* and *Chedda Cheez*.)

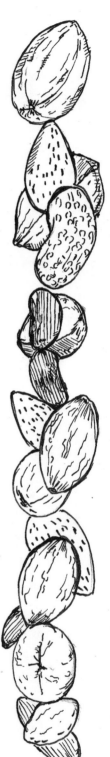

GRATED CHEDDAR AND PARMESAN TYPE CHEESE

1) Use the *Chedda Sauce* (page 210) recipe: Spread the sauce out on a dehydrator tray, lined with Teflex, and dehydrate. Then, crumble up the resultant "cheese".

2) *See Pine Nut Parmezan* or *Three Nut Parmezan* (page 226 or 231).These are made by soaking, sprouting, and then drying the nuts in the dehydrator. The dried nuts are then ground and stored in the refrigerator, to be used as needed.

SAUERKRAUTS, VEGGIE KRAUTS
AND FERMENTED VEGETABLES

Most of the recipes out there for making your own sauerkraut start out with, "Take six large cabbages and . . . " Well, that's as far as anyone gets, because who has such a large family nowadays that they would want to make six cabbages worth of sauerkraut!!? Also, a lot of the recipes called for pounding the cabbages, but that was before we had wonderful machines like the Champion and Green Power juicers which make the job a whole lot easier.

I've scaled my recipes down to "reality" size. Sauerkrauts and all fermented vegetables will keep for a couple of months in the refrigerator. There are hundreds of combinations you could try. In this section you'll find one of my favorites, *Hungarian Sauerkraut - see* page 228.

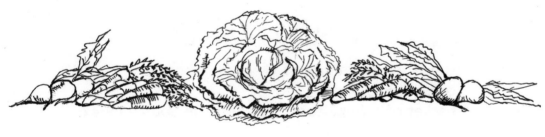

REJUVELAC
(Once Known as Poor Man's Beer)

Rejuvelac is a fermented beverage (non-alcoholic) which is super rich in enzymes, nutrients and other beneficial factors. It is made by putting sprouted grains into a quantity of filtered water and left to ferment for approximately 3-4 days at room temperature. (In a warm climate, it will probably take only 2 days.) *Rejuvelac* can be made with sprouted wheat, rye, barley, etc. or a combination. When fermented, it has a kind of tart, lemony flavor. For some people it may be an acquired taste.

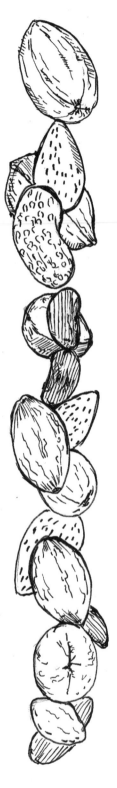

WALNUT-PINE YOGURT

2 cups walnuts, soaked overnight
1 cup pine nuts, soaked overnight
12 oz. filtered water (or *Rejuvelac* - *see* page 227)
additional filtered water for soaking

1) Soak the nuts overnight in filtered water.

2) Drain, rinse and drain the nuts again. Put all ingredients into a blender and blend well into a fine cream.

3) Pour the cream into a muslin bag and squeeze out all the liquid. (Save the pulp for another use.) Put the liquid into a wide-mouthed glass jar, cover with muslin or cheesecloth and let sit at room temperature for 8 hours.

   After 8 hours you will see the solids rise to the top and the liquid whey settles on the bottom. Sometimes with this yogurt (because of the walnuts), you get very little or no whey. Put the jar into the refrigerator and let the yogurt solidify more.

4) When ready to use, just spoon the yogurt off the top.

   Yield: 2 cups. Keeps for up to one week in the refrigerator.

SUGGESTION: Use this yogurt to make *Lassi* (*see* page 246).

ALMOND KEFIR

2 cups sprouted almonds
2 cups filtered water
1 packet of kefir culture (*see* "Kefir" in Source Index)

1) Put the sprouted almonds and filtered water into a blender and blend to a fine cream.

2) Pour the mixture through a muslin bag or cloth and squeeze out all of the liquid. (Save the pulp for *Mommy's Almond Cookie Surprise*, *see* page 260)

3) Pour the liquid back into the blender and put in the contents of one packet of Kefir culture. Blend well.

4) Pour the liquid into a wide-mouth glass jar, cover with a lightweight cotton cloth and let sit at room temperature for 6-8 hours. You can serve *Almond Kefir*, utilizing just the creamy part that rises to the top; or you can blend the mixture together and serve either plain or blended with fresh fruit or soaked dried fruit.

   Yield: more than 1 pint. Plain *Almond Kefir* keeps for up to 5 days in the refrigerator.

ALMOND YOGURT

2 cups sprouted almonds, blanched (*see* Glossary)
10 oz. filtered water (or *Rejuvelac* - *see* page 227)

1) Put the sprouted almonds into a blender with the water (or *Rejuvelac*) and blend to a fine cream.

2) Pour the cream into a muslin bag (*see* Source Index) and squeeze out all the liquid. You should have approx. 10 oz. Put this liquid into a wide-mouth glass jar, cover with muslin or cheesecloth and let it sit at room temperature for 8 hours. The yogurt will separate from the whey, which stays on the bottom of the jar.

3) When done, put the jar into the refrigerator and let the yogurt solidify more. To serve, scoop out the yogurt from the top CAREFULLY, so as not to mix it with the whey.

   Makes approximately 6 oz. of yogurt. Keeps for up to 5 days in the refrigerator.

NOTE: Save the leftover pulp to make *Mommy's Almond Cookie Surprise* (*see* page 260).

ALMOND SOUR CREAM

Double the ingredients in the *Almond Yogurt* recipe (see above) and take it one step further to make a rich and thick sour cream.

4 cups sprouted almonds, blanched
20 oz. filtered water (or *Rejuvelac* - *see* page 227)

1) Follow the recipe for *Almond Yogurt* (blend it in two batches, as it won't all fit in the blender). Once the yogurt is made, put it into the refrigerator for 3 hours to solidify more.

2) Set a double cheesecloth lined colander (use a colander with feet) into a bowl and carefully pour the *Almond Yogurt* through (discard the whey or save it for another use). Now you will have the almond solids sitting in the cheesecloth. Fold the cheesecloth over the almond cream (solids) and set the whole thing into the refrigerator overnight.

3) By morning, the yogurt will have released more liquid and solidified into a sour cream. Transfer the cream to a glass jar.

   Yield: 9 oz. Keeps for up to a week in the refrigerator.

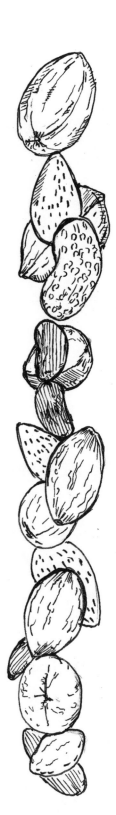

PINE NUT YOGURT

2 cups pine nuts
7-8 oz. filtered water (or *Rejuvelac* - *see* page 227)
additional filtered water for soaking

1) Soak pine nuts overnight in filtered water. Drain, rinse, and let sprout for 8 hours.

2) Rinse again. Put the nuts into a blender with 7-8 oz. filtered water or *Rejuvelac* and blend to a fine cream.

3) Pour the cream into a muslin bag and squeeze out all the liquid. There should be approx. 12 oz. of liquid. Put the liquid into a wide-mouth glass jar, cover with cheesecloth or muslin cloth, and let sit at room temperature for 8-12 hours (5-7 hours in hot weather). You will see the whey separate from the cream, which rises to the top.

4) When it is done, put into the refrigerator for about 3 hours, so the cream solidifies more. To serve, scoop out the yogurt carefully as needed from the top, leaving the whey on the bottom of the jar.

Yield: approx. 1 cup of a very rich and tasty yogurt. Keeps for up to 5 days in the refrigerator.

PINE NUT CHEESE

2 cups pine nuts
1/2 cup filtered water (or *Rejuvelac* - *see* page 227)
additional filtered water for soaking

1) Soak pine nuts overnight. Drain, rinse, and let sprout for 8 hours.

2) Rinse again and put into a blender with 1/2 cup of *Rejuvelac* or water. Blend to a fine cream.

3) Pour cream into a cheese bag (*see* Kitchen Equipment) and squeeze out a little of the liquid (about 3-4 ounces—this is *Pine Nut Cream*). Then hang the bag over the sink (or hang somewhere with a bowl underneath) and let drain and ferment at room temperature for 8 hours. If you leave it out longer, the cheese will develop a stronger flavor.

4) Transfer cheese to a glass storage jar and refrigerate.

Yield: approx. 1 1/2 cups. Keeps for up to a week in the refrigerator. Can be used as a good substitute for cream cheese once you get accustomed to the flavor.

ALMOND RICOTTA
with Veggie Chips
This Recipe Was Generously Shared by Elysa Markowitz, a Master Live-Food Chef and Hostess on TV of "Elysa's Raw & Wild Food Show"

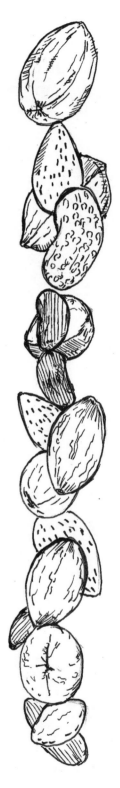

ALMOND RICOTTA: 2 cups almonds
2 cups purified water

VEGGIE CHIPS: 2 stalks celery
1/2 red bell pepper
2 slices purple cabbage

1) Soak almonds 12 hours, then blanch. (*See* "Almonds" in the Glossary for blanching instructions.)

2) In a blender: Blend blanched almonds with 2 cups water, pour into a pie plate and dehydrate at 105° F* for 6-8 hours—until "cream cheese" consistency.

3) **VEGGIE CHIPS:** Slice celery, bell pepper, and cabbage into chip shapes.

4) Serve "cheese" warm on a platter, surrounded by chips.

Yield: 4-6 servings. Keeps approx. 5 days in the refrigerator.

SUGGESTIONS:

• When blending the almonds with the water, you can spice them up with any one or a combination of the following: basil, dillweed, garlic, onions, or curry—but it tastes so fine plain, like ricotta cheese. Try variations and find your favorites. The thicker you make the *Almond Ricotta* (by using less water), the less time it takes to dehydrate.

• Try making *Luscious Lasagna Primavera* (*see* page 149).

*NOTES FROM RHIO:

The almond blend can also be dehydrated at 95° F and it works fine.

ALTERNATE WAY TO MAKE THE CHEESE WITHOUT USING THE DEHYDRATOR:

After blending the almonds and water, pour into a wide-mouth glass jar, cover with a cotton cloth (so it can breathe) and allow to sit at room temperature for approx. 15-20 hours. Then refrigerate.

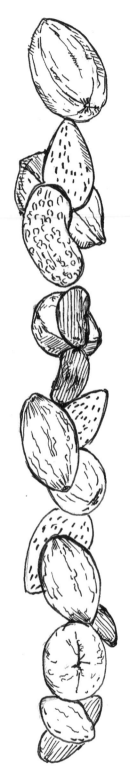

PINE NUT CREAM

1 1/2 cups sprouted pine nuts
3 oz. filtered water

1) Put the pine nuts and water into a blender and blend to a fine cream.
2) Pour the cream into a muslin bag and squeeze out all the liquid. Save the pulp for another use.

Yield: approx. 1 cup. Keeps for 1 day in the refrigerator.

CULTURED CREAM: Put it into a glass jar, cover with a clean tea towel and let sit at room temperature for 8 hours. Then refrigerate. Keeps for up to 5 days.

PINE NUT PARMEZAN

2 cups pine nuts

1) Soak the pine nuts in filtered water for 8 hours. Rinse, drain and sprout for 8 hours.
2) Rinse the pine nuts, then place on a mesh dehydrator tray and dehydrate at 95° F for 24 to 36 hours, or until thoroughly dry.
3) Grind the pine nuts in a coffee/nut mill. Store the *Parmezan* in the refrigerator.

Yield: a little more than 2 cups. Keeps for up to a month in the refrigerator.

ALPINE YOGURT

2 cups sprouted almonds, blanched (*see* Glossary)
3/4 cup sprouted pine nuts
3/4 cup sprouted sunflower seeds
1 3/4 cups filtered water (or *Rejuvelac - see page 227*)

1) Put all ingredients into a blender and blend to a fine cream.
2) Pour the cream into a muslin bag and squeeze out all the liquid.
3) Pour the liquid into a wide-mouth glass jar, cover with a tea towel and let sit at room temperature for 8-12 hours. You will see that the yogurt goes to the top and the whey settles on the bottom.
4) When done, put into the refrigerator to solidify more. Serve by scooping from the top.

Yield: approx 10 oz. Keeps up to 5 days in the refrigerator.

REJUVELAC

Rejuvelac is a beverage full of enzymes, friendly lactic acid bacteria (lactobacilli), aspergillus oryzae, B vitamins, vitamins E and K, proteins in the form of amino acids, carbohydrates (already broken down into the simple sugars, dextrines and saccharines) and minerals, among other good things. *Rejuvelac*, in olden times, used to be called "Poor Man's Beer" (non-alcoholic). *Rejuvelac* can also be used to help ferment seed cheeses and loaves, and to keep energy soups from oxidizing so they will last the whole day.

BASIC RECIPE

1/2 cup of sprouted grain
2 quarts of filtered or spring water

For the sprouted grain (*see* chapter on sprouting) you can use whatever combination tastes good to you. Try 1/2 cup of organic soft white wheat berries or 1/2 cup of rye and wheat combined or 1/2 cup of rye, or barley. Experiment and see what combination you can create to suit your taste. My favorite is 1/2 cup sprouted soft white wheat berries and 1/4 cup of sprouted rye.

METHOD #1

1) Take 1/2 to 3/4 cup of sprouted grain and put into a wide-mouthed, 2 quart mason jar, fill to the top with filtered water and cover with a cotton cloth (so it can breathe). Let sit at room temperature for approximately 3-4 days. In hot weather it may take 2-3 days. It is finished when it has a slightly lemony flavor.

2) Strain the *Rejuvelac* into another jar and refrigerate. Keeps in the refrigerator for up to 5 days.

3) To make more, you can re-use the same grain 2 more times. Just refill the original jar with water and grain and allow to ferment again. Usually, the *Rejuvelac* is ready much sooner the second and third time around.

METHOD #2

1) All the instructions are the same as in Method #1, but begin by putting 1/2 cup of sprouted grain into the blender with 1 cup of water and blend for a few seconds. This breaks up the grain a bit and helps start the fermentation process. It works especially well during the winter months in New York (and other cold climates) by helping the mixture to ferment more quickly. These blended grains can only be used once.

CAUTION: If the *Rejuvelac* has an off taste, throw it out and start again. This can happen occasionally if some of the wrong bacteria get in. Why? How? Sometimes the grain is old or moldy and you are not aware of it. Sometimes there may be contamination from something the sprouts have come in contact with. Sometimes the weather may be too humid. Don't despair, just try again and you will get the knack of it. Usually, if you start out with good, fresh grain seed, you won't have a problem. **Try to sample the flavor of a good *Rejuvelac*, so you have a basis for comparison when you make your own.**

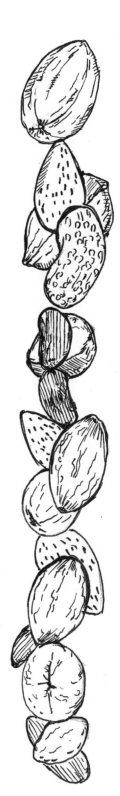

HUNGARIAN SAUERKRAUT

1 medium green cabbage
1/2 medium red cabbage
2 small muslin bags* with 2 tsp. caraway seeds
    in each
a few bay leaves
1/2 quince or 1 apple
small bunch of grapes or 1/2 cup raisins
1 tsp. Celtic sea salt

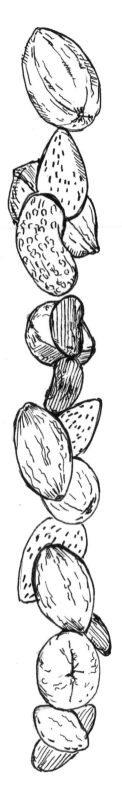

1) Peel the outer leaves from the cabbages and set them aside. You'll need about 5 or 6 large leaves.

2) Cut the green cabbage and put it through the Champion (or equivalent) juicer with the blank (homogenizer) in place. Cut the red cabbage and juice it, using the juice screen. Mix the red cabbage juice and the red cabbage pulp (left over from making the juice) together. Then with your hands, blend the two cabbage mixtures together and add in the Celtic sea salt (salt is optional). This method saves a whole lot of trouble. In the olden days, you would have had to grate and pound the cabbage to get it to mush up and release the juices. The Champion (or Green Power) juicer now does the same job easily.

   If you want more texture or crunch in your sauerkraut, grate or shred part of the cabbage (about two cups) and add it into the above mixture.

3) In a large glass bowl or crock, put in one layer of the cabbage mixture about 2 inches high. Slice the quince (or apple) into thin slices and lay a few pieces on top of the cabbage, add a few raisins (or mashed grapes), then place one of the bags with the caraway seeds on top, along with 3 bay leaves. Put another layer of cabbage on top and repeat the same thing (quince, grapes, caraway bag and bay leaves). Add a final layer of cabbage on top and then cover the mixture with the large cabbage leaves you saved in the beginning. Push the mixture down firmly to get rid of any air pockets. Put a cotton cloth over the cabbage leaves in the bowl.

4) Set this bowl into a larger bowl and then take a one gallon plastic water jug and fill with water, cap the top and set the jug on top of the cotton cloth. You need to have weight on top of the cabbage so that it will ferment properly. Put a cotton towel over the whole thing and set this out at room temperature for about 6 days (half as long in warmer weather), after which time you will have some wonderful sauerkraut. When it's ready, take the cabbage leaves off and discard. Also spoon off any dark or off-color spots or white scum that may be on top of the sauerkraut. This is a harmless yeast called kahm.

5) Put the sauerkraut (minus the quince, bay leaves and caraway bags) into a large glass jar and store in the refrigerator. This recipe makes over a quart, and it will keep for a couple of months in the refrigerator. To receive the

benefits of the live lactobacillus bacteria, consume the sauerkraut as soon as possible. After a short period of time the bacteria will die out. There are also other benefits from consuming sauerkraut (*see* below).

NOTE: When you have it available, try to have at least one tbsp. of this sauerkraut each day. It is wonderful and strengthening for the digestion, full of lactic acid (which regenerates the bowel flora), all kinds of enzymes, live lactobacillus bacteria, choline, acetylcholine, vitamin C, B-complex vitamins (including B12), and other good things. Unfortunately, the sauerkraut available at the supermarket is pasteurized, so it does not give you the same health-promoting benefits. There are a few companies who provide unpasteurized sauerkraut (Rejuvenative Foods is one brand), which can be found in the refrigerated section of some health food stores. Always read the labels carefully.

*Small muslin bags can be purchased by mail order from OrganzaBagg.com (*see* Source Index).

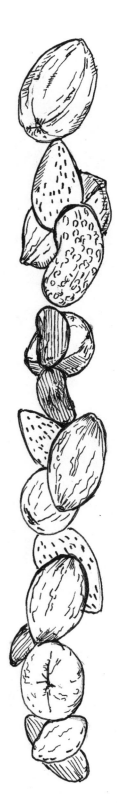

RICH YOGURT
"Rich" in Essential Fatty Acids

3/4 cup soaked walnuts
3/4 cup soaked pecans
3/4 cup sprouted and blanched almonds (*see* Glossary)
1/4 cup sprouted pine nuts
2 cups filtered water (or *Rejuvelac* - *see* page 227)
additional water for soaking

1) Soak the walnuts and pecans overnight. The almonds and pine nuts can be soaked overnight and then sprouted for one day.

2) Rinse all the nuts. Put into a blender with 2 cups filtered water or *Rejuvelac* and blend well into a fine cream.

3) Pour the cream into a muslin bag and squeeze out all the liquid. You should have about 20 oz. of liquid. Put the liquid into a wide-mouth glass jar, cover with muslin or cheesecloth and let sit at room temperature for 8 hours. After 8 hours you will see the solids rise to the top of the jar and the liquid whey settles to the bottom. Put the jar into the refrigerator and let the yogurt solidify more.

4) When ready to use, just spoon the yogurt carefully off the top.

Yield: 2 cups. Keeps for up to 5 days in the refrigerator.

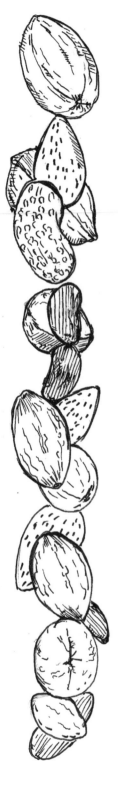

FLAXSEED "BUTTERMILK"

1 cup sprouted pine nuts (or soak overnight)
4 tbsp. flaxseeds (soak overnight in 4 oz. water)
filtered water
lemon juice, to taste

1) Soak the seeds and nuts (separately) overnight.

2) Next morning, put the soaked flaxseeds (which have now jelled) into the refrigerator to be used later.

3) Drain and rinse the pine nuts, put them into the blender with 4 oz. of water and blend to a fine cream. Pour the mixture through a muslin bag or cloth and squeeze out as much liquid as possible. Save the pulp for making *Pulp Gems* (*see* Recipe Index).

4) Put the pine nut liquid into a small glass jar, cover with a clean tea towel and let sit out at room temperature all day to ferment (approx. 8-12 hours or 5-7 hours in hot weather). You will end up with a pine nut yogurt which concentrates at the top of the jar, but instead of just using the creamy part, we are going to utilize the whey also. The whey is the liquid which settles on the bottom of the jar.

5) Put the pine nut yogurt, including the whey, into the blender, add in the flaxseeds that have soaked overnight along with 12 oz. filtered water and blend for 20 seconds. Then pour the mixture through a muslin bag or cloth and squeeze out all the liquid. Discard the pulp.

6) Flavor the "buttermilk" to your taste with a few drops of lemon juice.

   Yield: 1 pint. Keeps for more than a week in the refrigerator. After the third day, it becomes more tart, but not as tart as store bought dairy buttermilk. Shake well before using.

CREAMY TOFU

1 1/2 cups sprouted soybeans
1/2 tsp. Celtic sea salt

1) Put the soybeans through the Champion (or Green Power) juicer with the blank in place. Transfer to a small bowl, add Celtic sea salt and mix in by hand. Cover with a lightweight cotton tea towel and let sit at room temperature for 8 hours. Refrigerate.

SERVING SUGGESTIONS: Try making *Herbed Tofu Dip* (*see* page 215) or *Cheezy Tofu Dressing* (*see* page 186).

THREE NUT PARMEZAN

1 cup soaked macadamias   **1 cup soaked pine nuts**
1 cup soaked pistachios

1) Soak the nuts overnight. Rinse, drain and put into the dehydrator., set to 95° F, until thoroughly dry. This may take two or three days.

   Yield: 3 cups. Store in the refrigerator for up to a month.

BRAZIL SUN CHEESE

1/2 cup soaked Brazil nuts
1/2 cup soaked sunflower seeds
1/2 cup soaked pine nuts
1/2 cup soaked almonds, blanched
1 cup filtered water

1) Soak the nuts and seeds in filtered water overnight.

2) Drain and rinse the nuts and seeds. Put into a blender with 1 cup of filtered water and blend well to break the nuts down into a fine cream.

3) Pour into a cheese bag (*see* Kitchen Equipment) and squeeze out approx. 1 oz. of liquid. Then hang the cheese bag over a sink or bowl (additional liquid will drip out) and let ferment at room temperature for approx. 8 hours.

4) Transfer the *Brazil Sun Cheese* to a bowl, mix with the following seasonings and blend well.

   2 tbsp. minced scallions
   1/4 jalapeño, minced
   1 tbsp. minced dill
   1 tsp. olive oil (extra-virgin)
   Celtic sea salt, to taste

Yield: 1 pint. Keeps for up to 5 days in a covered container in the refrigerator

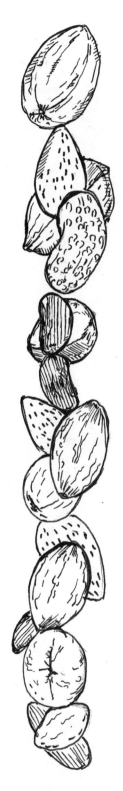

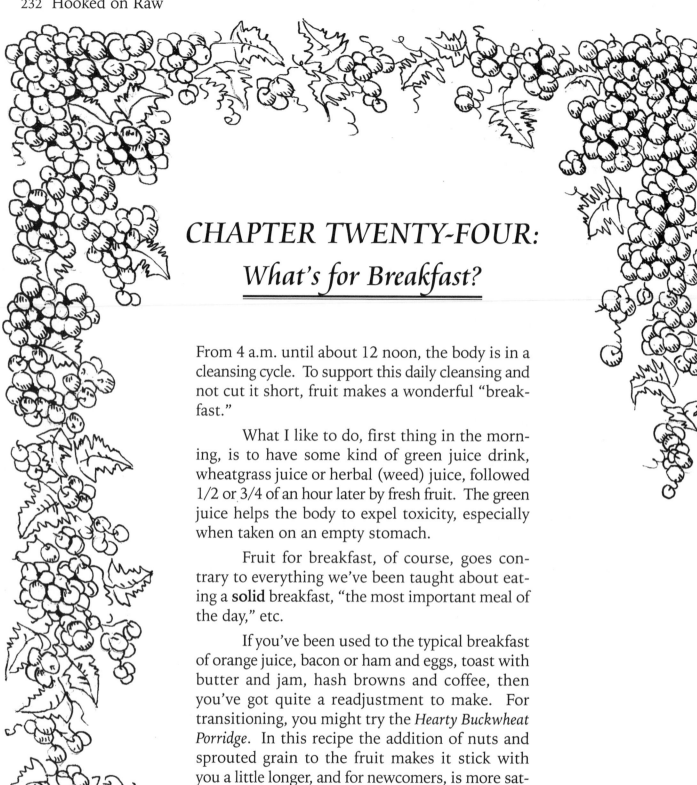

CHAPTER TWENTY-FOUR:
What's for Breakfast?

From 4 a.m. until about 12 noon, the body is in a cleansing cycle. To support this daily cleansing and not cut it short, fruit makes a wonderful "breakfast."

What I like to do, first thing in the morning, is to have some kind of green juice drink, wheatgrass juice or herbal (weed) juice, followed 1/2 or 3/4 of an hour later by fresh fruit. The green juice helps the body to expel toxicity, especially when taken on an empty stomach.

Fruit for breakfast, of course, goes contrary to everything we've been taught about eating a **solid** breakfast, "the most important meal of the day," etc.

If you've been used to the typical breakfast of orange juice, bacon or ham and eggs, toast with butter and jam, hash browns and coffee, then you've got quite a readjustment to make. For transitioning, you might try the *Hearty Buckwheat Porridge*. In this recipe the addition of nuts and sprouted grain to the fruit makes it stick with you a little longer, and for newcomers, is more satisfying.

For more ideas, *check* under Fruit Salads; also, Fruit Shakes and Smoothies.

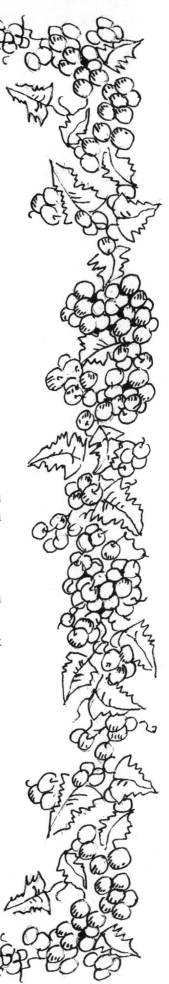

A "REGULAR" SHAKE

1 very ripe plantain (halfway to black skin)
8 soaked prunes, pitted (do not discard pits*)
3/4 cup nut or seed yogurt (use any of the
**   yogurt recipes)**

1) Put all ingredients into a blender and blend well.
   Serves 1 or 2.

WAKE-UP GRUEL

1 cup sunflower sprouts (or sunflower seeds—
**   soaked overnight)**
1/2 cup sprouted whole oats (or rolled oats—
**   soaked overnight)**
1/2 cup prunes (soaked overnight and pitted*)
2 oranges, juiced
1 tbsp. raw, unheated honey
squeeze of lemon

1) In a blender, blend the sunflower sprouts, oats, orange juice, lemon
   juice and honey. Then, add in the prunes and blend again. You can
   blend to either smooth or chunky.
   Serves 1-2.

NOTE: You could add sliced fruit (such as banana, mango or papaya) on
top.

*Chew a few of the seeds found inside the prune pits, along with the shake. Just crack
the pit lightly with a hammer, and out comes a delicious seed.

GREAT NUTS CEREAL

For each serving of Great Nuts Cereal:
**   1/2 cup *Buckies* (see page 256)**
**   1/2 banana**
**   1/2 cup cherries or other fruit**
**   1 heaping tbsp. raisins**
**   1 cup *Almond Milk* (*see* page 249)**
**   honey, to taste (optional)**

1) Combine all ingredients in a bowl, and dig in!

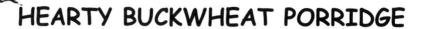

HEARTY BUCKWHEAT PORRIDGE

1/4–1/2 cup hulled raw buckwheat (see Glossary)
10–15 almonds, soaked overnight
1/4 cup raisins or currants, soaked overnight
1 banana (or 1/2 ripe plantain)
1 small mango (or other fruit, like papaya)
1/2 cup filtered water
additional filtered water for soaking

1) At night, soak 1/4 to 1/2 cup buckwheat in one cup of filtered water. Also soak almonds and raisins separately, using just enough water to cover.

2) In the morning, strain and rinse the buckwheat well. It will release a mucilaginous liquid, but keep rinsing until the water is clear. Drain and rinse the almonds. Strain the raisins through a colander, reserving the raisin water.

3) Heat up 1/2 cup filtered water on the stove only to the point where you can still put your finger in, and then turn off the flame. Pour the hot filtered water into the blender, add in the rest of the ingredients and blend to a cream. Thin out with some of the raisin soak water, if necessary.

Serves 1.

VARIATIONS:

- This recipe can also be made with hulled, sprouted buckwheat, which is the way I prefer, because sprouting increases the nutrient content.

- Use sprouted quinoa or amaranth instead of buckwheat.

MELON FRAPPÉ

1/2 cantaloupe,* honeydew, Persian, muskmelon, cran-
shaw or any other melon (or a combination)
1–2 tsp. raw honey (optional)

1) Cut the melon into chunks and put into the blender with honey (not necessary if melon is sweet) and a couple of ice cubes. Blend to a frappé.

Serves 1 or 2.

*Try to peel the cantaloupe very close to the skin. There is a green chlorophyll layer just under the skin of most cantaloupes and some other melons. Take advantage of this by including it for optimum nutrition. Save the seeds for *Melon Nectar* (see page 245).

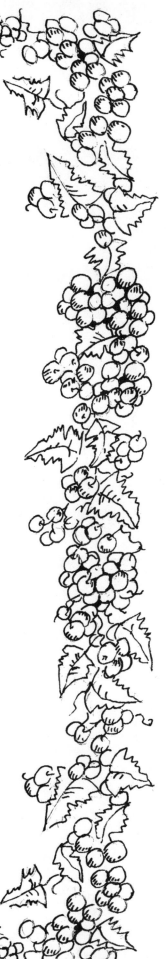

ORANGE-APRICOT MARMALADE

1 cup dried apricots, soaked overnight
2 small honey tangerines (peel and take the seeds out)
1 tbsp. tangerine peel, minced or grated
8 dates, pitted
1 1/2 tsp. psyllium seed powder
1 tsp. agar-agar flakes

1) Put all ingredients into a food processor with the "S" blade and blend well.

   Makes approx. 10 oz. Keeps for 2 weeks or longer in the refrigerator.

NOTE: Spread on *Brazil Nut Wafers* (*see* page 256).

ROSY ORANGE DAY

3 oranges
2 dates, soaked and mashed
1 tsp. rosewater* (edible)
1/2 tsp. cinnamon

Use only organic sweet oranges. Non-organic oranges may be too acidic—it's best to stay away from them.

1) Peel and slice the oranges into thin wheels. Put into a bowl.

2) Mash the soaked dates and mix with the rosewater and cinnamon. Toss the oranges gently with this aromatic mixture and then dig in.

   Serves 1-2. Use in the same day.

SERVING SUGGESTIONS:

- Serve as a light, refreshing, between-meal snack.
- It is also delicious when dehydrated at 95° F for 2 days.

*Available in some health food stores, or Indian grocery stores.

WATERMELON & FRAPPÉ

A delightful way to start the day is with watermelon. Just cut off a nice big chunk and enjoy! Or you could make a *Watermelon Frappé* by blending watermelon chunks and some ice together in a blender. Save the watermelon seeds for *Melon Nectar* (*see* page 245).

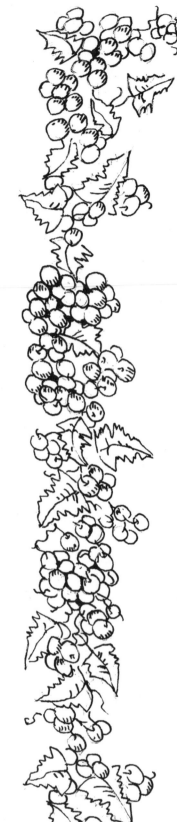

PEAR-PINE CANAPÉS

1 pear
few sprinkles of lemon juice
1 cup pineapple, finely chopped
1 oz. *Pine Nut Cheese* (*see* page 224)

1) Make *Pine Nut Cheese* a day ahead of time.

2) Finely mince the pineapple and mix with 1 oz. *Pine Nut Cheese*. Slice the pear and sprinkle lemon juice over the slices to prevent them from getting dark. Spread the pineapple mixture on top of each slice.

Serves 1.

NOTE: Peaches, nectarines or fresh apricots can be substituted for the pineapple.

SERVING SUGGESTIONS:

- Serve as hors d'oeuvres for parties or as a dessert.

- Dehydrate at 95° F for 24 hours and it will taste like cobbler.

CHEWY FRUIT & NUT CHEESE CREPES

1 recipe *Pear Fruit Roll* (*see* page 259)
1 portion of *Pine Nut Cheese* (*see* page 224)
1/2 pineapple, minced

1) Prepare the *Pear Fruit Roll* (a fruit leather) and the *Pine Nut Cheese*.

2) Cut the fruit leather into 2" by 3" strips. Spread 1 tsp. of *Pine Nut Cheese* over the leather, put 1 tsp. of minced pineapple on top and roll the fruit leather.

This makes a whole lot. But it does not keep well as the leather will become soggy from the juices in the fruit. Serve immediately.

VARIATION: Soak dried apricots or figs until soft. Then blend in the blender or food processor to a jam consistency. Use instead of the pineapple. Or use blended or mashed mango. Use your imagination!

POLLEN POWER

1 tbsp. pollen
2–3 tbsp. *Sprouted Sweet Brown Rice* (*see* page 153)
2 tsp. currants

1) Mix ingredients together in a small bowl.

Serves 1.

PANCAKES WITH FRUIT & CREAM
**You'll Have to Plan a Day or Two Ahead for This Breakfast,
But it's—Mmm, So Good!**

1 recipe *Brazil Nut Wafers* (check #1 below for
    slightly different instructions) (*see* page 256)
1 recipe *Almond Yogurt* or *Macadamia Cream* (*see*
    page 223 or 217)
1 recipe *Pancake Syrup* of your choice (*see* page
    273)
1 pint blueberries
1/4 cup soaked dates
strawberries, or mango

1) Make the batter for the *Brazil Nut Wafers*. When you pour it onto the Teflex-lined dehydrator trays—instead of making it into cookie shapes—spread it out bigger like pancakes. Do this by tilting the tray slightly, all the way around. (The batter will spread out.) It should make 9 pancakes.

2) Make the *Almond Yogurt* or *Macadamia Cream* and the *Pancake Syrup*.

BLUEBERRY JAM:

3) Put the blueberries and soaked dates into a blender and blend to a jam consistency. Set aside.

4) When you're ready to serve, layer onto a plate as follows:

    Pancake

    Blueberry jam

    Fresh sliced fruit (strawberries, mango, or your choice)

    Almond Yogurt or *Macadamia Cream*

    Pancake

    Blueberry jam

    Fresh sliced fruit, etc.

5) On the top layer, drizzle the *Pancake Syrup* that you prepared.

Serves 2. Serve immediately.

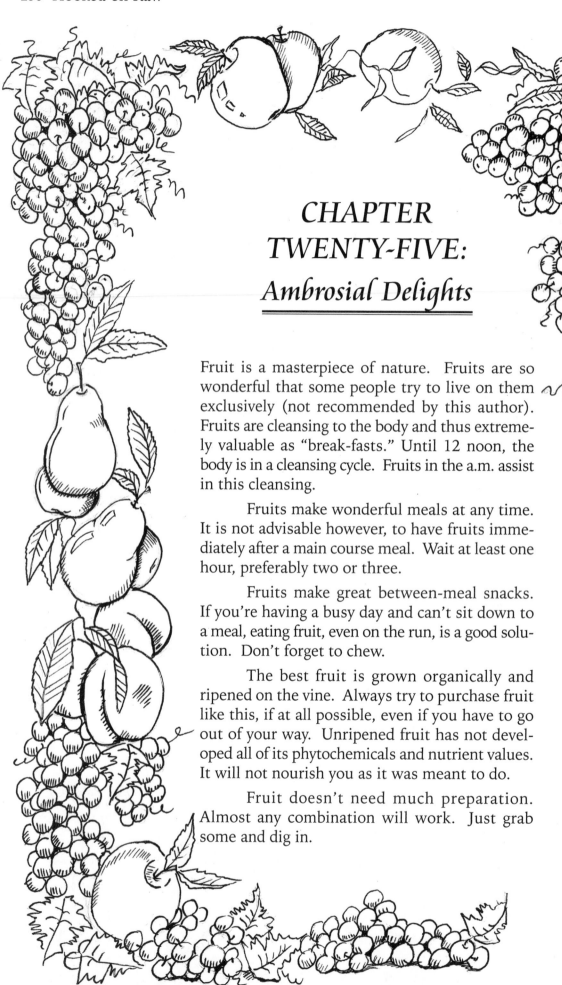

CHAPTER TWENTY-FIVE:
Ambrosial Delights

Fruit is a masterpiece of nature. Fruits are so wonderful that some people try to live on them exclusively (not recommended by this author). Fruits are cleansing to the body and thus extremely valuable as "break-fasts." Until 12 noon, the body is in a cleansing cycle. Fruits in the a.m. assist in this cleansing.

Fruits make wonderful meals at any time. It is not advisable however, to have fruits immediately after a main course meal. Wait at least one hour, preferably two or three.

Fruits make great between-meal snacks. If you're having a busy day and can't sit down to a meal, eating fruit, even on the run, is a good solution. Don't forget to chew.

The best fruit is grown organically and ripened on the vine. Always try to purchase fruit like this, if at all possible, even if you have to go out of your way. Unripened fruit has not developed all of its phytochemicals and nutrient values. It will not nourish you as it was meant to do.

Fruit doesn't need much preparation. Almost any combination will work. Just grab some and dig in.

AUTUMN SALAD
with Orange Bavarian Cream Sauce

1 apple, diced
1 pear, diced
small bunch of Concord grapes* (or other grapes)
squeeze of lemon

1) Dice the apple and pear and squeeze lemon juice over them.

2) Take the grapes off the stems. Mix fruits together gently and put on a plate.

ORANGE BAVARIAN CREAM SAUCE:

   4 oz. tangerine juice
   2 oz. pine nuts soaked
   2 dates, chopped
   1 tsp. agar-agar flakes
   1/2 tsp. fresh grated tangerine zest

3) Put all ingredients into a blender and blend well. Pour over the fruit.

   Serves 1. Best when eaten freshly made.

*Use Concord grapes when in season. They have a unique flavor, like no other.

FRUITS & ROOTS

   1 medium jicama
   1/2 mango, chopped small
   3 kiwi, chopped small
   2 oranges or tangerines, chopped small
   juice of 1/2 orange or tangerine
   1/3 cup currants

1) Peel the jicama and shred, using a mandolin or grater. Set aside in a large bowl.

2) Add the chopped fruit and currants to the bowl and toss with the orange or tangerine juice.

   Serves 3-4. Keeps for 2-3 days in the refrigerator.

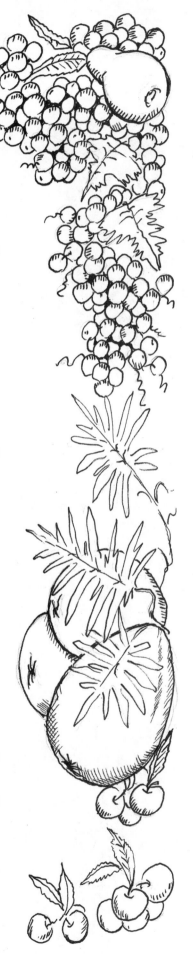

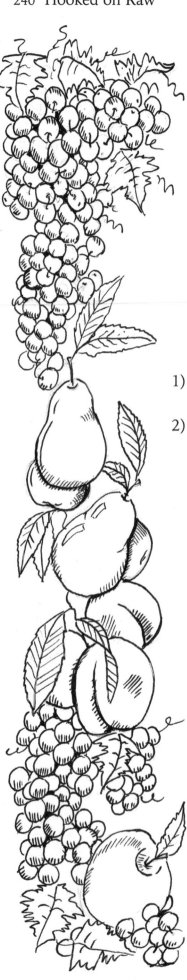

COOL & SPICY

1/2 cantaloupe or muskmelon, diced
1/2 Persian melon, diced
1 cucumber, sliced
1 tangerine, separate the sections—then chop
1 banana, sliced
1 cup tangerine juice
1/2 cup soaked dates
1/4–1/2 tsp. *Chat Masala* **(*see* page 292) or use**
store bought

1) Combine all the fruit, except tangerine juice and dates, in a bowl. Set aside.

2) In a blender, blend the tangerine juice, soaked dates and chat masala until creamy. Pour over the fruit and toss.

Serves 4. Best when eaten freshly prepared.

UNSTEWED FRUIT

4 sweet, ripe apricots   **1/2 pint blueberries**
4 ripe plums   **1/2 pint raspberries**
1 ripe plantain, sliced   **1/2 pint blackberries**
1/2 avocado   **1 pint strawberries**
1/2 cup dates, pitted   **1/2 pineapple, diced**
3/4 cup dried apricots,   **1 cup tangerine**
soaked   **juice**

1) Remove the pits from the apricots, plums and avocado. Chop, and put into a large bowl. Add in sliced plantain and strawberries, diced pineapple and berries.

2) Combine the dates, dried apricots and tangerine juice together in a blender, and purée.

3) Pour the purée over the fruit and gently toss.

Serves 8. Keeps for 2 days in the refrigerator.

MELON AMBROSIA

1 cantaloupe
1 honeydew melon
1/4 watermelon
1 Mexican papaya
1 cup pitted cherries

1) Cut the cantaloupe and honeydew in half and scoop out the seeds. Save them for *Melon Nectar* (*see* page 245). With a melon baller, carve out all the melons and the papaya. Mix in a serving bowl with the pitted cherries.

Serves 2-4. Best when eaten freshly made.

APPLE-WALNUT SALAD

2 apples, grated
1/2–3/4 cup soaked walnuts, chopped a little
1/2 cup soaked raisins
1/4–1/2 lemon, juiced
1 orange, juiced

1) Grate the apples, peel and all. Sprinkle the grated apples with lemon juice and toss. This helps prevent oxidation. Chew at least some of the apple seeds for complete nutrition.

2) Combine first three ingredients in a bowl, pour in the orange juice and toss the salad.

Serves 1-2. Serve immediately.

FRUIT & NUT SAUCES

If you want to dress up plain fruit or fruit salads with some delicious sauces, try the following recipes:

Apricot Butter (page 213)
Carob (the Un-Chocolate) Sauce (page 283)
Coconut Cream (page 276)
Creme Brulée (page 284)

Filbert Sun Sauce (page 214)
Mango Salsa con Clase (page 214)
No-Maple Syrup (page 273)
Orange Date Syrup (page 273)

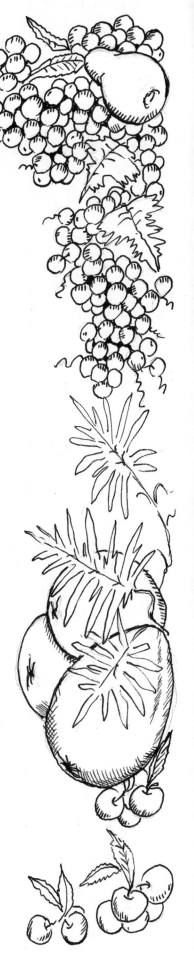

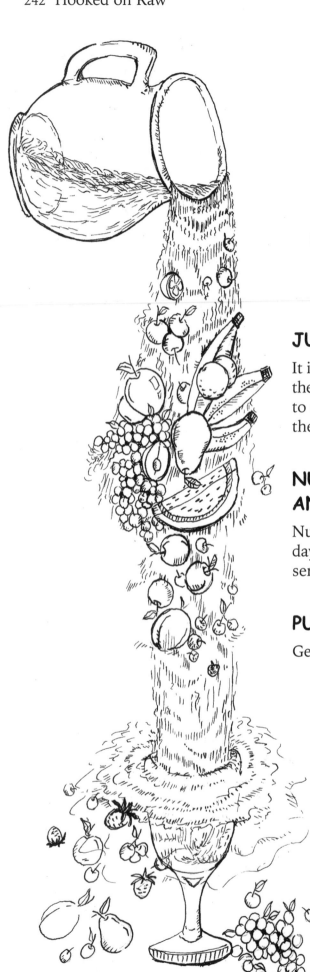

CHAPTER TWENTY-SIX:
Nectars of Life

JUICES AND SMOOTHIES

It is best to consume juices and smoothies right after they are freshly made. Do not keep juice from one day to another. If you want to take it to work with you, then put the juice into a glass-lined thermos.

NUT MILKS, SEED MILKS AND CREAMS

Nut and seed milks and creams generally last a few days. Store in the refrigerator and shake well before serving.

PUNCH

Generally keeps for 2 to 3 days in the refrigerator.

CABBAGE-TOMATO DELIGHT

1 thick slice or chunk of green cabbage
1 thick slice or chunk of red cabbage
1 large tomato
1 lemon, peeled (leave as much of the white pith on as
**   possible)**
dash of Celtic sea salt (optional)

1) Put all ingredients through a juicer. A dash of Celtic sea salt can be added, if desired.

    Serves 1.

CARROT WALLOP

3 carrots
1 fennel stalk
1 apple
4-inch piece of daikon radish
2-inch piece of burdock root
1/2 lemon

1) Juice everything and serve.

    Serves 1.

JICAMA, BEET & PEAR JUICE

1 small yellow beet (if you can't find yellow, use red)
1/4 jicama, peeled
1 pear

1) Scrub the beet and cut out any blemished parts but don't peel. Peel the jicama.

2) Put all ingredients through a juicer.

    Serves 1.

NOTE: This combination of ingredients also makes an excellent quick salad. Chop the vegetables and fruit into a small or medium dice.

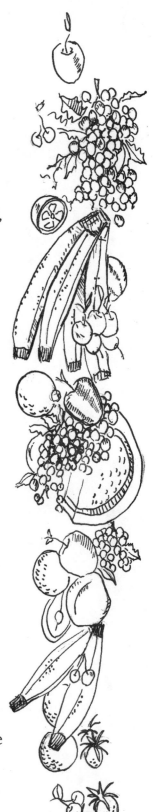

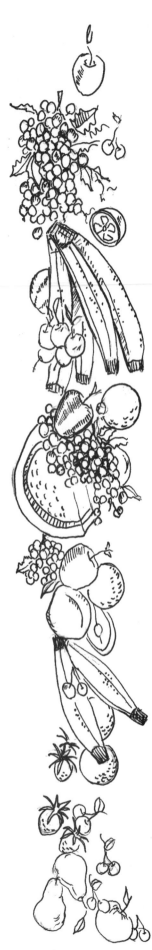

BURDOCK ROOT TONIC
Blood Purifier

1/2 cup carrot juice
1/2 cup sweet potato or yam juice
3-inch piece of burdock root, juiced

1) Scrub the burdock root with a vegetable brush, but don't peel. Do the same with the carrots and sweet potatoes. Only remove parts which look blemished.

2) Prepare 1/2 cup carrot juice and 1/2 cup of sweet potato juice and mix with the burdock juice. You could add a little nut milk or nut cream, if you have it available.

Serves 1.

DR. KIRSCHNER'S GREEN DRINK
In an Out of Print Book by Dr. Kirschner, I Found This Wonderful Recipe, which I've Modified a Little

1 pineapple, juiced
15 almonds, soaked and sprouted
4 dates, soaked and pitted
2 heaping tbsp. of sprouted sunflower seeds
1–2 large handfuls (or more) of green leaves (see below)
1/2 tsp. kelp powder

1) Juice 1 pineapple, then put into the blender with all the other ingredients and blend well.

Makes approximately 1 quart of a delicious and nutritious drink. Best consumed the same day.

NOTE: The green leaves can be one or a combination of watercress, parsley, spinach, arugula, carrot tops, beet tops, etc. or you can use edible weeds if you can get them. Dr. Kirschner had his own garden of wild edible weeds, such as lamb's quarters, purslane, comfrey, chickweed, filaree, malva, dandelion, etc.

VARIATION: This drink can also be made with just the pineapple juice blended with the green leaves.

MELON NECTAR

seeds from 1 cantaloupe or honeydew melon*
8 oz. fresh orange juice
1/2 to 3/4 cup filtered water
raw honey to taste (optional)

1) Cut 1 melon in half and scoop out the seeds. Save the melon for another use. Rinse the seeds, removing the pulpy mass in which they are embedded. Put the melon seeds into the blender with water and blend well. Then put the mixture through a colander. This gives you melon seed milk. (Discard the ground-up husks.)

2) Mix the seed milk with the orange juice, honey, 1 or 2 ice cubes and blend in the blender.

Makes 1 or 2 servings. Use the same day.

ALTERNATE VERSION: In the blender, blend seeds from 1 melon with 1 1/2 cups filtered water. Strain the mixture through a colander. Put the seed milk back into the blender with 1/2 tsp. *Vanilla Powder* (*see* Glossary) and honey to taste. Blend.

*NOTE: If you want to save seeds from melons to make the *Nectar* at another time, rinse them well, removing them from the pulpy mass in which they are embedded. Drain and store in the refrigerator. Keeps for up to 1 week. (If you don't remove the pulpy mass, they will ferment.)

CARROT-APPLE ZINGER

2 large carrots
1 apple
1 medium beet
1 one-inch slice of fresh ginger

1) Put all ingredients through a juicer.

Serves 1.

GRAPEFRUIT-PRUNE JUICE

1 cup grapefruit juice
6 prunes, soaked overnight

1) Put fresh grapefruit juice into the blender, add pitted prunes and blend well. Serves 1.

NOTE: This is an unlikely combination, but it tastes good and is very moving!!!

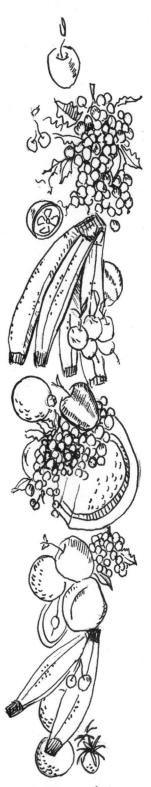

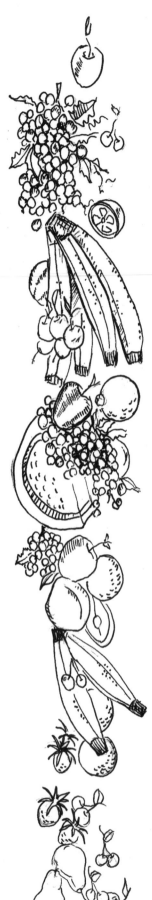

PLAZMA
Electrolyte-Charged Water

1 or 2 green water coconuts

These coconuts are much bigger than the little brown coconuts that most of us are familiar with. They are green or sometimes yellow on the outside, and have a wonderful and refreshing water inside of them. They are much consumed on the islands where they grow. In Puerto Rico these coconuts are swiftly cut open with a machete. But machetes create a dilemma for most of us, because we were never trained in their use. And because we fear using the machete, we end up not utilizing this wonderful water.

An easier and safer way to open cocos at home is to slice off a chunk of the husk on one side (not the end) with a large sharp knife. Then cut a hole through the skin and pour out the water. **Caution:** This only works with young and fresh coconuts. When the coconuts are old, you cannot slice into them because the husks become tough, begin to petrify, and then become hard as a rock.

Coconut water is a most refreshing drink. *Plazma!* In many parts of the world it is known for its healing properties, especially for the kidneys

NOTE: Sometimes these coconuts have a custard-like coconut meat inside. In order to get to this, you have to whack the coconut in half with a machete (only suggested for those who know how to use it).

ALTERNATIVE: 1 or 2 *light* brown coconuts

These coconuts are a lighter brown color than the dark brown ones we usually see in the markets. The light brown ones are younger coconuts. On one side of the coconut you will find three "eyes." One of these eyes is soft. With a flathead screwdriver, punch through the soft eye, widen the hole a little bit and then pour out the water (sometimes called juice or milk).

LASSI

1 cup *Walnut Pine Yogurt*, including the whey (*see page 222*)
1/2 pint strawberries
1 banana
6 dates

1) Blend all the ingredients in a blender.
   Serves 1. Enjoy!

NOTE: You could use other combinations of fruit. Experiment.

RHIO'S HOT DRINK

   2 tomatoes
   1 cucumber
   1 green bell pepper
   1 red bell pepper
   1 small onion
   1/2 lemon, juiced
   1/4 fresh jalapeño pepper, seeded (or to taste . . . start
      out with less)
   1–3 tsp. olive oil and flaxseed oil (mixed)

1) Put all ingredients, except the oil, through a juicer. Then add the oil and stir. Or for a thicker drink, blend everything in a blender.

   Serves 1.

NOTE: This is a good aid for losing weight if you have it as your dinner.

GO-GO GOUTWEED

If You Can Get A Hold of Some Goutweed, This Drink Gives a Lot of Energy

Goutweed is a wild, edible plant with distinctive green leaves and an unmistakable aroma. If you live in New York City, Wildman Steve Brill (*see* Source Index), a naturalist who leads walks in the parks to teach people how to identify wild plants that are good for eating, can show you where to find some goutweed. Every area of the country has people who are knowledgeable about wild, edible plants and are willing to pass this valuable information along to newcomers.

Using *Rhio's Hot Drink* recipe (see above), eliminate the jalapeño pepper and blend in a handful or two of goutweed.

POTASSIUM DRINK

   3–4 large carrots
   3 stalks celery
   1 cucumber
   large handful parsley
   large handful spinach

1) Wash the vegetables but don't peel. Use a vegetable brush on the carrots. Try to get unwaxed cucumbers.

2) Put all ingredients through a juicer.

   Serves 1.

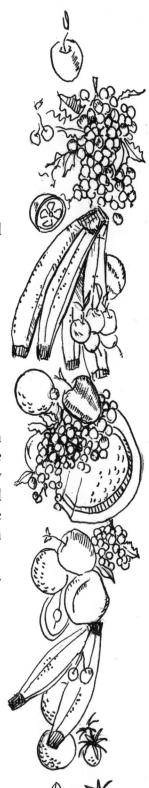

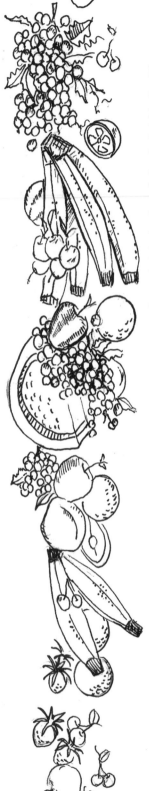

WHEATGRASS JUICE

fresh wheatgrass (*see* Glossary)

1) In a wheatgrass juicer, juice up some wheatgrass. Start with small quantities of juice until you get used to it. One-half to 1 ounce is good to start and then, according to your needs, you could build up to 3 to 4 oz.

NOTE: Wheatgrass juice is not my favorite; and I've never been able to actually like the flavor. But I do drink it—for its good effects—first thing in the morning on an empty stomach and then it's over with for the day. Wait at least 1/2 to 3/4 of an hour before having breakfast. I suggest you do a course of three to four weeks in which you drink wheatgrass juice every day on an empty stomach. Then leave off for three weeks. Then do another course. This is for maintenance. During the three weeks off, I would substitute another juice first thing in the morning, usually a green drink. If I can get a hold of some wild edible weeds, I juice them instead.

If you are trying to re-establish good health, then I suggest you drink wheatgrass juice more regularly (more than once a day), until you see results.

TIP: Some people can down it easier with a little ginger juice added.

FENNELICIOUS

1 carrot
1 green apple
1 thick slice of Mexican papaya or 1/2 of a
    Hawaiian papaya
1 stalk fennel
1/2 lime

1) Juice everything and enjoy.

    Serves 1.

ORANGE JULIETTA

6 oranges
3–6 dates
1/2–3/4 cup walnuts, soaked overnight (or at least
    2 hours)
1/4 tsp. *Vanilla Powder* (*see* Glossary) or cut a 2-inch
    piece of vanilla bean into tiny pieces

1) Put all ingredients into a blender with a few ice cubes and blend until smooth and frothy.

    Serve immediately. Serves 1-2.

ALMOND MILK

1 cup sprouted almonds, blanched (*see* Glossary)
3 1/2 cups filtered water

1) Process almonds in the blender with 1/2 to 1 cup of water until well blended, then add balance of water and blend again.

2) Pour into a cotton or muslin bag or cloth and squeeze out all the milk. This is simple, plain almond milk. This milk can be enjoyed as is or flavored in various ways (*see* suggestions below).

   Yield: almost a quart. Keeps for up to 5 days in the refrigerator. The *Sweet Almond Milk* (*see* below) keeps 1–2 days. After storage, the milk separates—so shake well before using. Save the leftover almond pulp to make *Mommy's Almond Cookie Surprise* (*see* page 260).

SWEET ALMOND MILK

1) Take plain almond milk, put into a blender with soaked dates and a little ground vanilla bean (*see* Glossary) and blend well. Make with as many or as few dates as you like. Some people like it sweet and others prefer just a hint of sweetness.

   You can also try adding freshly ground lemon rind, pumpkin pie spice, nutmeg or cinnamon, or a combination. With experimentation you will hit upon a flavor combination which will taste delicious to you.

CREAMY OAT MILK

For Those Who Shy Away From Almond Milk Because They Think it Has Too Much Fat—This is The Answer!

1 1/2 cups sprouted oats
2–2 1/2 cups filtered water or coconut water

1) Put the oats and water into a blender and blend very well.

2) Pour the liquid through a cotton or muslin bag and squeeze out all the milk.

3) You could flavor this milk like the *Sweet Almond Milk* recipe (*see* above), but I kind of like it plain.

   Makes over a pint. Keeps for 3 days in the refrigerator. Shake well before using.

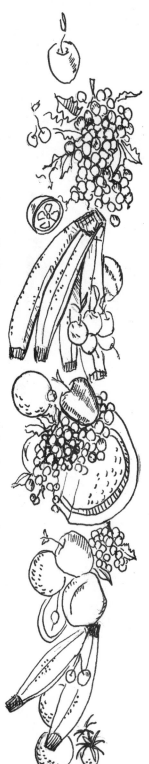

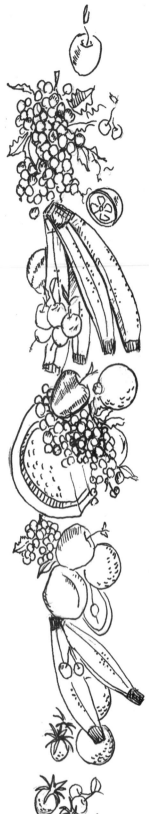

CONCORD SANGRIA

4 lbs. Concord grapes (or other grapes in season)
2 quarts filtered water
1–2 heaping tbsp. of dried hibiscus flowers
1 tangerine, diced
1 nectarine, diced
1 peach, diced
2 apricots, diced
1/2 cup diced pineapple
1/2 pint strawberries, diced
1/2 pint blueberries

1) Fill a 2 quart jar with filtered water and add in 1 or 2 heaping tablespoons of dried hibiscus flowers.* Let sit at room temperature for approx. 3 hours or until the water turns a wonderful shade of pink. Then strain the flowers out.

2) Juice the 4 lbs. of Concord grapes. Transfer to a punch bowl, adding in the hibiscus tea.

3) Add all the fruit. Let chill before serving.

Serves 2-4. Keeps for 2 days in the refrigerator..

*Sunorganic Farm offers organically grown hibiscus flowers. (*See* Source Index.)

RED CHARD STEM JUICE
(This Tastes Better Than it Sounds)

red chard stems (leftover from making marinated red chard ribbons—*see* recipe for *Marinated Collard Ribbons,* page 206)
handful of parsley
2 stalks celery

1) Put all ingredients through a juicer.

Makes 2 servings of 1/2 cup each.

NOTE: This is energizing to have first thing in the morning on an empty stomach. It has a mildly salty flavor.

HIBISCUS PUNCH

Hibiscus is a flower which is dried and much used in Mexico as a refreshing beverage. This punch could be the original Kool-Aid. If kids ask for Kool-Aid, try giving them this instead.

FOR 2 QUARTS OF PUNCH:

> **1 1/2 quarts of filtered water**
> **1/4 cup dried hibiscus flowers**
> **1 pint of mixed fresh fruit juices (try 1 cup of a mixture**
> **of orange and tangerine juice with a squeeze of lime,**
> **and 1 cup of pineapple juice)**
> **3 tbsp. raw honey or to taste**
> **garnish with a few grapes**

1) Put the dried hibiscus flowers into 1 1/2 quarts of filtered water, stir and let sit at room temperature overnight or for at least 3 hours. The water will become a beautiful shade of pink.

2) Drain the flowers and discard. Transfer the hibiscus water to a punch bowl, add the other ingredients and blend well. Refrigerate until cold.

3) When ready to serve, float grapes in the punch bowl. Serve with a slice of tangerine on the rim of each glass.

   If you want a gallon, double the recipe. Keeps for 3 to 4 days in the refrigerator.

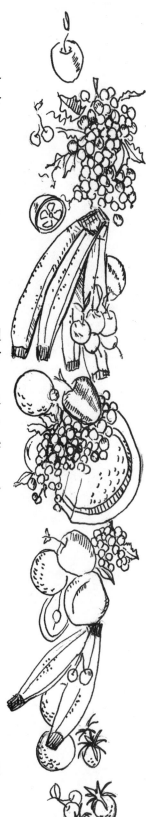

CHIA LIMEADE

A Delicious Surprise!

> **3 cups filtered water**
> **1 lime, juiced**
> **2 oz. mild flavored raw honey (or more, to taste)**
> **2 tbsp. chia seeds (*see* Glossary)**

1) Put the water, lime juice and honey into a blender and blend well.

2) Then pour into a quart jar, add the chia seeds, put the top on the jar and shake well. Let cool in the refrigerator for an hour before serving.

   Makes 1 quart. Keeps for 2 days in the refrigerator.

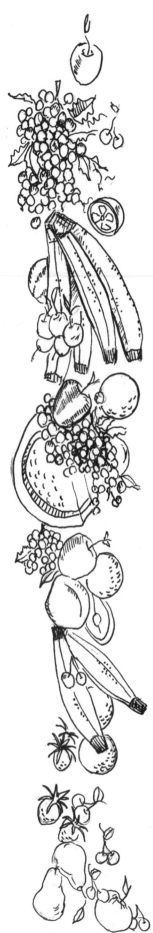

PUMPKIN SEED SHAKE

2 apples
2 stalks celery
small bunch of grapes
1 lemon, peeled but including the white pith
small piece of lemon peel (undyed)
1/4 cup pumpkin seeds, soaked
1 banana

1) Juice the apples, celery, lemon and grapes.
2) Put the juices into the blender and blend with pumpkin seeds, small piece of lemon peel and banana.

Serves 2.

GREEN DRINKS

Green drinks are used at the raw/live food institutes lavishly to optimize regeneration and rejuvenation. The following are just samples; create your own out of a variety of green leaves and vegetables. Put all ingredients into the blender and blend well, adding water only if necessary. Alternately, juice in a juicer.

1 cucumber
1 small tomato (optional, but adds flavor)
1–2 handfuls buckwheat lettuce
1–2 handfuls sunflower greens
handful dill
handful parsley
1 chard leaf (cut out the rib)

2 stalks celery
1 cucumber
1 small tomato (optional, but mellows the flavor)
1 garlic clove
2 handfuls wild greens
lemon, to taste (optional)

1 cucumber
1 small tomato (optional, but adds flavor)
1–2 handfuls buckwheat lettuce
1–2 handfuls sunflower greens
1 green onion
2 heaping tbsp. *Hungarian Sauerkraut (see page 228)*

1 cucumber
1 box of a mixture of spicy sprouts
1 small tomato
1/2 lemon (optional)
1 garlic clove
pinch of cayenne

DR. SCHULZE'S SUPER-TONIC

fresh hot chili peppers, including cayenne
raw, unpasteurized apple cider vinegar
fresh ginger   **fresh garlic**
fresh onion   **fresh horseradish**

1) Fill a blender 3/4 full with equal amounts of coarsely chopped chili peppers, ginger, onion, garlic and horseradish. There is no need to peel the vegetables or to remove seeds from the chili peppers. Pour in apple cider vinegar to cover.

2) Blend on high speed until "applesauce" consistency.

3) For maximum potency make the tonic on the day of the new moon and let sit either at room temperature or in the refrigerator for 14 days, until the full moon. (Of course, you don't have to wait 14 days to drink or eat some.)

4) This tonic can be consumed either as a beverage or as a sauce. The sauce is ready once it is blended. To make a beverage, put some sauce through a colander, discarding the pulp.

Dr. Schulze says you can store the tonic at room temperature or in the refrigerator. It lasts a long time and gets better with age. In the *Save Your Life Videos* (*see* Source Index), Dr. Schulze states that this tonic is good for the common cold and flu, and even for serious problems like heart disease and cancer. He recommends 10-15 spoonfuls a day. The tonic kills germs, boosts circulation and builds up strength.

SERVING SUGGESTION: Goes well with any dish for which you would like a little hot sauce.

WHOLESOME TODDY

1–2 heaping tbsp. *Dr. Schulze's Super-Tonic* (*see* above)
1–2 garlic cloves, pressed
2 heaping tbsp. *Vegetable Seasoning & Broth* (*see* page 291)
1–2 tbsp. minced Greek, sun-dried black olives, desalted (*see* Glossary)
16 oz. filtered water
1/4 tsp. flaxseed oil
1 tsp. Nama Shoyu

1) Put all ingredients except water into a large mug. Heat up the water (don't boil) and pour over the ingredients. Stir, and enjoy.

Serves 1.

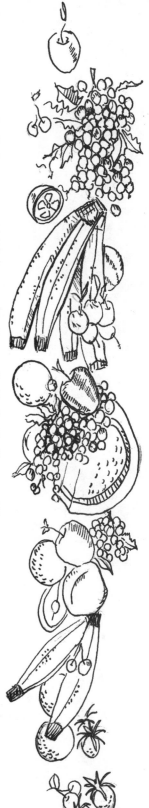

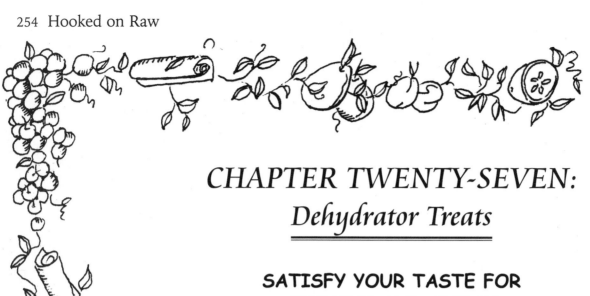

CHAPTER TWENTY-SEVEN:
Dehydrator Treats

SATISFY YOUR TASTE FOR CRUNCHY AND CHEWY

Some of the recipes in this section satisfy our desire to eat something crunchy—like chips or crackers—and chewy—like cookies and fruit leathers.

I dehydrate most foods at 95° F (to be on the safe side), in case the equipment is not calibrated just right. It takes slightly longer, but I feel better about it. At 105° F, some foods start losing enzymes, and at 118° F, the life force is mostly extinguished.

You cannot go wrong making fruit leathers. Almost any combination of fruits will come out good, when liquefied in a blender. Taste it, and if it tastes good in its liquid form, it will taste good as a leather. Sometimes, but not always, you might need to make it sweeter than you think it should be, because it may lose a little sweetness after dehydration. Whole fruits, on the other hand, when sliced and dehydrated, concentrate their sweetness, i.e., they get sweeter. Fruit Leather is a wonderful, natural snack for children and they love it. It contains high fruit sugar, yes, but with all the other natural, intrinsic factors that keep sugar working **for you** instead of against you.

Fruit leathers can be stored at room temperature. I roll them, put them into a cotton cloth or bag, and then store them in a covered container.

When storing dehydrated crackers or chips at room temperature, make sure they are thoroughly dry or they may get moldy. After you remove them from the dehydrator, to allow for condensation, let the crackers or chips sit a while to cool down, before storing in a cookie jar.

Any foods which are moist, like dehydrated veggie burgers, must be stored in the refrigerator.

Dehydrated foods are an excellent choice when traveling, or going on camping trips. The dehydration of fruits and vegetables for winter use is an ancient method of food preservation. If you have extra fruits and veg-

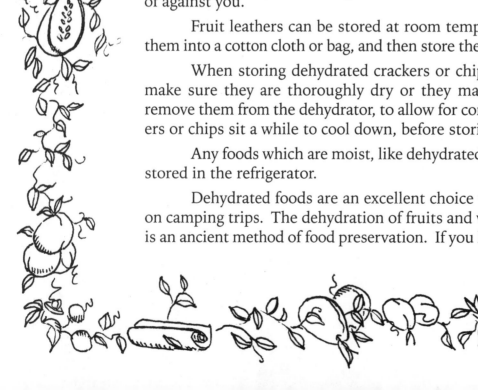

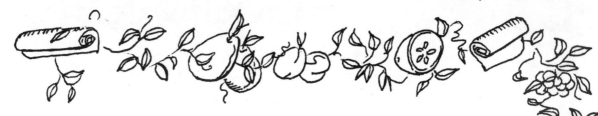

etables from your garden that you're not going to eat promptly, utilize your dehydrator to preserve them.

Unless you have a source for low-heat dried fruits, it's best to dry your own. If you do purchase them, however, check your sources carefully and ask, "At what temperature was this fruit dried?" Other questions to ask are: "Was this fruit fumigated?" and, "Was this fruit processed with any additives or did it go through any treatments before or after being dehydrated?"

Two mail order catalog companies that offer some **sun-dried** fruit are Sunorganic Farm and the Living Tree Community (*Check* Source Index).

Lora Lee of Sunorganic Farm told me she "refrigerates, not fumigates," to prevent insect damage.

At home, I dry most of my fruits and vegetables at 95-100° F.

SPROUTED PEA CHIPS

2 cups sprouted whole peas
2 cups carrots (cut into chunks to measure)
1/2 medium red onion
1/3 cup Kalamata olives, desalted (*see* Glossary)
1/2 cup raw sesame tahini
1 tsp. mellow white miso
1/2 tsp. Celtic sea salt

1) Put the carrots and sprouted peas through the Champion (or equivalent) juicer, with the blank in place.

2) Mince the red onion and Kalamata olives, and add them into the pea mixture, along with the sesame tahini and Celtic sea salt. Mix well. (It doesn't taste too good at this point, but once it's dehydrated, it takes on a different flavor.)

3) Spread the mixture onto a dehydrator tray lined with Teflex. Spread it out about 1/4-inch thick with the back of a large spoon. Dehydrate at 95° F for approx. 20 hours. Once dry, break it apart into chips. For more chips, double or quadruple the recipe. Keeps for 2 weeks in a cookie jar.

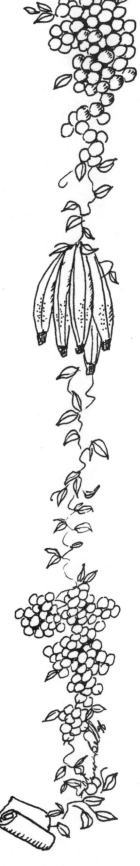

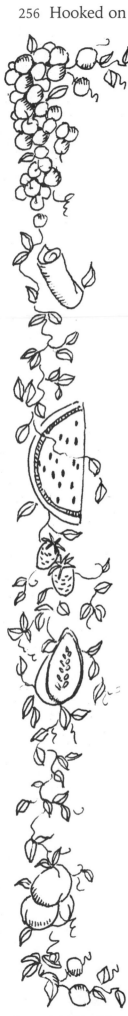

BRAZIL NUT WAFERS

2 cups Brazil nuts, soaked overnight
3 bananas (or 2 ripe plantains)
cinnamon
***Rejuvelac*, mild (see page 227) or filtered water**

1) Rinse and drain Brazil nuts. Put Brazil nuts in the blender with just enough *Rejuvelac* or water to cover. Blend, adding more liquid if necessary, until you have a smooth batter. Don't make too thin. Then blend in bananas, adding cinnamon to taste.

2) Pour the batter, in the shape of round cookies, onto dehydrator trays lined with Teflex sheets (*see* Glossary). Dehydrate at 95° F for 1 or 2 days.

   Yield: 18 wafers. Don't worry about storage—they'll be gone fast!

BUCKIES

1 quart sprouted buckwheat

1) Spread the sprouted buckwheat onto mesh dehydrator trays and dehydrate for approx. 4 hours at 95° F.

   Store the thoroughly dried *Buckies* in a covered container at room temperature.

SERVING SUGGESTIONS:

- Use in *Great Nuts Cereal* (*see* page 233).
- Add into soups or salads—for crunch.

MACAROON CHEWS

2 cups coconut pulp (left over from making *Coconut Cream* - *see* page 276)
10 large dates, pitted and cut in half
2 cups of filtered water
sprinkle of *Vanilla Powder* (*see* Glossary)

1) Put the coconut pulp, dates and *Vanilla Powder* into the blender with the water and blend well.

2) Spoon onto dehydrator trays (lined with Teflex), in the shape of round cookies and with the back of a spoon, flatten to approx. 1/4" thickness. Dehydrate at 100° F for approx. 24-36 hours.

   Makes 18 large chews or 36 small ones. Leigh says this tastes like the baked macaroons that are sold in the stores, except of course, they have no wheat or additives and were dehydrated instead of cooked.

ESSENE BREADS

SOUR DOUGH RYE BREAD:

    4 cups sprouted rye
    2 cups sprouted sunflower seeds
    2 1/2 tsp. dill seeds
    2 1/2 tsp. caraway seeds
    1/2 tsp. Celtic sea salt

1) Put all ingredients through a Champion or Green Power juicer with the blank (homogenizer) in place.

2) You will now have a pliable bread dough. With your hands, knead the dough for a couple of minutes to blend all the ingredients evenly.

3) Form the dough into a round ball and then flatten it to approx. 1 1/2 inches high, keeping the edges even. Place the loaf on a mesh dehydrator tray and dehydrate at 95° F for approx. 20–24 hours. The outside will be crusty and the inside moist. Store in a covered container in the refrigerator.

Serve with *Buttah* (*see* page 213) or *French Lentil Tapenade* (*see* page 209).

RAISIN SWEET BREAD:

    3 cups sprouted barley
    1 cup almonds, blanched (*see* Glossary)
    1 cup sprouted sunflower seeds
    1 med. mango, seeded and diced
    1 tbsp. olive oil (extra-virgin)
    1 1/2 cups raisins, soaked for 10 minutes

1) Put barley, almonds and sunflower seeds through the Champion or Green Power juicer, with the blank screen in place. Transfer to a bowl and add in the other ingredients, mixing well.

2) Divide the dough into 2. When shaping each portion into a loaf, first place the dough onto a Teflex-lined dehydrator tray and then shape the loaf there. If you shape the loaf on your work counter and then try to transfer the loaf, it will be too moist to lift and place onto the tray, without breaking apart.

Dehydrate for approx. 24-36 hours. Store in a covered container in the refrigerator. Serve with *Apricot Butter* (*see* page 213).

Yield: 2 loaves. *Essene Breads* keep for approx. 1 1/2 to 2 weeks in the refrigerator.

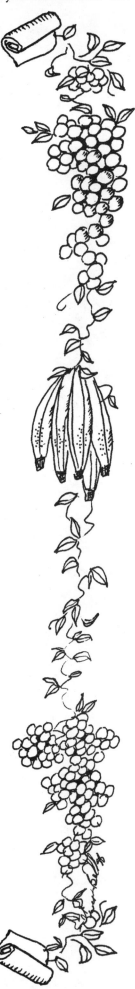

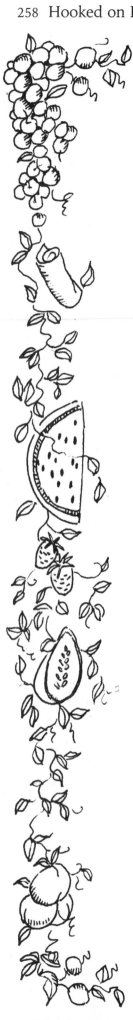

BLUEBERRY MUFFINS

2 cups soaked and/or sprouted barley   2-4 tbsp. honey
1 1/2 cups soaked Brazil nuts   2 tsp. cinnamon
1/4 cup golden flaxseed, ground   1 tbsp. extra-virgin olive oil
2 cups Hunza raisins, soaked and strained
(this will swell so you will have more than 2 cups)
2 fresh dates (or 4 dried, soaked)
1/2 vanilla bean, ground (approx. 1/2 tsp.)

1) Put the first 3 ingredients into a food processor with the "S" blade and blend as finely as possible. You might have to do this in batches. Transfer to a bowl.

2) Put dates, 2 cups of the raisins, honey, olive oil, cinnamon, and vanilla bean into the food processor and using the "S" blade, blend very well. Add to the bowl. Also add in 1/2 cup raisins (soaked, whole, unblended) and mix everything very well by hand.

3) Put the blueberries into the food processor and utilizing the "S" blade, pulse chop to break them up a little bit. Add them to the ingredients in the bowl and mix well.

4) Form into round flat muffins approx. 1/2" high (not your traditionally shaped muffins) and place on Teflex-lined trays and dehydrate at 100° F for 24 hours, or until muffin consistency. Half-way through, turn the muffins onto mesh screen.

Yield: 20 muffins. Keeps in covered container in the refrigerator for 2 weeks or more.

RYE PRETZELS

4 cups sprouted rye   1 tbsp. onion powder
1 tsp. Celtic sea salt   2 cups sprouted sunflower
1/2 cup soaked or sprouted   seeds
   caraway seeds

1) Measure all ingredients into a bowl and with a large spoon mix them.

2) Feed the ingredients through a Green Power juicer utilizing the pretzel making attachment.* As the dough comes out of the machine, it will be in the shape of a long, continuous breadstick. Place this dough gently on a table. Then you can cut it into breadsticks, or you can braid two of them together or create other interesting pretzel shapes. Place the *Pretzels* onto a mesh dehydrator tray and dehydrate at 95° F for 24 to 48 hours.

Yield: 14 braided *Pretzels*. When thoroughly dried, they can be stored at room temperature. The *Pretzels* can also be dehydrated to the chewy stage. These must be stored in the refrigerator.

*If you don't have the Green Power juicer, you can make the dough in a Champion juicer with the blank in place and then shape the dough by hand into pretzel shapes.

PEAR FRUIT ROLL
A Fruit Leather

3 pears, coarsely chopped
2 apples, coarsely chopped
3–6 dates, pitted
1/4 tsp. cinnamon
1/8 tsp. nutmeg
1/2 tsp. *Vanilla Powder* or 1-inch piece of vanilla bean, cut
into tiny pieces (*check* the Glossary for *Vanilla Powder*)

1) Purée pears and apples (with seeds and skin—do not peel) in blender, adding a little water only if necessary. Add the next four ingredients and blend well.

2) Pour onto dehydrator trays, lined with Teflex (*see* Glossary). With the back of a large spoon spread out to 1/8" to 1/4" thickness. Dehydrate for approx. 12 to 15 hours at 95° F, or until the fruit peels away from the Teflex sheet easily. This is fruit leather. Makes 2 sheets approx. 12" x 12".

3) With a sharp knife cut leather into 2" x 3" wide pieces. Then roll pieces.

NOTE: This recipe can be used as the basis for *Chewy Fruit & Nutcheese Crepes* (*see* page 236).

PRUNE-BANANA LEATHER

1 1/4 cups soaked, pitted prunes (include a couple of prune pit seeds,* if available, after discarding the hard shell)
1/4 cup soakwater
2 bananas
1–2 tbsp. lemon juice

1) Put ingredients into a blender and blend well.

2) Pour onto a Teflex-lined dehydrator tray and, with the back of a large spoon, spread out to 1/8" to 1/4" thickness. Dehydrate at 95° F for approx. 15-20 hours or until the leather peels away from the Teflex sheet easily.

Makes one 12" x 12" fruit leather.

*Prune pit seeds are delicious. I always feel cheated when I buy already pitted prunes. Try to get prunes with the pits, then tap the pit lightly with a hammer and inside you will find a delightfully flavored seed.

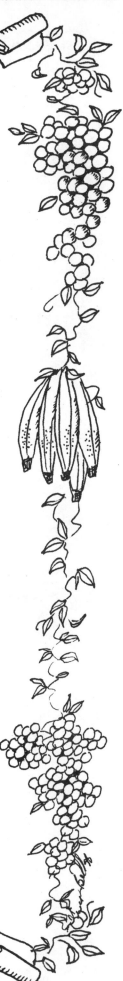

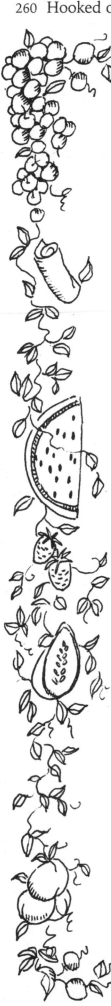

MOMMY'S ALMOND COOKIE SURPRISE

**2 cups almond pulp (left over from making *Almond Milk*
   or *Yogurt*)**
1/2 cup sprouted almonds,* blanched (*see* Glossary)
1 cup raisins, soaked
1/2 cup dried papaya, rehydrated and chopped
1/2 tsp. *Vanilla Powder* (*see* Glossary)
2 tbsp. raw, unheated honey (*see* Glossary)

1) Soak the raisins overnight (preferably), or at least 3 hours, in just enough water to cover. (When they plump up they are easier to blend.)

2) Drain the raisins and save the soak water. Put all the ingredients, except the papaya and 1/4 of the raisins, into a food processor and using the "S" blade, blend to smooth, adding some of the raisin soak water, if necessary. Transfer to a bowl, add in the whole raisins and papaya and mix well.

3) Form into cookie shapes and dehydrate at 95° F for approximately 24 to 48 hours, until chewy or crispy.

   Yield: approximately 26 cookies. Store in a covered container in the refrigerator.

*A small amount of **whole** almonds are added to impart flavor and nutriment. Don't forget that the almond pulp (when making milk or yogurt) has been squeezed of practically all of its essence.

PLANTAIN CHIPS

1) Take any amount of ripe plantains,* peel and cut diagonally into thin slices. (Just cut down on an angle to create oblong slices.) Lay the slices on a mesh dehydrator tray and dehydrate at 95° F for 24 hours.

NOTE: These are wonderful! Serve as an accompaniment to any Latin style dish, or as a snack. If you dehydrate them longer, they become crispy. At the 24-hour stage, they are chewy.

*For ripe plantains—wait until the skin gives a little when you push with your finger. The skin will be from halfway to almost all black. At that point, the starch, which is hard to digest, will have turned to sugar, which is easy to digest.

CHIA CRISPS

Chia is a Thirsty Little Seed and Very Economical Too.
1 Cup of Chia Seed Makes 57 Cookie Size Crisps

1 cup chia seed*
2 cups pear or apple juice (or a combination)
3 cups filtered water
1 tsp. pumpkin pie spice
sprinkle of extra cinnamon
a few edible flowers

1) Put the chia seeds into a deep bowl. Pour the water, juice and spice over the seeds and stir until most of the lumps are out. Cover and let sit in the refrigerator overnight. The chia seeds will soak up the liquid and become a gelatinous mixture.

2) With a tablespoon, spoon the mixture onto dehydrator trays, lined with Teflex, and flatten into round cookie shapes. You can coax the mix into shape with the back of the tablespoon. Place flower petals on top of each cookie (optional) in pleasing designs. Dehydrate at 95° F for approx. 24 hours, then peel the crisps off. Remove the Teflex, turn the crisps over and place directly onto the mesh screen and dehydrate until completely dry.

Yield: 57 crisps.

*Chia seed is not a big seller at health food stores. As a consequence, it may have been sitting around for a long time before you purchase it. It is always fresher from a mail order source. *See* "Sunorganic Farm" in Source Index.

SPINACH FLATBREAD

This bread reminds me of the flat bread served in Ethiopian restaurants where the bread is used to scoop up the food, in place of silverware.

1 recipe *Creamed Spinach* (*see* page 207)

1) Prepare the *Creamed Spinach*.

2) Divide the mixture into generous 1/2 cup portions. Pour each portion onto a Teflex-lined dehydrator tray and spread out in a circle to approx. 1/4-inch thickness. Dehydrate at 95° F for 24 to 36 hours. About three-quarters of the way through, peel the bread off the sheet, turn over and lay directly onto the dehydrator's mesh screen. Continue dehydrating until dry but pliable.

Yield: 6–7 slices.

NOTE: For a flaky type of flatbread, dehydrate the *Spicy Indian Spinach Soup* (*see* page 196).

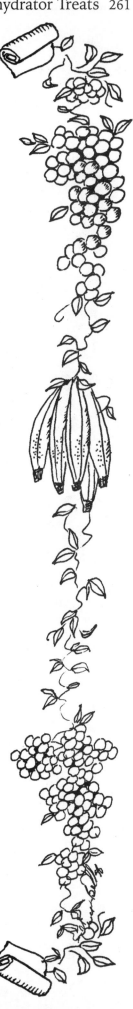

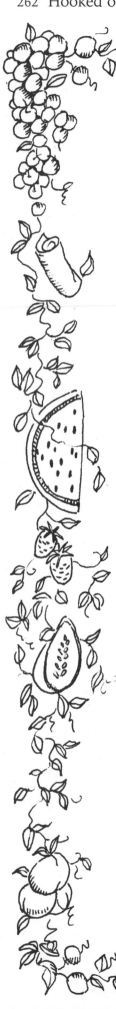

RICE CRACKERS

1 cup brown rice, soaked and sprouted
1 cup walnuts, soaked overnight
1 tbsp. slippery elm powder (*see* Glossary)
filtered water for soaking rice and walnuts

Believe it or not, brown rice, if it's not too old, does sprout. I have taken pictures of it because no one wants to believe me. I learned the secret one hot, humid, summer day in New York when some previously soaked rice, much to my surprise, sprouted. I surmised from this that rice, in order to sprout, needs to have some warmth.

1) Soak one cup of brown rice for 24-36 hours, changing the soak water 2-3 times. Then rinse and let sprout for 2-3 days, rinsing 2 times per day. Sink water is OK for the rinsing.

2) When the rice is ready, put the rice and the drained, rinsed walnuts into a bowl and mix them. Then put the mixture through the Champion (or Green Power) juicer, with the blank in place. The reason you mix the rice and walnuts together in the bowl first is because, as you put the mixture through the machine, the walnuts, which have more moisture, will help to grind the rice, which has less moisture. This way, you don't have to add any additional water.

3) Once the mixture comes out of the Champion (or Green Power), add in the slippery elm powder and mix well. With your hands, form into round, flat cookie shapes, and dehydrate at 95° F for approximately 20 hours.

Makes approximately 12 crackers. When thoroughly dry, this stores very well at room temperature in a cotton or muslin bag. It lasts a long time.

AROMATIC PECAN-RICE CRACKERS

Using the same recipe as above, substitute 1 cup of pecans (soaked 1 hour) for the walnuts and add 1/2 tsp. pumpkin pie spice.

DRIED COCONUT SHREDS

1, 2 or more coconuts—look for the ones that have a light brown shell and rubbery meat, they are younger & fresher, or use the meat from young Thai coconuts (for more information on coconuts, see Glossary)

1) Punch a hole in one of the eyes of the coconut and drain out the coconut water. (With Thai coconuts, slice off the top to open.) Drink the water straight or use in making nut milk or smoothies.

2) Break the coconuts with a hammer and separate the coconut meat from the shell. (With Thai cocos, make the hole on top big, then separate the meat from the shell with the back of a large spoon.) Wash the coconut and grate or slice the meat into very thin shreds. (I do not peel the coconut skin, but you could if you like.)

3) Once all the coconut is grated or sliced, spread it out on dehydrator trays lined with Teflex, and dehydrate at 95° F until very dry. Approx. 2-3 days.

   Store thoroughly dried coconut in a glass bottle in the refrigerator. It keeps for up to 6 months.

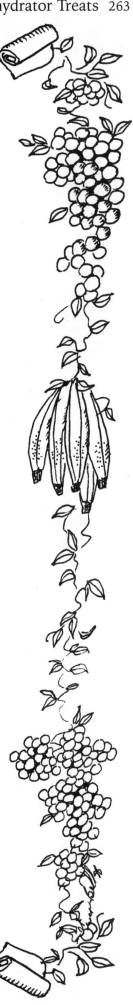

SAVORY NUT CRACKERS

1/2 cup soaked walnuts
1/2 cup soaked pine nuts
2 cups sprouted sunflower seeds
1/2 cup Jerusalem artichokes (sprinkle with lemon juice)
1/2 cup carrots
1/2 cup parsley
1 garlic clove
dash of Celtic sea salt or Nama Shoyu

1) Rinse the nuts and seeds and drain. Process all ingredients through a Champion or Green Power juicer with the blank in place.

2) Mix well with a spoon or your hands. Form into round, flat patties and place onto mesh dehydrator trays. Dehydrate at 95° F for 1 to 2 days.

   Makes 18 crackers. When thoroughly dry, they will keep a long time at room temperature. I keep mine in a bowl with a muslin cloth on top.

NOTE: If you can't find Jerusalem artichokes (also known as sunchokes), substitute with more carrots.

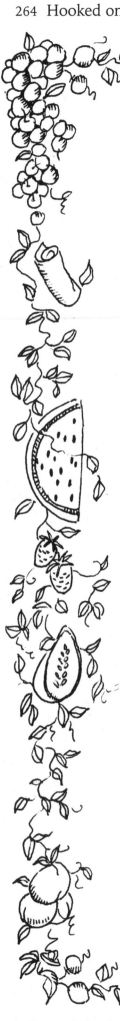

INDIAN CHIPS

6 cups chipped fresh coconut (*see Glossary*)
1 date, soaked and mashed
1 tbsp. date water (water in which dates have soaked)
1 tbsp. olive oil (extra-virgin)
1 tbsp. Nama Shoyu
1 tbsp. lemon juice
1/4 tsp. Celtic sea salt
1/2 tsp. ground cumin
1/2 tsp. ground brown mustard seed
1/2 tsp. garam masala
1/4 tsp. turmeric
pinch of asafoetida

1) For this recipe, use **firm** coconut meat, from slightly older coconuts. A coconut has 3 indentations on one end. Find the soft one and punch a hole in it with a flathead screwdriver. Widen the hole with the screwdriver, drain out the coconut water and drink or save it for later. Break open the coconut with a hammer.

2) Utilizing a kitchen utensil that makes potato chips (like the Salad-Shooter®) or a food processor with a chip grating attachment, make 6 cups of coconut chips. It's not necessary to peel the brown skin. Set aside in a large bowl.

3) In a small bowl, mash the date with a fork and mix well with the rest of the ingredients. Pour over the coconut chips and toss so the chips are well coated. Spread the chips onto mesh dehydrator trays (don't overlap the chips) and dehydrate at 95° F for approx. 2 days. (Put a piece of parchment paper under the lowest tray to catch any drippings, for easier clean-up.)

Yield: 5 cups. Keeps for up to a month. Store in a sealed container in the refrigerator.

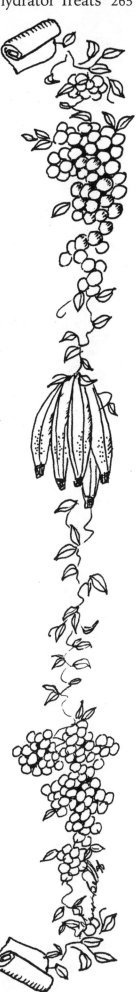

JAMEY & KIM'S FLAX CRACKERS

**This Recipe is Delicious and was Generously Shared by
Jameth Sheridan, N.D. and Kim Sheridan, N.D.
of Healthforce Nutritionals***

**1 cup flaxseeds (do not blend—oils are fragile and may
    become rancid—keep whole)
1 1/2 cup purified water
3/8 cup celery juice
3 tbsp. fresh-squeezed lemon juice
4–5 cloves garlic (or to taste)
Celtic sea salt, to taste (optional)**

1) In a blender, blend garlic into 1 1/2 cups water. Pour garlic water over the flaxseeds, stir and let soak at room temperature for about 5 hours. You will then have a gelatinous mixture.

2) Add the celery and lemon juices into the mixture. Stir until thoroughly mixed.

3) Scoop mixture onto a mesh** dehydrator tray, and spread out to an approximate 1/8" to 1/4" uniform thickness. To make individual crackers, rather than one giant cracker, it is helpful to create "perforations" before drying. Using a butter knife or the edge of a spatula, slice lines through the flax mixture to make desired cracker shapes (such as squares). Criss-crossing lines across the entire tray works well for this. Repeat this criss-cross slicing about 45 minutes to 1 1/2 hours later to help make the perforations deeper and the crackers easier to break apart when dry.

4) Dehydrate at 110° F for 24 or more hours (or until fully crispy). When the cracker is partially dry, turn it over and continue dehydrating. When done, break at perforated lines into individual crackers. Enjoy!

Yield: Approximately 2 dozen.

NOTES FROM RHIO: I have dehydrated the crackers at 95° F. You could also shape the mixture, with a spoon, into individual crackers as you go along, in case you don't have time to come back later to make the perforations. **I also line the mesh trays with Teflex sheets, because I find that putting the mixture directly onto the mesh trays doesn't work for me.

VARIATION: Blend in 1/2 cup soaked sun-dried tomato, 1/4 cup onion and 1 tsp homemade Italian Seasoning (see page 292).

*For information about their unique catalog of products, *check* the Source Index.

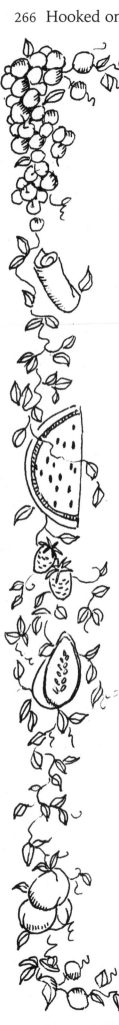

POTATO CHIPS

4 med. size potatoes (waxy type potatoes are best)
1 recipe *Some Like It Hot Marinade*, without the cilantro
   (*see* page 270)
distilled water

1) Scrub the potatoes with a vegetable brush and cut out any blemishes, sprouting parts or greenish parts. It's not necessary to peel. Slice the potatoes very thin with a V-Slicer or a SaladShooter® (*see* Kitchen Equipment), utilizing the chip blade. Put chips into a large bowl. Fill the bowl with distilled water and the juice of one lemon, stir and refrigerate overnight.

2) Make *Some Like it Hot Marinade* without the cilantro

3) Drain the potatoes and rinse well. (You may notice they have lost some of their starch, as evidenced by a white residue in either the bottom of the bowl or in the water.)

4) Pour the marinade over the potatoes and toss very well, so all the potatoes are coated. Taste and adjust flavors. Cover and let sit for two hours at room temperature.

5) Drain the marinade,* and put the potatoes in a single layer (don't overlap) onto mesh dehydrator trays and dehydrate at 95° F for 24 to 36 hours.

   Yield: 5 cups. When chips are thoroughly dehydrated, they'll keep for 2-4 weeks in a cookie jar.

NOTE: These are as tasty as the chips which advertise "you can't eat just one!" Save for times when you truly have the urge for potato chips. Of course you will have to plan your urge 24 hours in advance!

*With the exception of potatoes, leftover marinades can be used for salad dressings, etc. With potatoes, however, starch drains into the marinade and then it doesn't have a good flavor for other uses.

LEMON/CHILI PEANUTS

1 cup raw Valencia peanuts
1 lemon, juiced
1 tbsp. olive oil (extra-virgin)
1/2 tsp. fresh Serrano chili, minced
Nama Shoyu or Celtic sea salt, to taste

1) Combine the lemon juice, oil, Nama Shoyu or Celtic sea salt and chili. Pour over the peanuts and toss well. Let sit at room temperature for one hour.

2) Can be eaten as is or dehydrated at 95° F for 12 to 24 hours.

Yield: 1 1/4 cups. Keeps for up to 2-3 weeks refrigerated.

ALTERNATIVE: Before preparing the recipe, dehydrate the peanuts for 24 hours at 95° F. Then make the recipe, using Step #1 only.

PULP GEMS

This recipe is excellent for making good use of the carrot and beet pulps left over from making juice as well as the pulp left over from making nut and seed yogurts and milks.

1 1/2 cups carrot pulp (or carrot and beet pulp)
1 1/2 cups pulp left over from making seed and nut
    yogurts, milks or sour cream. (If you don't have any
    of this pulp, just take some pine nuts, almonds, and/or
    walnuts and blend with some water to a thick paste.)
2 cups sprouted sunflower seeds
1 cup celery with leaves
1/2 cup Greek, sun-dried black olives or Kalamata olives,
    desalted (*see* "Olives" in Glossary for instructions)
1/2 cup parsley
1/4 cup fresh basil
1–3 garlic cloves
2 oz. lemon juice
1/4–1/2 tsp. Celtic sea salt

1) Combine the vegetable and nut/seed pulps in a large bowl and set aside.

2) Put the rest of the ingredients into a food processor, and using the "S" blade, process as fine as possible. Add this mixture into the pulps, and with your hands, mix very well.

3) Form into flat, round cookie shapes and dehydrate at 95° F for approx. 24 to 36 hours.

Makes 32 *Pulp Gems*. When thoroughly dry, keeps for approx. 2–3 weeks in a cookie jar.

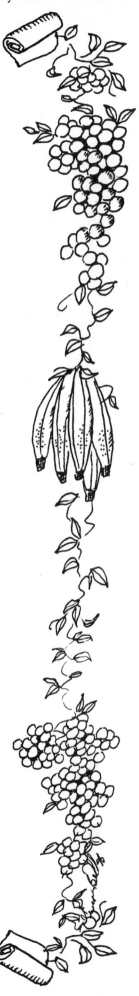

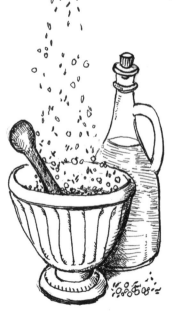

CHAPTER TWENTY-EIGHT:
Marinades, Condiments, Appetizers & This n' That

This chapter is all about flavor! By using some of the recipes in this section, you will maximize the flavor of your raw food meals.

Marinades are useful in bringing out the really delicious flavors of what I like to call "the heavy greens": kales, collards, chards, etc. What a little tasty marinade can do for these vegetables is wonderful.

Condiments are savory additions which serve to complement main courses.

Some appetizers can be found here, but most of them are located in other sections of the book. These include: *Honey of a Pistachio Spread, Indian Chips, Lemon/Chili Peanuts, Plantain Chips, Veggie Sushi Rolls, Potato Chips, Collard Rolls, Stuffed Grape Leaves, Sprouted Pea Chips* and *Pear-Pine Canapés*. To find these recipes, *check* the Index.

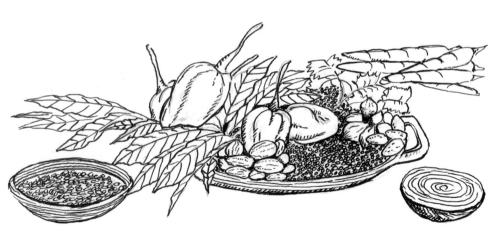

APPLE-CRANBERRY RELISH

1 cup dried unsweetened cranberries, soaked overnight
1 large apple
8 large dates, soaked overnight
1/2 cup walnuts, soaked overnight
2 oz. raisins or currants, soaked overnight

1) Cover the cranberries with filtered water and let sit at room temperature overnight. This should almost double the amount.

2) In three separate bowls soak dates, walnuts and raisins (or currants) with just enough filtered water to cover. In the morning, drain and rinse. (Save the date and raisin soakwater for another use.)

3) Put everything, except the raisins (or currants), into the food processor and blend well using the "S" blade. Take completed relish out of the food processor and stir in the raisins or currants. Store in a glass jar.

Yield: approx. 3 cups. Keeps in the refrigerator for up to two weeks.

SERVING SUGGESTIONS:

- Use as a topping over any of the seed or nut yogurts, or cheeses.
- Goes well with *Pecan-Wild Rice Loaf* (*see* page 161).
- Makes good dehydrated wafers. Shape into cookie shapes with your hands and dehydrate at 95° F for 2 days.

MANGO CHUTNEY

A Delicious Chutney Recipe Generously Shared by
Sarah Tuttle, Raw Chef Extraordinaire

2 cups of fresh, ripe mango pulp
1 cup of fresh coconut pieces
1 Serrano green chili
3/4 cup lemon juice
1/2 cup fresh mint (optional)
1 tsp. Celtic sea salt (optional)

1) Grind all the ingredients together in a food processor, using the "S" blade. Serve with raw crackers.

Yield: 2 1/2 cups. Keeps for 5 days in the refrigerator.

WASABI MOUSSE

2 tsp. wasabi powder (*see* Glossary)
4 tsp. *Pine Nut Cream* (*see* page 226)

1) Mix together by hand until finely blended. Make fresh each time.

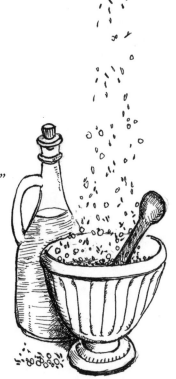

SOME LIKE IT HOT MARINADE

2 lemons, juiced
2 oz. olive oil (add a dash of flaxseed oil for the
 benefits)
2 garlic cloves, pressed
1 tsp. cumin powder
1/8–1/4 tsp. cayenne (or to your own taste)
2 tbsp. fresh minced cilantro (optional, but good
 with eggplant)
Nama Shoyu and/or Celtic sea salt, to taste

1) Mix all ingredients together in a bowl.

SERVING SUGGESTIONS:

- This is excellent for marinating very thin sliced eggplant (*see* recipe for *Eggplant Marinade* - opposite page).

- You can also marinate the following thinly sliced vegetables for a couple of hours at room temperature or overnight in the refrigerator:

Broccoli   Potatoes   Brussels sprouts
Cauliflower   Winter squash   Celery root
and try sprouted beans and legumes also.

- Very tasty as a salad dressing (with or without the cilantro and the cayenne).

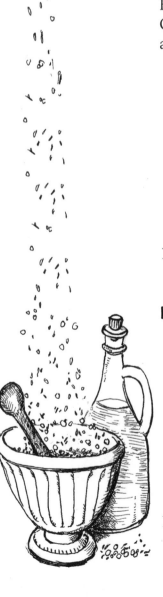

PRUNE PASTE

1/2 cup pitted prunes, soaked overnight or at least
 2 hours
4–5 tbsp. apple cider vinegar
1 tbsp. prune soak water

1) In a food processor using the "S" blade, blend ingredients to a paste.
 Yield: 1/2 cup. Keeps up to a month in the refrigerator.

NOTE: Crack open the prune pits and eat the delicious seeds inside.

BEET RELISH

1 med. beet, grated
1 cup sprouted French lentils
6 tbsp. *Prune Paste* (see above)
1 tbsp. olive oil (extra-virgin)
Celtic sea salt, to taste
sprinkle of freshly ground white pepper

1) Put all ingredients into a bowl and blend well together
 Yield: approx. 3 cups. Keeps for a week in the refrigerator.

SUN-DRIED TOMATO TAPENADE

**1/2 cup Kalamata olives (or Greek, sun-dried
    black olives*)**
1/2 medium onion
**1/2 cup soaked sun-dried tomatoes (soak 1 hour in just
    enough water to cover)**
1 garlic clove
2 tbsp. capers (soak overnight in distilled water)
1/2 lime, juiced
1 1/2 oz. olive oil (extra-virgin)

1) Pit the olives and soak overnight at room temperature in distilled water, to remove most of the salt. Also, in a separate little bowl, soak the capers. Next day rinse and drain the olives and capers.

2) Put all ingredients into a food processor and process as fine as possible using the "S" blade. Taste and adjust flavors.

    Yield: 2 cups. Keeps well for up to a month in the refrigerator.

SERVING SUGGESTIONS:

- Try in the *Unbaked Beans* (page 157) and *Sloppy Joes* (page 139) recipes.
- A little of this tapenade goes a long way and can be added into some of the other recipes for flavor.

*Available from Sunorganic Farm (*see* Source Index).

EGGPLANT MARINADE

I got this idea from listening to chefs on the TV Food Network saying that you could "cook" fish in a lemon or lime juice marinade. So I thought, why not apply a marinade to eggplant to see if it would take the bitterness out and soften it up enough to enjoy raw . . . and it works beautifully.

    1 eggplant
    1 recipe of *Some Like It Hot Marinade* (*see* page 270)

1) Make 1 recipe of *Some Like it Hot Marinade*.

2) Slice 1 peeled or unpeeled eggplant very thin with a Mandoline, V-Slicer (*see* Kitchen Equipment) or similar kitchen utensil. Dip each slice of eggplant into the marinade to coat both sides, then place into another bowl. After dipping all the eggplant, pour the rest of the marinade over the eggplant. Let marinate at room temperature for 2 hours, then refrigerate until ready to use. If you're not going to use it within the same day, then drain the marinade out after 4 or 5 hours, otherwise the eggplant gets soggy and all its flavor drains out.

    Serves 2. Keeps for 2 days in the refrigerator.

NOTE: The drained marinade liquid can be used as a base for salad dressings or sauces and it's very tasty just on its own.

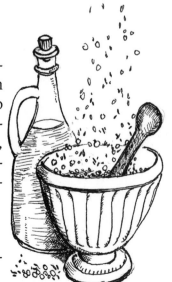

WILD STUFFED TOMATOES

3–4 boxes large cherry tomatoes
1 cup sprouted wild rice
1 cup sprouted barley or oats
1/2 cup soaked English walnuts (soak 1 hour)
1/2 cup soaked black walnuts, chopped (soak 1 hour)
1 cup parsley
3/4 cup minced shallot or onion
1/2 cup raisins or currants
1/4 cup pine nuts
Nama Shoyu and/or Celtic sea salt, to taste

1) To prepare the tomatoes for stuffing, de-stem them and cut off a thin sliver from the top. With a small serrated spoon, scoop out the tomato pulp. Save for another use, such as juice or salsa.

2) Put the sprouted wild rice, 1/2 cup of the sprouted barley or oats and the parsley into a food processor, and process with the "S" blade for about a minute. Transfer to a bowl and set aside.

3) Put the remaining 1/2 cup of barley or oats and the English walnuts through the Champion or Green Power juicer with the blank (homogenizer) in place. Scrape the resulting paste out of the juicer housing (almost all of this small amount will be stuck in there). Add this paste into the wild rice mixture in the bowl.

4) Add in the rest of the ingredients and mix well. Stuff the tomato cups.

Makes approx. 60 stuffed tomatoes. Best the first day, but keeps for two.

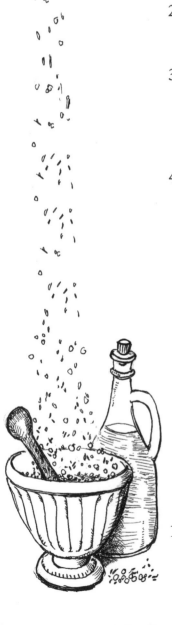

DIM SOME

4 avocados
1 cup Greek, sun-dried black olives, desalted
  (see Glossary)
1/2 cup, or more, of diced onion
1/2 lemon, juiced
1/4 tsp. Celtic sea salt (opt.)
1/2–1 tsp. *Creole Spice* (see page 293)
2 medium turnips or rutabagas
8 sheets of nori

1) Pit the avocados and scoop out the pulp into a large bowl. Squeeze the lemon juice over the avocados. Set aside.

2) Mince the olives and onions and add to the avocados in the bowl. Add *Creole Spice* and Celtic sea salt and mash the contents of the bowl with a wire whisk or fork until it becomes the consistency of guacamole.

3) With a V-Slicer or mandoline, slice the turnips or rutabagas into very thin circles. Cut each nori sheet in half and then in half again creating 4 square pieces per sheet. Dip the pieces briefly in filtered water and place them on the counter. Put a heaping tsp. of the avocado mix in the center of each nori piece and then fold up the sides of the nori creating a little pouch. Place each pouch on a turnip or rutabaga slice and serve.

Yield: approx. 30 pieces.

PANCAKE SYRUPS

ORANGE DATE SYRUP:

> 2/3 cup dates, soaked
> 1 cup orange juice
> 1/2 tsp. *Vanilla Powder* (*see* Glossary)
> 1/2 rounded tsp. agar-agar flakes

1) Soak the dates in just enough filtered water to cover. Let sit in the refrigerator overnight.

2) Next day, pit the dates. Put dates, orange juice, agar-agar, and *Vanilla Powder* into the blender and blend well.

Yield: approx. 1 cup. Keeps for 2 days in the refrigerator..

NO-MAPLE SYRUP:

> 2/3 cup dates, soaked
> 1 recipe *Coconut Cream* (*see* page 276)
> 1/2 tsp. *Vanilla Powder* (*see* Glossary)

1) Pit the dates. Put all ingredients into the blender and blend well.

Yield: approx. 1 cup. Keeps for 2 days in the refrigerator. After storage, reblend to liquefy.

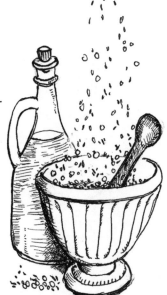

CHAPTER TWENTY-NINE:
Delectable Desserts

DESSERT—AN OCCASIONAL TREAT

The way I think about dessert is different. If I want dessert, I just make a meal of it.

If you eat dessert at the end of a meal, as is the conventionally accepted practice, then you are usually creating mixtures that are very difficult to digest. If you must have dessert after a meal, **at least wait**, hopefully an hour. Take a walk or something. But this short interval is still less than excellent for your digestion. The better way is to re-train yourself . . . and I know you can do it; otherwise, why would you be reading this book in the first place? Try to get out of the habit (that's all it is—a habit) of having dessert after a meal. Have healthy desserts as a meal (occasionally), or as a between-meal snack. This way you won't be piling food upon food, making mixtures that are difficult to digest, and creating flatulence, upset stomachs, acid indigestion and all those other things for which the television commercials are full of (questionable) remedies.

I'm not suggesting you have dessert for breakfast, lunch and dinner. I mean **occasionally**, or as a between-meal snack.

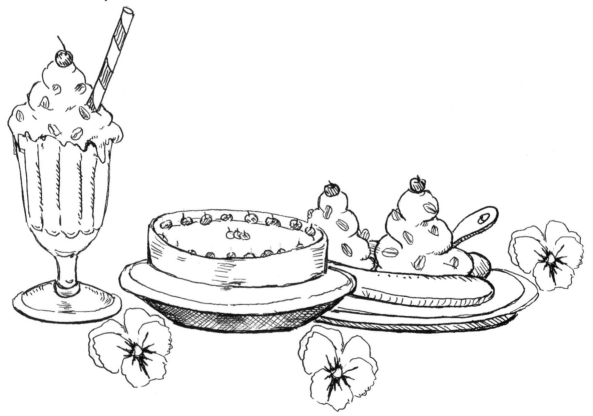

ALMOND ROCA

2 cups sprouted almonds
1/2 cup dried, shredded coconut
1/4 cup raw wildflower honey
1/2 vanilla bean, ground

1) Put all the ingredients, except coconut, into a food processor and process until mixture holds together.

2) Transfer to a bowl, add in the shredded coconut, and blend well by hand.

3) Form into small ball shapes, and refrigerate. These are very delicious, but don't overdo!

Makes 1 dozen. Keeps up to 2 weeks in the refrigerator.

CONNIE'S SPUMONI ICE CREAM

Inspired by my Lovely Niece, Connie

2 cups macadamias   **1/4 cup raw honey**
1 quart filtered water   **2 cups fresh cherries**
1/4 cup raw carob powder   **1 cup pistachios**
1 cup honey tangerine or orange juice
1 vanilla bean, cut into small pieces

1) Put the macadamias into the Vita-Mix blender with half the water and blend well. Add remaining water and blend again. (A regular blender can also be used, but it will only accommodate 1/2 of the nuts at a time.)

2) Pour the mixture through a muslin bag and squeeze out all the liquid. Save the pulp for making cookies.

3) Pour the macadamia milk back into the blender; add the orange or tangerine juice, honey, vanilla and carob, and blend well. Pour into ice cube trays and freeze overnight.

4) Pit and chop the cherries. Pulse chop the pistachios in a food processor with the "S" blade. Set aside in a bowl.

5) Put the frozen macadamia cubes through the Champion (or equivalent) juicer with the blank in place. Add cherries and pistachios to the ice cream and lightly blend in by hand. Serve immediately.

Yield: 1 1/2 quarts.

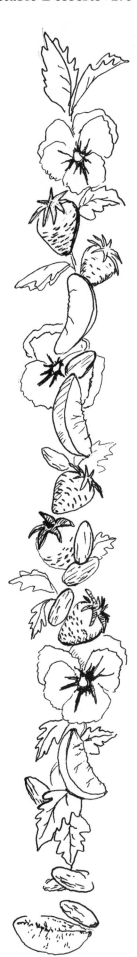

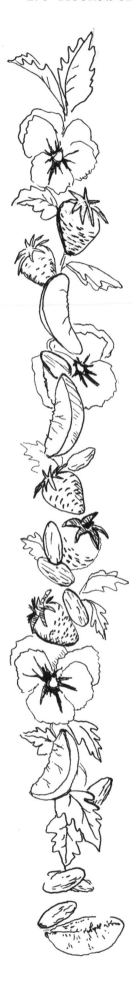

COCONUT CREAM

1 fresh coconut (look for a coconut with a light brown shell, as opposed to dark brown—it will usually be younger and fresher.) *See* Glossary for more information on coconuts

1) With a flathead screwdriver poke a hole into one of the "eyes" of the coconut and pour out the coconut water.* The coconut water is not used in this recipe, however, it is an excellent water to drink.

2) With a hammer, break the coconut open and separate the meat of the coconut from the shell. Rinse the coconut, then cut into pieces and put through the Champion juicer,** using the juice screen. You are making coconut juice, which comes out as a cream. If you are juicing more than two coconuts, keep checking the juicer because it has a tendency to overheat, and then you will be cooking your cream. If the juicer feels hot, turn it off and let it cool before proceeding.

One average coconut yields approx. 1/4 to 1/2 cup of *Coconut Cream*. To keep overnight, put into the refrigerator. If you want to keep it longer, freeze in ice cube trays.

NOTE: *Coconut Cream* can be used to make various ice creams and parfaits, and also some Caribbean style main course dishes, such as the *Caribbean Wild Rice* (*see* page 156). It is also good by itself or as a topping for fruit salads.

*Sometimes I've heard it called coconut milk, but it looks more like water to me. In Latin countries they call this "Agua de Coco" (water of the coconut). When it's fresh, it tastes slightly sweet or neutral, but if it's old, it can taste sour or soapy. You don't want to drink it then or use the coconut meat either.

**I find that the Champion juicer makes the *Coconut Cream* easier than the Green Power juicer. (When making *Coconut Cream* with the Green Power juicer, it's best to put the coconut through first with the blank (homogenizer) in place, then put the resulting pulp through again using the juice screen.)

BLUEBERRY JELLO

1 pint blueberries
2 bananas
1/2 lemon or lime, juiced

1) Blend all the ingredients in a blender. Pour into custard cups and chill. Makes 4 custard cups. Keeps for 2 days in the refrigerator.

HONEY VANILLA ICE CREAM

2 cups *Almond Milk* (*see* page 249)
1/2 vanilla bean (cut into tiny pieces)
2 1/2–3 tbsp. raw honey (choose a mild-flavored variety,
    like clover, so the flavor of the vanilla comes through)

1) Put all the ingredients into a blender and blend very well. Blend long enough so that the vanilla bean breaks up and releases its flavor, then pour the liquid into an ice cube tray and freeze overnight.

2) When ready to serve, put the cubes* through the Champion (or comparable) juicer with the blank (homogenizer) in place.

   Makes 1 pint.

*To get the cubes out of the ice cube tray, use a dinner knife (NOT a sharp knife) and gently pry around the edges of the cubes. A sharp knife will cut into the plastic of the tray, which I discovered when I saw a tray after someone had made some ice cream. You DON'T want plastic in your ice cream!

ORANGE SHERBET

1 cup *Almond Milk* (*see* page 249)
1 cup orange juice
2 tbsp. raw, mild clover honey

1) Put all ingredients into the blender and blend until smooth and the honey is dissolved. Taste it. You may need to add more honey if it is not sweet enough for you.*

2) Pour into an ice cube tray and freeze overnight. When ready to serve, put the cubes through the Champion (or comparable) juicer with the blank (homogenizer) in place.

   Makes approx. 1 pint.

*Use the juice of sweet organic oranges or tangerines because it is usually less acidic than the juice of conventionally grown citrus.

PEARS & CHEEZ

1–2 pears (or apples)
1/2 lemon or lime, juiced
1 recipe *Chedda Cheez* (*see* page 210)

1) Slice the pears and sprinkle with lemon juice. Put a slice of *Chedda Cheez* on top of each pear slice and serve.

   Serves 1.

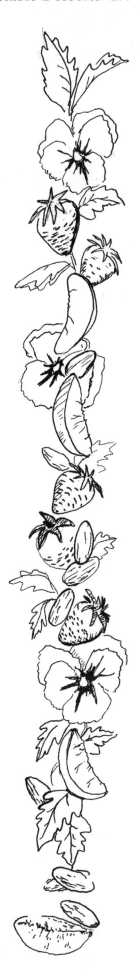

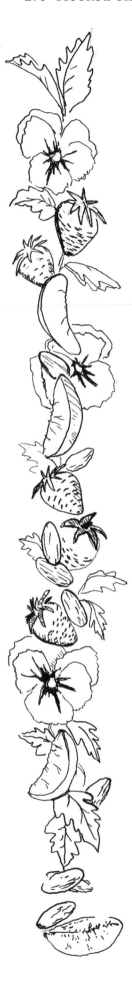

FRUIT SHERBET

With a Champion or Green Life juicer it is always super easy to make any number of fruit sherbets. These two juicers have a "blank" screen (attachment) that can be used for making sherbet.

1) The first step is to freeze the fruit. Cut the fruit, put it into a plastic container and place it in the freezer overnight. You could freeze strawberries, blueberries, chunks of pineapple, chunks of mango, bananas, kiwi, raspberries, cherimoya chunks (take the seeds out), tangerines, etc. You get the idea. You could use two, three or more varieties of fruits in your sherbet—it's really up to you. There's no way to make a bad sherbet, but I always use at least some banana or plantain in all the sherbets to make them creamier.

2) Once the fruits are frozen hard, you are ready to make the sherbet. Put the fruit through the Champion (or Green Life) juicer with the blank in place. Out comes the best sherbet ever –100% fruit with no additives of any kind!

In my house, we always keep some fruit frozen for when the urge hits!

PINEAPPLE SORBET

1 pineapple
1–2 tbsp. raw honey

1) Wash and peel the pineapple. Prepare fresh pineapple juice in a juicer.

2) Put the juice into a blender and blend with the honey. Pour the juice into ice cube trays and freeze.

3) When ready to make the sorbet, put the pineapple cubes into a food processor and process to a sorbet consistency. Serve immediately.

Serves 2.

RASPBERRY FRAPPÉ

2 cups frozen raspberries
3 frozen bananas, sliced into chunks
2 tbsp. raw honey blended with a little water

1) Put all the ingredients into a food processor and using the "S" blade, process to a creamy consistency. Serves 4.

MAGGIE'S WEDDING CAKE
This Recipe was Generously Shared by
Maggie J. Hodge-Neill, C.C.T., Natural Health Educator

> 3 large apples, grated (choose hard ones, not soft
> or mushy)
> 1 cup grated carrots
> 1 or 2 mangoes, mashed (optional, but makes the
> cake moister)
> 1/4 lemon, juiced
> 1 cup sunflower seeds
> 1 cup walnuts (or other nuts) coarsely chopped
> 1 cup raw carob
> 1 cup dehydrated shredded coconut
> 1 cup finely chopped dates
> 1 cup raisins
> 1/3 cup dried pineapple (opt.) soaked 1/2 hr. & cut
> into small pieces
> 1/3 cup dried papaya (opt.) soaked 1/2 hr. & cut
> into small pieces
> 1 heaping tsp. cinnamon

1) Put all ingredients into a large bowl. With clean hands, mix and squeeze through fingers. Blend it all together with lots of love.

2) Press the cake into a large glass Pyrex® loaf pan, approx. 1 1/2" high.

3) Refrigerate for 2-3 hours before serving.

Serves 12. Keeps up to a week in the refrigerator.

HONEYED NUTS

> 1/2 cup pistachios, chopped
> 1/2 cup black walnuts (or English walnuts), chopped
> 1/2 tsp. olive oil (or sunflower oil from Flora—*see*
> Source Index)
> 1 tsp. raw honey
> dash Celtic sea salt

1) In a small bowl, blend the honey, olive or sunflower oil and Celtic sea salt.

2) Next, mix the nuts with the honey mixture, blending together by hand.

Yield: 1 cup. Keeps for two weeks in the refrigerator.

NOTE: This makes a delicious nutty topping for any of the ice cream recipes—try over *Honey Vanilla Ice Cream* (*see* page 277).

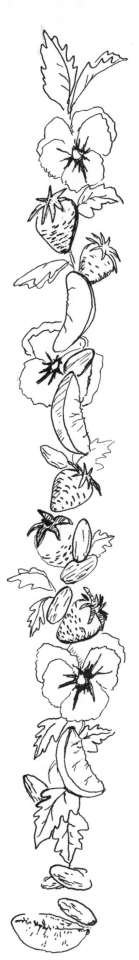

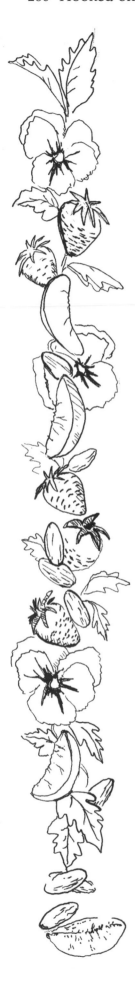

LEIGH'S CHERRY COBBLER
with Crumbly Crumbs

2 cups fresh pitted cherries
2 cups frozen mango (2 to 3 mangoes, depending on size)
2 large ripe bananas
1/2 cup pecans
1/2 cup almonds
1/2 cup sunflower seeds
5 large dates
1/2 cup raisins or currants

1) The night before you want to make this recipe, peel sweet, ripe mangoes and cut into chunks. Then put into a plastic container and freeze.

2) Put pecans, almonds, sunflower seeds and dates into a food processor, and with the "S" blade, process to a crumb texture. These are the crumbly crumbs. Set aside in a bowl.

3) Pit and coarsely chop cherries and set aside.

4) Put the banana and approx. 2 cups of frozen mango into the food processor and with the "S" blade, process to a smooth custard.

TO ASSEMBLE THE COBBLER:

5) In a glass pie pan, put a layer of crumbly crumbs, followed by a layer of the banana/mango custard. Then add a layer of cherries and a sprinkle of raisins. Keep layering in this way until you run out of ingredients. Top with a sprinkle of raisins, and it's ready to serve. You could also put it into the freezer for about an hour before serving if it's too soft.

Serves 6-8. Keeps for a week or longer in the freezer.

NOTE: If you want to make the pie but forgot to freeze the mango in advance, go ahead and make the pie with fresh, unfrozen mango. When the pie is made, put the whole pie into the freezer for an hour or two before serving.

BERRIES & CREAM

1 pint strawberries, blueberries, raspberries or
    blackberries (or a combination)
1 recipe *Macadamia Cream* (*see page 217*)
1 heaping tbsp. unheated honey or 2 oz. date syrup
    (made by blending soaked dates with a little water—
    keep it thick)

1) Divide berries into two bowls. If using strawberries, slice them. Add a large dollop of *Macadamia Cream* on top of the berries, and drizzle with honey or date syrup. Enjoy! Serves 2.

APPLE-STRAWBERRY-FIG PIE

**This Scrumptious Pie Recipe was Graciously Shared
by Cher Carden**

ALMOND-COCONUT CRUST:

> **3/4 cup almonds**
> **1/4 cup pecans**
> **1/2 cup sunflower seeds**
> **2 tbsp. shredded dried coconut**

1) In a food processor with the "S" blade, process the above ingredients until nuts are reduced to tiny granules. Put into a bowl and set aside.

APPLE-STRAWBERRY-FIG FILLING:

> **5 Granny Smith apples**
> **1/2 lemon, juiced**
> **1/2 cup raisins (soak in water for 1 hour)**
> **1 cup dates (soak in water for 1 hour)**
> **1 cup dried figs (soak in water for 1 hour)**
> **1 tbsp. cinnamon**
> **1 pint strawberries**

2) Core the apples and shred in a food processor using the shredder blade. Sprinkle with lemon juice and set aside.

3) Drain raisins and dates. Then process them with cinnamon in a food processor with the "S" blade, until a smooth, jam-like texture is reached.

4) Take 1/2 of this jam mixture and place in the bowl with the nuts previously set aside. Knead together until crust becomes like silly putty. Mold crust into a 9" pie plate using your hands to flesh out the crust across the plate. (Or place crust in between 2 sheets of wax paper and roll flat with a rolling pin. Peel off 1 wax sheet and place flattened crust over pie plate and gently press into place.) Set aside.

5) Blend the remaining jam with the figs and 1/2 pint of strawberries in the food processor. Process well. (This is strawberry-fig jam.)

6) Remove strawberry-fig jam from the food processor and mix with the shredded apples. Fill the pie crust and smooth out with a spatula.

7) Decorate the top of the pie with the remaining strawberries.

Serves 6-8. Keeps for 3-4 days in the refrigerator.

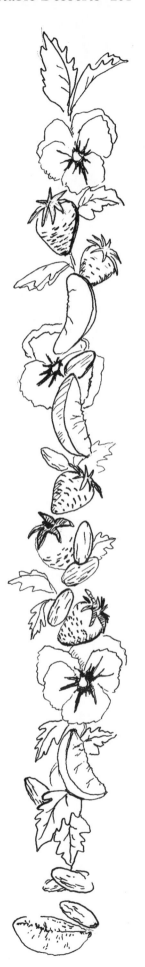

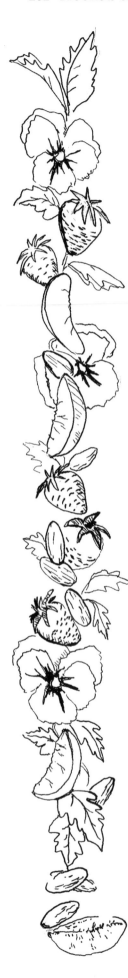

CELESTIAL PECAN PIE

5 bananas
1 papaya (or mango, or a pint of strawberries, sliced)
1 cup pecans (soaked in water for 1 hour)
1 1/2 cups pecans (don't soak)
6 oz. filtered water
5-10 dates, soaked
1/2 vanilla bean, cut into tiny pieces
1 heaping tbsp. raw honey (or to taste)
dash of Nama Shoyu

1) Soak one cup of pecans in filtered water. Set aside.

FRUIT CRUST:

2) In a 9-inch glass pie pan, arrange one layer of sliced bananas (2 1/2 bananas should do it). Lay the banana slices in a spiral pattern with one slice slightly overlapping the other until you have covered the entire pie pan. Also put a layer going up the sides of the pie pan. Next, cut the papaya into 1/4 inch thin slices and layer the papaya over the banana. Over the papaya, put another layer of slightly overlapping banana slices. Now with your hands, compress the fruit down evenly. Set aside.

PECAN CREAM FILLING:

3) In a blender, put 1 cup of soaked (drained) pecans, dates, 6 oz. filtered water and tiny pieces of vanilla bean and blend to a fine cream. Taste the cream, and if it is not sweet enough for your taste, add more dates.

4) Pour the *Pecan Cream Filling* over the fruit in the pie pan. Put the pie pan into the dehydrator and dehydrate at 95° F for 3 hours.

5) In a small bowl, blend the raw honey with just a little water and a dash of Nama Shoyu. Prepare the unsoaked pecans for the topping by tossing gently with the honeyed water to coat the pecans.

6) After 3 hours, take the pie out of the dehydrator and place one layer of the prepared pecans on top of the pie. Place them artistically radiating towards the center of the pie.

7) Chill the pie at least one hour before serving.

Serves 6-8. Keeps for a few days in the refrigerator.

NOTE: The *Fruit Crust* can be made with any fruit you choose to put between the two banana layers. Try mango, sliced strawberries, cherries, etc.

FUDGE X TASTY

2 cups pecans (soaked 1/2 hour)
1 cup dates, soaked and pitted
3/4 cup *Coconut Cream* (*see* page 276)
6 tbsp. raw carob powder
3 to 4 tbsp. raw honey (or to taste)
1/2 cup soaked walnuts, chopped (optional)
1/2 cup fresh grated coconut (optional)
1 tsp. *Vanilla Powder* (see Glossary)

1) Make the *Coconut Cream*. Set aside.

2) Drain the pecans and dates and put them through the Champion or Green Power juicer with the blank in place.

3) Add 1/2 cup *Coconut Cream*, along with the carob, vanilla and honey, to the pecan/date mixture and blend well by hand.

4) Add in optional ingredients. Mix well.

5) Spread mixture, about 1 1/2 inches thick, into a rectangular plastic container, and frost the top with the balance of the *Coconut Cream*. Score the fudge with a knife, dividing it into squares. Cover, and put it into the freezer.

   Makes about 15 fudge squares. Keeps for 2-3 weeks in the freezer.

CAROB (the Un-Chocolate) SAUCE

1 cup raw sesame tahini
1/4 cup raw honey
1/2 cup (or more) of raw carob powder
1/4 cup filtered water

1) Put all the ingredients, except the carob powder, into a bowl.

2) Begin stirring and add in 1/2 cup carob powder. Blend ingredients very well by hand, adding in more carob powder if desired. Let your own taste guide you. Also, add more water if you want it thinner, less water if you want it thicker.

   Makes approx. 1 1/2 cups. Keeps for up to a month in the refrigerator.

NOTE: For a chunky sauce, add in finely chopped black figs and pecans.

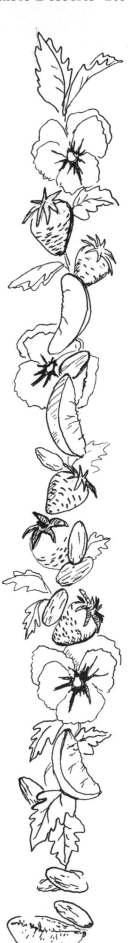

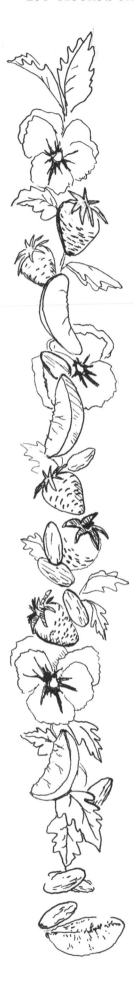

COCONUT-ALMOND LOG

1/2 cup sprouted almonds
1/2 cup dates
1 1/2 cups freshly grated coconut (or unpasteurized, dried coconut)
2 tsp. rosewater (edible)
1 tsp. raw honey
6 tbsp. grated almond

1) Put the sprouted almonds and the dates through the Champion (or equivalent) juicer with the blank (homogenizer) in place. Scrape the almond and date paste out of the juicer housing and put into a bowl. Add in the coconut and mix together.

2) Blend in the rosewater, honey, and 2 tbsp. of grated almond. Mix well with your hands and form into a log. Roll the log into the remaining grated almond to coat the whole outside of the log. Chill well before serving. Slice the log with a sharp knife as needed.

Serves 6-8. Keeps up to 1 month in a covered container in the fridge.

CREME BRULÉE

2 cups *Coconut Cream* (*see* page 276)
1 heaping tsp. agar-agar flakes
1 1/2 cups raisins
1 cup filtered water
1/2 tsp. *Vanilla Powder* (*see* Glossary)
1 tsp. Sundial honey*

1) 24-hours in advance of making this recipe, soak the raisins in 1 cup of filtered water. Keep in the refrigerator.

2) Make the *Coconut Cream* as per recipe.

3) Put the *Coconut Cream*, agar-agar flakes, *Vanilla Powder* and 4 to 5 ounces of raisin water into a blender and blend well. (Save the raisins for another use.) Pour the cream into custard cups and chill in the refrigerator for 1/2 hour. Before serving, drizzle lightly with Sundial honey.

Makes 4 custard cups. Keeps for 3 days in the refrigerator.

*Raw, unstrained, unheated, wild, black and organic honey from Africa. It tastes like chocolate with a hint of herbs. Very unusual. (Available from Sundial Herbs, 3609 Boston Rd., Bronx, NY 10466, (718) 798-3962.)

COOKIE-RAMA

GENERAL INSTRUCTIONS: Dehydrated cookies are very easy to make! Just take a combination of soaked nuts, seeds and dried fruits, drain the water, add a little spice such as vanilla or cinnamon, and process in a food processor until the fruits and nuts are mixed together. Then form into cookie shapes with your hands and place onto Teflex-lined dehydrator trays. If the mixture is not too wet, you can place the cookies directly on the mesh dehydrator trays. Dehydrate at 95° F for 12 to 36 hours, depending on how dry you want them. That's all there is to it. If the combination you choose tastes good to you after you blend it together in the food processor, it will taste good as a cookie too. (These can also be enjoyed without dehydrating.)

Following are a few of my favorite recipes, but use your imagination and invent some of your own. There are endless combinations. You can't go wrong. If the cookies are dried to the very dry stage, then they can be stored at room temperature in a covered container. If the cookies are dried to a moist, chewy stage, then they are best kept in a covered container in the refrigerator.

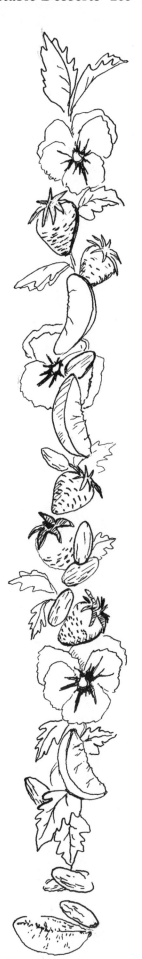

TOLEHOUSE

1 cup soaked pine nuts
1 cup soaked pecans
1 cup soaked dried apricots
1/4 cup soaked dates
1/4 cup raisins
1/4 vanilla bean, ground
1 tbsp. raw honey (optional)

SESAME BARS

1 cup soaked almonds
1/2 cup soaked sesame
1/2 cup soaked sunflower
8 dates
2 oz. unheated honey
juice of 1 orange

CHUNKY CHEWS

1/2 cup Brazil nuts (soaked or not)
1/2 cup Valencia peanuts (soaked or not)
1/2 cup sprouted sunflower seeds
1/2 cup dried coconut shreds
3/4 cup dates, pitted
unheated honey, to taste

Form the *Chunky Chews* into thick cigar shapes.

BANANA BABE

1 ripe plantain
2 cups soaked walnuts
1/2 cup soaked dates
1/2 cup soaked raisins
juice of 1/2 lemon
1/2 tsp. grated lemon rind

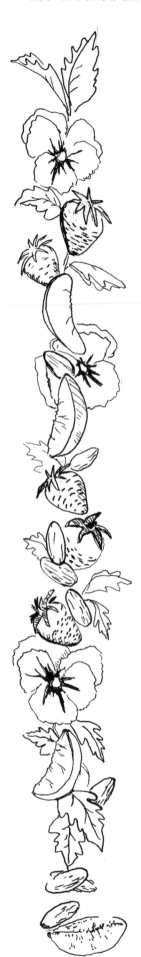

MANGO PUDDING PIE

FILLING:

> 2 mangoes (peel and remove pits)
> 1/2 cup sprouted almonds, blanched
> 1/2 lemon, juiced
> 1/2 tsp. rosewater
> 2 heaping tbsp. raw honey (or to taste)
> 4 tbsp. agar-agar flakes
> 2 cups filtered water

1) Bring the water to a boil, add the agar-agar and gently simmer for 3 to 5 minutes, stirring until the agar-agar is completely dissolved. Take off the stove and set aside to cool a bit.

2) This recipe works best using the sweetest mangoes you can find (not the tart ones). Put the mango pulp, 1/2 cup almonds, lemon juice, honey and rosewater into a blender and blend to a cream. Once the agar-agar mixture is cool enough so that you can stick your finger in, add the agar-agar mixture to the mango mixture in the blender and blend well. Taste it and if it's not sweet enough for you, add additional honey.

3) Pour mixture into an empty glass pie plate and refrigerate for 1/2 hour or until it hardens. In the meantime make the pie crust.

ALMOND PIE CRUST:

> 2 cups sprouted almonds, blanched
> 3/4–1 cup dates
> grated lemon rind to taste (from undyed lemons)

4) Process the almonds, dates and grated lemon rind in a food processor with the "S" blade. Then press the mixture into a 9-inch glass pie plate.

5) After the filling gels, put it back into the blender and blend it again, then pour this mixture into the pie crust. (This RE-BLENDING is very important because otherwise, you will get a gelatin-type dessert instead of a creamy pudding.)

TO DECORATE TOP OF PIE:

> 1 mango and a few sprouted, unpeeled almonds

6) Cut the mango in half the long way. Peel, and slice thin, long pieces. Decorate the top of the pie by placing slices all the way around, like a flower. Put a few almonds in the center.

Serves 6-8. Keeps for 3-4 days in the refrigerator.

ORANGE PUDDING

1 cup raisins, soaked overnight (or minimum 2 hours)
1/2 cup almonds, soaked overnight & blanched
   (*see* page 302 for instructions on blanching without
   cooking)
1 tbsp. pine nuts, soaked overnight
2 oranges
1/4 tsp. *Vanilla Powder* (*see* Glossary)

1) Drain soaked raisins (reserve water for other uses) and put into a
   blender with the juice and pulp of the oranges, blanched almonds, pine
   nuts, and the *Vanilla Powder*. Blend well and put into custard cups. Chill.

   Serves 4. Best served the same day, but will keep for 2 days in the refrigerator. For storage, cover with plastic wrap. (Instead of plastic wrap,
   you could use small demitasse saucers as covers for the custard cups.)

SWEET BROWN RICE PUDDING

1 cup sprouted sweet brown rice
1/2 cup sprouted almonds, blanched
1–1 1/2 cups filtered water
4 dates
3 tbsp. raw honey
1/2 tsp. *Vanilla Powder* (*see* Glossary)
2 rounded tsp. psyllium powder
raisins
cinnamon

1) Use the variety of rice known as "Sweet Brown Rice." Soak for 24 hours
   and then sprout for 24 hours.

2) Put the sprouted brown rice and sprouted almonds into a food processor with the "S" blade and process as finely as possible. Stop the
   processor and scrape down the sides a couple of times.

3) Add in 1 cup of water, dates, honey, *Vanilla Powder* and psyllium. Process
   until dates are blended. Add in more water, if needed, and process again.

4) Pour into custard cups. Put a few raisins in each cup with a dusting of
   cinnamon powder. Let set in the refrigerator for 1 hour before serving.

   Makes 7 custard cups. Keeps for 3 days in the refrigerator.

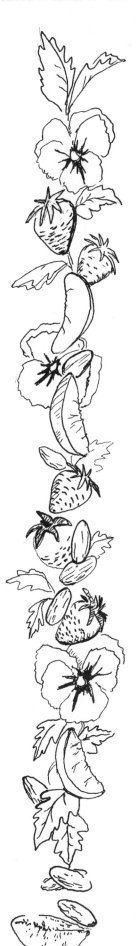

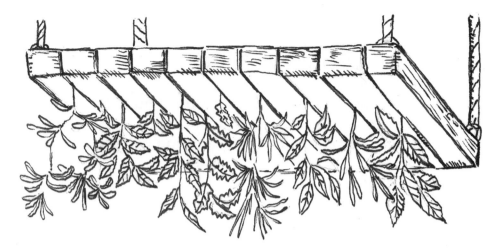

CHAPTER THIRTY:
Spice Blends From Scratch

SPICE WORLD

Looking at spices and inhaling their mysterious aromas has always conjured up, for me, an exotic world lush with tempting possibilities.

I've included these recipes for those who have the time and inclination, for those who may get inspired and want to create their own "from-scratch" blends, and for professional chefs who may wish to experiment with some of the ideas in this book. Spice blends last a good year before needing to be replaced.

Most of these blends can be purchased. Some store-bought items, however, may have been toasted or roasted (like garam masalas, for example). Also be aware that many spices have been irradiated, so look for the words "non-irradiated" on the label.

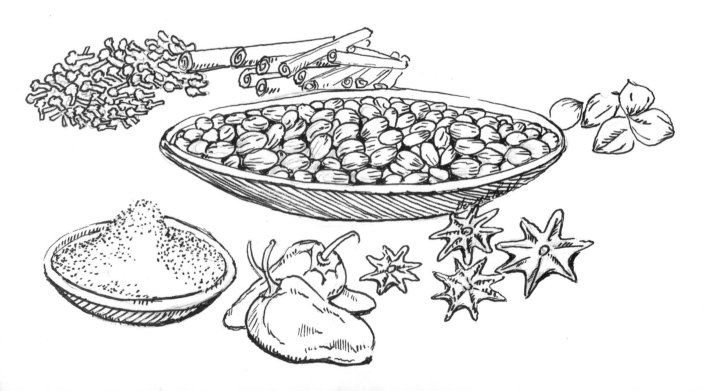

GARAM MASALA
(Hot & Spicy)

It's best to make Garam Masala yourself because the prepared Garam Masala you buy may be roasted. Use raw ingredients as follows:

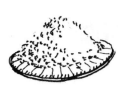

1/2 cup green cardamom pods
1/4 cup coriander seeds
1/4 cup whole cloves
1/4 cup cumin seeds
1/4 cup white peppercorns
3 three-inch cinnamon sticks*

1) Grind all the ingredients in a blender or nut grinder and blend well. If you use a blender, put the cinnamon sticks into a paper bag first and hammer them a little (because they can be very hard) before putting into the blender with the other ingredients.

2) Keeps for one year in a dark glass container. Best kept in a cool, dark place. Try to find the coolest place in your kitchen to store spices; a pantry is ideal.

NOTE: You can make a milder Masala by doubling the amount of coriander and cumin.

*If you can get the Mexican cinnamon, which is long and very soft, use 1 ground tbsp.

HERBS DE PROVENCE

1) Grind to a powder 1 tbsp. of each of the following:

basil	**oregano**
fennel	**rosemary**
lavender	**savory**
marjoram	**thyme**

2) Keep in a glass jar in a cool, dark place.

Makes approx. 4 oz.

JAMAICAN JERK SEASONING

1 tsp. ground allspice   **1/2 tsp. ground white pepper**
1 tsp. garlic powder   **1/2 tsp. cayenne**
1 tsp. dried thyme   **1/4 scant tsp. ground nutmeg**
1/2 tsp. cinnamon

1) In a small bowl combine all the ingredients. Store in a dark glass jar in a cool place. **Always add 1 tsp. honey per tbsp. of this seasoning when preparing a recipe.**

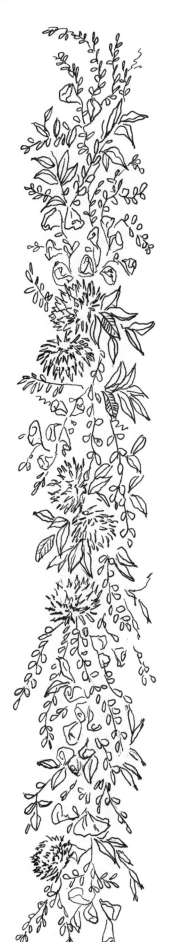

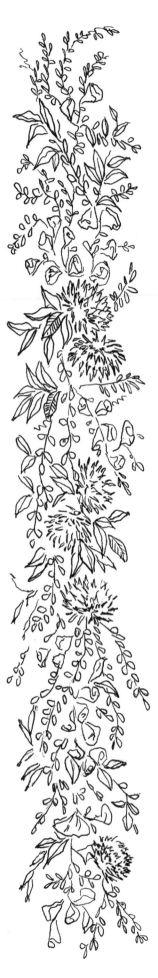

RED BELL PEPPER POWDER

5 red bell peppers

1) Cut out the stems and core the peppers but leave half of the seeds. Coarsely chop the peppers and put into the food processor. Process to a mush utilizing the "S" blade.

2) Spread the pepper mush on a Teflex-lined dehydrator tray, as if it were a fruit leather. Spread it out with the back of a spoon to 1/8 to 1/4" thickness. Set dehydrator to 95° F. Dehydrate until dry (1 1/2 to 2 days). Two thirds of the way through the drying process, peel the pepper sheet off of the Teflex, turn it over and place it directly onto the mesh dehydrator tray to continue drying.

3) When completely dry, grind to a fine powder in a nut or coffee grinder. This gives you 4 oz. of red bell pepper powder. This red bell pepper powder will compact after a while (which does not allow you to sprinkle it), but you can break it up with a fork and then measure out the amount you want. The fact that it compacts does not damage it in any way, and in fact, you will be able to tell it's good by the aroma. It smells great! The best way to store red bell pepper powder is to put it into a glass jar with a mouth wide enough to insert a spoon. Store in a cool place at room temperature. Keeps for a very long time. Once it loses its fragrance, toss out the powder and make another batch.

NOTE: I have not found red bell pepper powder in the stores, except for some herb shops. Paprika doesn't have the same flavor. Frontier Herbs sells red and green bell pepper flakes, which you can grind to a powder, but this could be expensive. Since I find red bell pepper powder to be such a good flavoring ingredient, once a year I buy a large amount of red bell peppers, dehydrate them all, then grind them to a powder as needed. Then I have plenty for the year. Extra bell peppers from my garden also get dehydrated. You can also purchase dried, diced red bell peppers from the Sunorganic Farm mail order catalog (*see* Source Index), and grind them to a powder.

"ORGANIC VEGETABLE MIX"

Available from Sunorganic Farm's mail order catalog. This mix of organic, low-heat dehydrated vegetables* is delicious as a quick soup, or when ground, as a flavorful seasoning for many dishes.

VEGETABLE SEASONING & BROTH

1 cup organic Vegetable Mix* (from Sunorganic Farm—
see Source Index)

1) In a coffee or nut grinder, grind the Vegetable Mix to a powder. Store in a glass jar in a cool and dark place.

*Contains organic celery, broccoli florets, mushrooms, carrots, spinach flakes, parsley and tomatoes.

INDIAN SPICE SEASONING

6 tbsp. ground *Dehydrated Lime***
4 tbsp. ground cumin
2 tbsp. ground coriander
2 tbsp. curry powder
2 tbsp. turmeric
2 tbsp. paprika
2 tbsp. cinnamon (use Mexican cinnamon if you
can find it)
1/4 tsp. ground nutmeg

1) In a small bowl mix all the ingredients.

Yield: 1 cup. Store in a dark amber bottle in a cool place. Keeps for up to 1 year.

**DEHYDRATED LIME: Thinly slice 5 organic limes and place them on the mesh dehydrator tray. Dehydrate at 100° F for 2 to 3 days, or until thoroughly dry. After letting them cool, store in an airtight container at room temperature. Grind as needed.

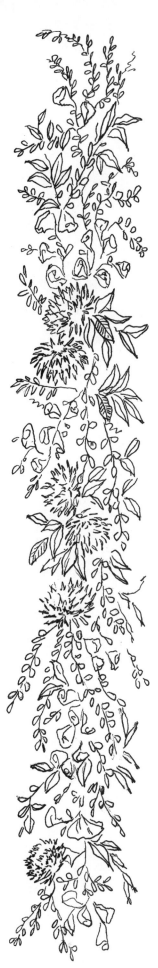

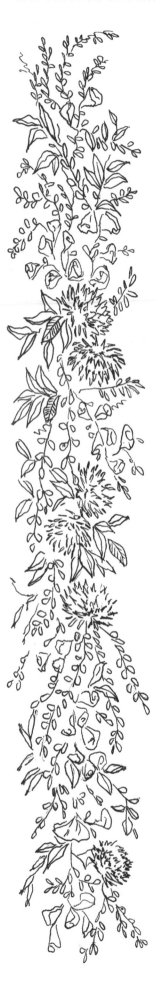

CHAT MASALA

3 tsp. amchoor (dried, unripe, mango powder)—can
    be found in a store that sells products from India
1 1/2 tsp. cumin seed
1/2 tsp. white pepper
1/2 tsp. ginger powder
1/2 tsp. cayenne pepper
1/4 tsp. asafoetida
1/8 scant tsp. dried mint flakes
1 tsp. Celtic sea salt

1) Grind all the ingredients in a coffee or nut grinder. Transfer to a bowl and mix well with a spoon.

Store in a dark glass container in the coolest spot in your kitchen. It will keep for approx. 1 year.

ITALIAN SEASONING

1) In a nut mill, grind to a powder 2 tbsp. of each of the following:

basil	bay leaves
celery seed	cinnamon
cloves	parsley seed
rosehips and seeds	white peppercorns
cayenne pepper	

(for a milder version, use 1, instead of 2, tbsp. of cayenne)

2) After grinding, mix together well and store in an amber-colored bottle in a cool place.

NOTE: You will be able to find most of the ingredients in a good herb shop. The one ingredient you might not be able to locate is parsley seed. I usually buy parsley seed from a seed supply house, which sells seeds for planting. **You must make absolutely certain, however, that the seed has not been treated in any way.** It would be best to buy organic seed. If you can't find parsley seed, leave it out.

DRIED LEMON & ORANGE ZEST

3 lemons
2 oranges

1) Use only undyed lemons and/or oranges. Peel the skin thinly and place the peelings on mesh dehydrator trays. Dehydrate at 95° F for approx. 2 days, or until thoroughly dry.

Store the lemon and orange zest separately in glass jars. Keep in a cool, dark place and grind as needed.

RED "HOT" SESAME OIL

8 oz. bottle sesame oil (Flora or Omega oils)
2 tsp. anatto seeds (look for them in Hispanic markets)
1/3 cup fresh hot chili peppers, habaneros or
**   jalapeños, minced**

1) Pour the bottle of sesame oil into a larger glass bottle. Add in anatto seeds and hot peppers. Let sit at room temperature for 4 hours, then refrigerator for 4 days.

2) Strain the oil (to remove the seeds and hot peppers) and rebottle. Keep it in the refrigerator and use it when you want to add a "hot" flavor to a dish. The anatto seeds impart a red color to the oil.

CREOLE SPICE

2 tbsp. Celtic sea salt   **1 tbsp. dried thyme**
2 tbsp. garlic powder   **1 tbsp. dried oregano**
2 1/2 tbsp. Hungarian paprika   **1 tbsp. cayenne**
1 1/2 tbsp. onion powder
2 tsp. ground white pepper

1) Grind the Celtic sea salt in a nut mill and measure out 2 tbsp. into a small bowl.

2) Add all the other spices and with a spoon, blend them well. Store in a dark glass container in a cool place.

Yield: 3/4 cup. Keeps for up to 1 year.

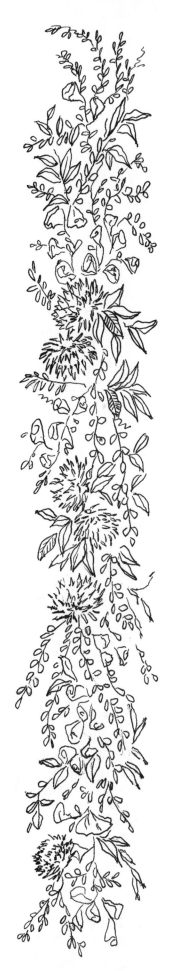

CHAPTER THIRTY-ONE:
Sample Menus

TIPS:

Take the time to plan your menus for each week. Make a shopping list of ingredients and save them in a permanent place. This way, you'll save time when you want to use the same menus again.

At least one weekend per month, prepare a variety of crackers, cookies and perhaps an Essene bread. Try to make enough to last the entire month. This economizes on your time and gives you lots of crunchies to eat. If you have children, try to get them involved in making these tasty treats. At the same time, make other things that you might want to use throughout the month, like *Pine Nut Parmezan* and *Prune Paste*. You might also freeze up some fruit for sherbets and prepare some ice cream mixes to freeze in ice cube trays. If you do this prep work once a month, then your daily preparation time is much shorter and easier.

If time is a major consideration, then use the menu plan every other day, or every third day, instead of every day. On the alternate days, substitute simpler menus made up of whole raw foods, such as fruits, soaked nuts and seeds, and vegetables, eaten plain or with avocados, nut butters, or quick dips.

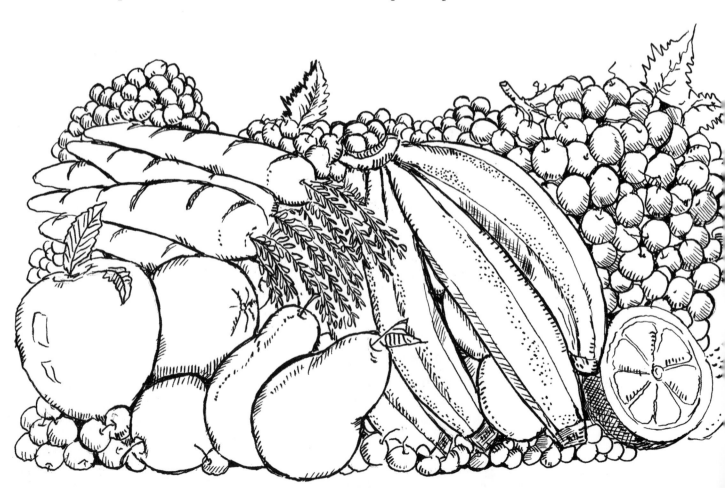

Breakfast each day starts with *Wheatgrass Juice* or a *Green Drink*, wait 1/2 hour, then *Fresh Fruit*, or *Hearty Buckwheat Porridge*, or *Great Nuts Cereal*, etc.

Lunch:	*Green Power Soup, Spinach Caesar*
Juice Break:	*Carrot Wallop*
Dinner:	*Toona, Crudité*

Lunch:	*Nori Rolls stuffed w/ Toona, sprouts, cucumber & tomato* *Gorgeous Greens Salad*
Juice Break:	*Cabbage-Tomato Delight*
Dinner:	*Lazy Man's Porto Pitza, Rainbow Super-Slaw*

Lunch:	*Leftover Rainbow Super-Slaw* *Leftover Marinated Collard Ribbons*
Juice Break:	*Melon Nectar*
Dinner:	*Indian Cole-Slaw, Spinach Salad—Indian Style*

Lunch:	*Watercress & Red Bell Pepper Salad, Jamie & Kim's* *Flaxseed Crackers with French lentil Tapenade*
Juice Break:	*Potassium Drink*
Dinner:	*Spicy Jamaican "Jerk" Veggies, Gorgeous Greens Salad*

Lunch:	*Borscht, Almond Yogurt,* *Tomatoes, Cucumbers, Avocados, Sprouts*
Juice Break:	*Jicama, Beet & Pear Juice*
Dinner:	*Curried Chick-Peas & Carrots* (use *Almond Yogurt* since you already have it) *Gorgeous Greens Salad*

Lunch:	*1 mango, 1 papaya & handful of soaked macadamias*
Juice Break:	*Fennelicious*
Dinner:	*Squaghetti w/Garlic & Oil, Fast & Tasty*

One day per week: Liquid Diet

SUGGESTIONS:

- *Coconut Water* from green water coconuts. Have a quart or two. OR
- *Organic Watermelon Juice,* including some of the green rind. Drink as much as you like. I like to drink the red and green juices separately. If you mix them together, the red juice will not taste as good. By keeping them separate, you can enjoy the flavor of the sweet red juice, and then take sips of the green juice also, which is full of chlorophyll.

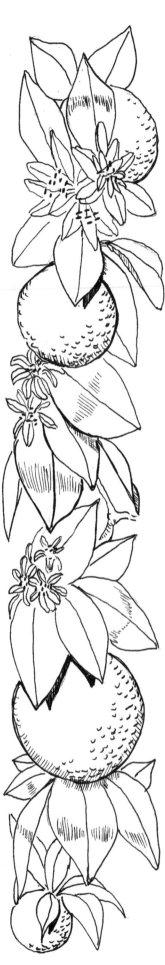

CHAPTER THIRTY-TWO:
A Few Kitchen Cosmetics

If you want the very best results for your face, hair and body, you'll make your own. Despite all the hype about cutting-edge products, most of them are made from toxic chemicals. Even many so-called natural products sold in health food stores contain toxic chemicals, additives and preservatives, or are contaminated with them in one way or another. If you want to learn the real low-down on the situation, please refer to a well-researched book on the subject entitled *Natural Organic Skin and Hair Care* by Aubrey Hampton.

Everything you put on your skin ends up in your bloodstream. People don't seem to believe this, because we've all been taught that the skin is a barrier. But think about it; how else could an insulin patch or any other kind of patch that delivers drugs into the system work? The substances get absorbed through the skin and into the blood, and the blood goes everywhere in the body, including into the brain. This is why I recommend that only truly natural products be used on the skin.

Retin-A has proven to be valuable as a face peel which, over time, shows impressive results in lessening deep facial wrinkles, but what are the potential effects on your health? And, why use something which could be a potential risk, when there are so many, many choices you could make to get the same effects without risk, such as the alpha-hydroxy acids derived from apples, grapes, citrus, and soured milk? Just the fresh juice from apples, grapes or citrus (citrus, only if your skin can handle it) patted onto the skin every evening will do the same thing over time, and without any potential side effects whatsoever.

Following are a few of my favorite kitchen cosmetic recipes. For more extensive ideas, information and recipes, please refer to the many excellent books on the subject.

---

[1]Retin-A, a vitamin A derivative, is synthetically produced. It also contains other additives, such as stearic acid, isopropyl myristate, butylated hydroxytoluene, polyoxyl 40 stearate, stearyl alcohol, etc.

BREWERS YEAST MASK

This mask brings the blood up to the face and really softens the fine lines around the eyes over time. It also tightens the skin. After using it, you will have roses in your cheeks for a while.

> **1 heaping tbsp. Kal unfortified, imported yeast (Saccharomyces Cerevisiae)**
> **1 drop wheat germ oil***
> **approx. 2–3 tbsp. filtered water**

1) Transfer some wheat germ oil to a dropper bottle. (These are obtainable at drug stores.) Keep the oil in the refrigerator.

2) Mix all the ingredients together to make a spreadable paste. You may have to add more or less water.

3) Spread this mask over the face and neck and let dry for approx. 45 minutes to an hour.** It will feel kind of tingly at first. While the mask is drying, you can lie down and relax or just go about your household chores.

4) To remove, rinse gently with tepid water using a washcloth. Pat dry and apply a thin layer of olive and peanut oil (mixed).

NOTE: A double or triple portion can be made ahead as it keeps for up to a week in the refrigerator.

* If you put in too much oil, then you get a mask that flakes off and won't tighten the skin.

** You could also leave this mask on for 1, 2 or 3 hours, if it doesn't bother you. Sometimes I just put it around my eyes (look like a raccoon) and sleep with it. It smoothes out the fine laugh lines. **Caution: Do a test first on a tiny section of skin to make sure you are not sensitive or allergic.**

WILLARD WATER FACIAL MIST

> **dark or clear Willard Water**
> **(see Glossary & Source Index)**
> **distilled water**

1) Prepare Willard Water according to the directions on the label. Dilute this prepared Willard Water again by mixing 1/2 Willard Water and 1/2 filtered water. Put this mixture into a small spray bottle.

2) Spray onto the skin after applying moisturizer and anytime throughout the day to refresh the skin. Does not need refrigeration.

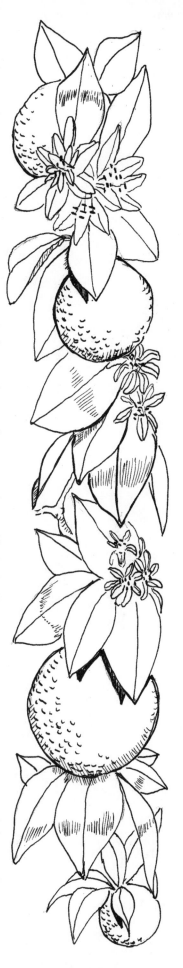

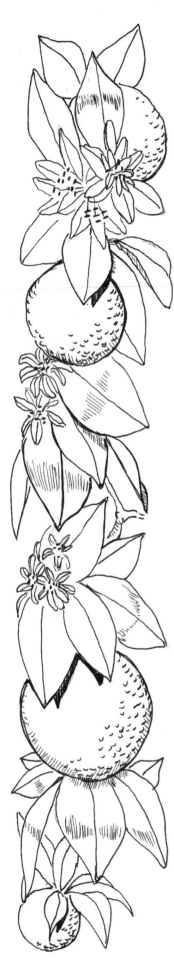

GREEN OLIVE MOISTURIZER/TONER

8 oz. piccholine olives

1) Pit the olives. Put the pitted olives into a bowl and cover with distilled water. This is to draw out the salt. Let them sit at room temperature for 15 hours.

2) Drain and rinse the olives well. Put the olives through a juicer to extract the olive juice, then strain the juice through a muslin cloth or bag. You now you have your *Green Olive Moisturizer/Toner*.

3) Use as a moisturizer/toner under makeup or for moisturizing before sleep, or anytime.

This keeps in the refrigerator for one month. Shake well before using.

NOTE: Olives contain an ingredient called squalene that is beneficial for the promotion of a healthy, beautiful skin. We produce about 10% squalene naturally in our sebum. Some cosmetic companies are adding squalene to their products, but they are getting the squalene from the Japanese, who are obtaining it from an endangered species of shark known as the Aizame. The sharks are killed and the squalene is then extracted from their liver. This seems to be a drastic way to get the same ingredient that olive trees offer to us freely. Olive trees have been known to live and produce for 1500 years! When the Aizame are gone, our planet will be irrevocably changed.

HOME-CURED GREEN OLIVE MOISTURIZER/TONER

This is similar to the previous recipe, except that, if you can get a hold of some raw green olives and home-cure them yourself, then the toner will have an even more tightening effect on the skin

12 oz. raw green olives*

1) Pit the olives, cover with distilled water and leave them at room temperature. Each day, change the water. At the end of approx. 15 days, the bitterness will be out of the olives. Rinse and drain well.

2) Put the olives through a juicer to extract the olive juice, then strain the juice through a muslin cloth. You now have your moisturizer/toner. This keeps in the refrigerator for one month or longer. Shake well before using.

Use as a moisturizer/toner under makeup or for moisturizing before sleep.

* Green olives, which are unripe olives, produce the skin-tightening effect. Ripe olives do not have this property.

MOISTURIZERS FROM FRUITS

You can find any number of excellent facial moisturizers in fresh fruits. Those which I've found to be excellent are fresh apple juice and grape juice. The grape moisturizer is very easy to prepare. Just take a grape, squish a little juice out of it and pat this onto the skin. One or two grapes should do it. With apples; grate approximately 1/4 of an apple on a fine grater and then put the pulp through a sieve. Pat the juice onto the face and let dry naturally. These two work very well for my skin type (which is not too dry and not too oily), but you can experiment with other fruits, such as the citrus family, which I've heard are good for oily skin.

Fruit moisturizers can be used in place of commercially prepared moisturizers. Give them a try. They are cheap, yes. . . but only in cost. Their value to the beauty of your skin cannot be beat. Most of what you pay for in fancy moisturizers is the advertising and the packaging anyway.

OATMEAL MASK
For Dry Skin

1/2 cup dry oatmeal, ground
2 tbsp. aloe vera gel*
1 tbsp. raw, unheated honey
1 tsp. raw apple cider vinegar
filtered water, enough to make a paste

1) Put all the ingredients into a bowl and stir with a spoon to blend well.

2) You may have to add more water or more ground oatmeal, to make a spreadable paste.

3) Spread evenly over the face and neck, even under the eyes. Let dry for 45 minutes to an hour. Rinse off with a washcloth and tepid water. Spread a thin layer of a combination of olive and peanut oil over the skin. Spray skin with *Willard Water Facial Mist* (*see* page 297).

*For best results, use fresh aloe vera leaf. Cut open the leaf and scoop out 2 tbsp. of gel. If you can't find the leaf, then look for an additive-free gel at your health food store.

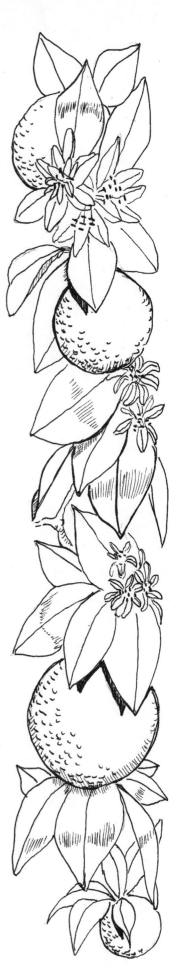

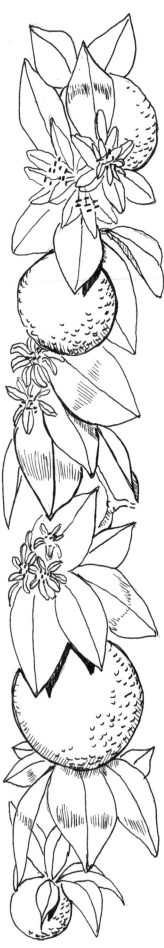

SEAWEED MASK

This mask tightens the skin, refines the
pores, and makes wrinkles seem to disappear

**1/4 cup. wakame (soak in water 5 minutes,
then drain)
3 tbsp. agar-agar flakes
1 3/4 cup filtered water**

1) Put all ingredients into a glass cooking pot with 1 3/4 cup filtered water and bring to a gentle simmer, until the agar-agar is dissolved. This takes approx. 3 to 5 minutes. (The wakame will soften but not dissolve.)

2) Take the mixture off the stove and let it cool down for a couple of hours, until it gels. Then put it into a blender and blend to a soft gel-like consistency. You may have to add a little water, but don't add too much. Then put the blended mixture into a glass jar and store in the refrigerator.

   Keeps for one month or longer. Sometimes a white film forms over the top; just scrape this off and discard. It will still be green and ready to use underneath.

3) **To use:** Spread a thin layer over your face and neck, and let dry for approx. 45 minutes to an hour. It is safe to use under the eyes. After it dries on the skin, rinse off with tepid water and apply *Green Olive Moisturizer/Toner* (*see* page 298). Let it dry. Then spray with *Willard Water Facial Mist* (*see* page 297). This locks the moisture into your skin. If you don't have an hour to devote to it, you can leave the mask on for 20 to 30 minutes, and even though it may not be dry when you rinse it off, it will still give your skin a very clean, refreshed look.

NATURAL DEODORANTS

The skin is the largest organ of elimination. Deodorants, and particularly anti-perspirants, interfere with the body's ability to purge toxins. When an anti-perspirant, as its name clearly implies, prevents you from perspiring, the toxins that would have been released don't just disappear. Instead, they are deposited into lymph nodes below the armpits. In time there is a buildup. Could this be one of the reasons for the high incidence of breast cancer among women? (Breast cancer tumors frequently occur in the upper outside quadrant of the breast area where the lymph nodes are located.) Men who use anti-perspirants are less likely to get a buildup of toxins because most of the anti-perspirant applied gets caught in their underarm hair.

Most deodorants and anti-perspirants also contain aluminum, which is something that we don't want to absorb into the body.

1) Apple Cider Vinegar makes an excellent deodorant. You only smell like a salad for about 2 minutes! I keep a small bottle in the bathroom. After bathing, I splash or spray the vinegar under my arms. Or you can saturate a small cotton pad and dab it under the arms. I like spraying best. Of course, do not use the vinegar after you've just shaved. Ouch! I know that for women, who have sparse underarm hair, the vinegar works well. I have not had enough men willing to test it though, so I can't say how it will work for men, who generally have more underarm hair.

2) Some of the liquid colloidal mineral products available, such as Toxoid Formula, or Willard Water, a unique catalyst-altered water (*see* Source Index), may also serve as effective deodorants.

3) A tablespoon of sprouted fenugreek seeds, eaten every day, is said to be a natural deodorant. After eating these seeds for a period of time, you will have a very pleasant, subtle odor emanating from your skin—your own natural perfume.

LEIGH'S HOMEMADE TOOTHPASTE

1/2 cup white clay (edible)
2–3 tbsp. Celtic sea salt
2 tbsp. vegetable glycerin
5 drops peppermint oil
4–5 tbsp. (or more) filtered water

1) Put all ingredients into a small glass bowl and add water to make a very thick paste. Stir well. At this point, you can adjust the thickness—if the consistency is too loose, add in more clay; if too stiff, add in more water.

Yield: 1/2 cup. Keep in a small jar in the bathroom.

NOTE: Why does toothpaste have to be used at all? Why not just clean the teeth with water and a brush only? Once you've been on a high-raw diet for a period of time, you will find this option very satisfactory. Typical morning bad breath will be a thing of the past.

You might want to brush with something because you want to maintain your teeth white. Highly colored fruits and vegetables have a tendency to stain the teeth. A suggestion is to rinse the mouth after eating. Also, I recommend Peelu Dental Fibers[1], a powdered tooth cleanser which gently whitens the teeth over time.

---

[1] Peelu is made from the microfibers, resins and cleansing compounds of the Salvadora Persica Tree.

GLOSSARY

ACID/ALKALINE BALANCE

(*See* Chapter 5, "Is Aging Inevitable?")

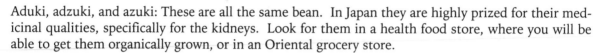

ADUKI

Aduki, adzuki, and azuki: These are all the same bean. In Japan they are highly prized for their medicinal qualities, specifically for the kidneys. Look for them in a health food store, where you will be able to get them organically grown, or in an Oriental grocery store.

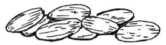

ALMONDS

Almonds are one of the nuts that have an alkaline reaction in the body. Many nuts produce an acid reaction in the body, which is not to say we can't use them, but we must be aware of the 80/20 principle. Try to have your diet composed of 80% alkaline producing foods and 20% acid producing foods.

Since 2009, almonds in the US are required by law to be either pasteurized or treated with a toxic fumigant called ethylene oxide. Truly raw almonds can only be purchased at a farmer's market or directly at the farm.

ALMOND SPROUTS:

When sprouting almonds, soak overnight, and sprout for 1 or 2 days. You will not be able to see the actual sprout unless you remove the skin, and then you will see it very clearly. Store them in the refrigerator in filtered water and change the water every two days to prevent fermentation. Keeps for up to a week.

DEHYDRATED ALMOND SPROUTS:

Soak and sprout almonds, then blanch (*see* below). Put the blanched almonds into the food dehydrator, set to 95° F. Remove when they are thoroughly dry, approximately 2 days. These can be used as a "crunchy" snack, also try the *Too Much Crunch* recipe.

BLANCHED ALMONDS:

To blanch almonds (without cooking them), first prepare a large bowl of cold water into which you have added two trays of ice cubes. Then heat up some other water to a boil, turn off the flame, and put in the sprouted almonds for 7 seconds. Time the 7 seconds, and **stay with the pot**. If you move away to do something else, you might not come back to your almonds in 7 seconds, and then you will have cooked them. Drain the almonds quickly through a strainer and plunge the strainer into the ice water. This stops the process of cooking immediately. The almond skins will then pop off easily when you push them between your thumb and forefinger.*

* If you see that the almond skins pop, after just soaking them, then you can be sure that you, unfortunately, have purchased treated almonds.

WHY IS IT NECESSARY TO REMOVE ALMOND SKINS?

Almond skins have a high concentration of tannic acid. Research has indicated that tannic acid may interfere with the body's uptake of iron. When you eat a lot of almonds, it might be a good idea to remove the skins. (If you are just having a handful, then you don't need to skin them.) The Merck Index states that tannic acid is highly soluble in water. Once the almonds have been soaked, I suspect a lot of the acid is leached out, but I have not had my theory tested.

REMOVING ALMOND SKINS WITHOUT BLANCHING

Almond skins can also be removed, without blanching, by peeling sprouted almonds with your thumbnail. This is a tedious process which most people will probably not do; however, this is the way it's done at the Ann Wigmore Institute. If you're going to remove the skins this way, a tip is to soak the sprouted almonds in filtered water for 24 hours (in the refrigerator). This loosens the skins and makes the job a little easier.

APPLE CIDER VINEGAR

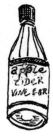

Always look for raw, unpasteurized, apple cider vinegar, made from **whole** apples. Apple cider vinegar is the only vinegar I recommend. None of the other vinegars that I know of are available raw. Apple cider vinegar contains beneficial malic acid, and when used judiciously, has many positive effects. It also contains minerals, including an extraordinary amount of potassium, which helps the system to achieve harmony and calm. Apple cider vinegar is antiseptic, and anti-inflammatory. It improves digestion by stimulating the secretion of digestive juices. Even though vinegar acts as a preservative, once opened, I like to store it in the refrigerator.

ASAFOETIDA

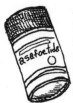

Asafoetida is a strong smelling (some say foul-smelling), resinous exudation from a plant that is a member of the carrot family. Its odor derives from acrid sulfur compounds, called mercaptans. (I like the way it smells though—kind of stinky, but mysterious too.) It tastes something like onions and garlic and is much used in Indian and Iranian cuisines. A pinch is all that is needed. It can be obtained in powder form in a health food store or in Indian grocery stores.

BALSAMIC VINEGAR

Balsamic vinegar is a wonderfully flavorful vinegar. It is seldom used in the living foods lifestyle, however, because all vinegars, except apple cider vinegar, have been found to negatively impact red blood cells. Balsamic vinegar also contains naturally occurring sulfites. Severe reactions can occur in sensitive individuals when they ingest sulfites.

BANANAS

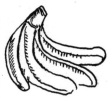

The banana is one of our most popular fruits. In the USA, the most prevalent type of banana, the Cavendish (commonly sold everywhere) should be speckled with black dots before it is eaten. This indicates that the starch has turned to sugar and then the banana is a lot easier to digest and more nutritious. In Puerto Rico, however, I've seen many kinds of native bananas ripen without speckling. I don't know what accounts for the difference. Since bananas are picked when green, they are treated with ethylene gas to ripen them. I've read that this process causes the bananas to speckle. I've seen supposedly untreated bananas, however, also develop speckling.

The bananas of today are not the bananas of my childhood. I remember, as a child, that the bananas had many tiny black seeds all through the center of the fruit. These bananas had a full, rich banana flavor. Our bananas now, which most people eat while the skin is still yellow, do not compare to them. While we weren't looking, somebody stole the seeds—and the flavor. Hybridization was again carried to an extreme.

BARLEY

Three kinds of barley are generally available; pearled barley, hulled barley and unhulled barley. Pearled barley has been refined (not recommended). Hulled barley is unrefined and can be used in recipes, after soaking and sprouting. It will develop a little sprout, but will not grow into grass. Unhulled barley is used for growing barley grass.

BRAGG LIQUID AMINOS

This is a liquid amino acid product made from soybeans. It is not fermented. It was developed by Paul Bragg, a pioneer in the health field. Bragg Liquid Aminos is high in naturally occurring sodium, so use it sparingly. Some of the guest recipes include Bragg as an ingredient, but try to wean yourself off it if you can, or learn to use as little as possible. A good way to do this is to put it into a spray bottle and lightly spray onto the food as needed.

I used to use Bragg myself but, in the last year, switched to other forms of seasoning. My reason is that Bragg will not commit to using only organically grown soybeans. When you speak to Patricia Bragg or other representatives of the company (as I have done), they say that they use only organically grown soybeans or transitional soybeans. If that is true, then I see no reason why they cannot state it clearly on the label, which they refuse to do. The question of whether the soybeans used in Bragg are grown with pesticides, herbicides, insecticides and fungicides, while of concern, is not so important to me as the question of whether the soybeans used are genetically engineered. In the past I could live with the fact that perhaps Bragg wasn't organic. If all the rest of my meal was organically grown and then I seasoned it with a tsp. of Bragg, I did not find that ratio too objectionable. But for me, consuming a product of genetic engineering is another matter (*see* Chapter 9, "Frankenfoods: Biotechnology and Genetically Engineered Foods"). At this time, the only way to know for sure that you are not eating genetically engineered products is to verify that the label reads "organic" or "organically grown."

Another objection that many raw fooders have voiced about Bragg is that it may be produced using chemicals. Information about the process is couched in secrecy, since it is considered proprietary. The issue of whether Bragg contains monosodium glutamate (MSG) has never been cleared up either. At one time, the label stated "NO MSG," but they dropped that designation. I've seen some independent test results, which were inconclusive because the test did not distinguish between free glutamic acid (an amino acid needed by the body) and glutamates.

BUCKWHEAT

Botanically, buckwheat is not a cereal grain because it belongs to a different family (Polygonaceae instead of Gramineae). Practically though, it's considered to be in the grain category because it looks like a grain, it tastes like a grain, and it can be used like a grain. When you buy buckwheat, look for raw buckwheat groats or whole buckwheat groats. Buckwheat that has been roasted is known as Kasha.

CANOLA OIL

I am convinced that canola oil is not a favorable oil for the body. First of all, unlike first-pressed, extra virgin olive oil, it has not withstood the test of time. Canola used to be called rapeseed and was found to be toxic to pigs. Then apparently, it was renamed and repackaged for humans. I am also suspicious of its quality because, when I go to the supermarket and find the cheapest oils available (whose label simply reads "vegetable oil"), many times canola oil is the ingredient listed. (Other oils sold under the "vegetable oil" catchall are cottonseed and soybean oils. Cottonseed oil is not beneficial either. Since cotton is not grown primarily as a food crop, huge amounts of pesticides are allowed to be sprayed on this plant, much higher than are allowed on "food" plants. Cotton by-products do, however, end up in the food supply in the form of oil and as feed for animals, which are then consumed by humans. Soybean oil is not recommended because a large percentage of soybeans are now grown from genetically engineered seeds.)

Most canola is grown using genetically engineered seeds. According to researchers at the Laboratory of Comparative Invertebrate Neurobiology in France, early results of a three-year study showed that genetically altered rapeseed plants were lethal to insects feeding on them. As reported in "Healthy & Natural Journal," April 1998, "bees fed a sugar solution made with the altered plants died 15 days earlier than did bees fed on normal sugar solutions. Rapeseed is particularly important to bees since it is the first plant to bloom in the Spring."

CAPERS

Capers are the immature flower buds of a Mediterranean shrub that have been pickled. To get some of the salt out of prepared capers, soak the portion you are going to use overnight in distilled water.

CAROB POWDER

Carob, sometimes called St. John's Bread, is the fruit of an evergreen tree which can grow to heights of almost 50 feet. Straight from the tree, the fruit looks like a big brown pod. After harvest, it is dried and powdered. Be careful to purchase it raw, because it is generally roasted. Carob has a flavor similar to chocolate, but without all the negative effects of chocolate. Of course, chocolate aficionados are not going to be convinced, but if you *want* to switch, this is a good substitute and you can learn to like it very much. Carob contains Vitamin A and B-complex, minerals, proteins and carbohydrates. Raw carob is not generally available in health food stores so you must send for it by mail. Sunorganic Farm carries it (*see* Source Index).

 ## CASHEW NUTS

"Raw" cashew nuts are cooked. When you go to buy cashews you will find that some are classified as raw, but they are not raw because of the processing they have undergone to remove the nut from the shell. The cashew nut has a double shell, and between the two shells there is a toxic liquid which most processors burn off, cooking the cashew in the process. Then the interior shell (which is really a skin) is removed. You can get the story in almost any good encyclopedia.

"Raw" cashews are classified as "raw" to distinguish them from roasted cashews. Roasted cashews, of course, have been cooked again. A good substitute for cashews is pine nuts, macadamias, or pecans.

TRULY RAW CASHEWS ARE AVAILABLE, BUT NOT ON THE US MAINLAND

Jeremy Safron, co-author of *The Raw Truth*, told me that in Hawaii and other parts of the world, like India and Ecuador, there is a natural way to process the cashew nut so you end up with a truly raw cashew. Jeremy, who lives in Hawaii when he's not traveling and lecturing on living foods, says that he has used this method himself. After harvesting the cashews, the nuts are placed on tarps on the ground and then allowed to sit in the hot sun for 1 to 2 weeks, which dries up the toxic liquid between the outer shell and inner skin. The inner skin is then peeled off, releasing the nut and the nuts are then put into the sun again to cure for a few days. Result: Raw, viable nuts. Unfortunately, these cashew nuts are not available on the US mainland.

CELERY ROOT

In the United States we are not too familiar with celery root (aka celeriac). People think it has a harsh taste (maybe, because of its appearance, as it is big, gnarled and kind of rough), but it really is very pleasant and mild tasting. Give it a try.

My father checked himself out of a hospital once, over the objection of the doctors, when his body swelled up because they had injected him with a drug, to which he was allergic. He thought he would do better on his own; so he came home and made celery root soup, because he had read it would help pass kidney stones. Sure enough; in short order, the kidney stones came out as gravel. Hippocrates said "Let your food be your medicine."

CELTIC SEA SALT
(pronounced Keltic)

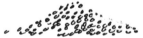

This salt is harvested from the ocean in a 9,000-acre pristine area of Brittany, in northwestern France. The area has been protected by the French government as a historical site so that the ancient traditions can be preserved for future generations.

To produce the salt, ocean water is channeled into a series of shallow ponds. The sun and wind evaporate the water, leaving a mineral-rich brine. The salt farmers (known as paludiers) then hand rake the brine with wooden tools, and within hours, crystals form and are gathered by hand. The method used for the whole process is a 2000-year-old tradition in Brittany. This salt is unheated and unrefined. It is light gray in color and moist to the touch. It consists of 14% trace mineral elements and 84% sodium chloride. Refined table salt by contrast contains 97.5% sodium chloride and no trace minerals.

There are three Celtic salts available. The Light Grey Celtic salt (also called Celtic Grey Sea Minerals) and the Flower of the Ocean are sun-dried and unheated. **Caution: The Fine Ground Celtic sea salt has been heated to 200° F** before grinding on natural granite stones. I would not recommend this one. The Light Grey Celtic sea salt can be put into a coffee/nut grinder to grind it. Of course, it will not pour, but we can accustom ourselves to the difference. You could measure out what you want with a spoon or take a pinch between your fingers to sprinkle. (*See* "The Grain & Salt Society" in the Source Index.)

When you eat seaweed, there is sea salt in it. I believe that using small quantities of unrefined Celtic sea salt is OK. Individualities come into play here and some people cannot handle any salt, unrefined or not. (It is best **not** to use salt if you have a health "challenge.") Celtic salt is the only sea salt I have researched at this time. Great care is taken in its production. There are other sea salts around, but I would not use them. First, I do not know how they are produced and secondly, they are very white, which makes me suspicious.

CHIA SEED

Chia is an ancient seed which was treasured by the Incas for producing endurance. It was also favored by the Southwestern Native Americans, as food and medicine. It is the seed of a common, rough, sage plant, which is high in protein (24%), omega 3 and fiber. In order for it to sprout, you must obtain it very fresh. Since it is not very popular now, it tends to hang around health food stores for long periods of time. Mail order is best.

COCONUTS

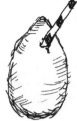

In the United States, you will usually find only brown coconuts for sale. In some states, in the Hispanic communities, you can find what is known as a **green or yellow water coconut**, so called because it has a lot of water inside, sometimes more than a pint. This water is known to be excellent for cleansing the kidneys. I have fasted on this water for many days with good effect. In Puerto Rico, everywhere you go, vendors sell chilled "Agua de Coco" (coconut water). They hack off the top with a machete and put a straw in it. Mmm . . . after the first sip, you feel so refreshed!

Inform yourself as to how a really fresh brown coconut should taste. You can usually tell by the water inside the coconut, sometimes called coconut milk. (For the purpose of this book, I'm calling it coconut water.) If the water tastes soapy or sour, then the coconut is old. If the water tastes fresh and slightly sweet or neutral, then it's good. In very young coconuts, the coconut meat is soft like custard. In slightly older coconuts, the meat is of a soft rubber consistency, not hard like we usually see here in the USA. A younger coconut has a lighter brown shell (not dark). You really have to be careful about getting coconuts which are still good, because most supermarkets and fruit vendors do not refrigerate coconuts, and they need to be refrigerated.[1]

Since the early 1960s, dried, shredded coconut sold in stores has been submitted to pasteurization. The coconut industry,[2] following the pattern of the dairy industry, made this decision to "protect the public." The only thing they really protected however, is their own commercial interests; because blanched, pasteurized, dried coconut will stay on the supermarket shelves indefinitely, without spoiling. It is very easy to dehydrate your own *Dried Coconut Shreds* (*see* page 263).

The United States is not a heavy coconut-consuming nation. People in places like India, Thailand, the Philippines, Indonesia and Malaysia consume a lot more coconuts than we do and consider them an important food in their diet. Of course, the coconuts grow right there, because the climate is right.

I think one reason we don't value the coconut is because of our obsession with being thin in this country. We somehow think coconuts are fattening. While coconuts do contain a high percentage of fat, you couldn't eat enough in any one recipe to put on fat. (The ice creams, made with coconut cream, might be an exception, **if you overdo.**)

COLD-PRESSED

WHAT SHOULD "COLD-PRESSED" REALLY MEAN?

When you go to the health food store and look in the oils section, you may see a lot of oils labeled as cold-pressed. But most, if not all, of those oils are not really cold-pressed. Cold-pressed should mean that the oil was extracted in such a way that it was not subjected to heat, and additionally, that heat was not generated in the process of the oil being extracted. If a little heat **is** generated, it should be **below** the temperature at which the value of the oil is destroyed. **Genuinely** cold pressed oils have all their nutritional value intact, including enzymes, Omega 3's and 6's, and other known and unknown factors. These oils must be refrigerated to preserve their freshness.

IN PRACTICE, WHAT DOES COLD-PRESSED MEAN?

Most cold-pressed oils have been heat treated. Seeds that are going to be mechanically pressed are usually cooked first to increase their yield. This means they are heated to 248° F for up to two hours. This

---

[1]They do look very hardy; maybe if they were perceived to be perishable like lettuce, they would be refrigerated.

[2]*A Century of Coconuts* by Andrew M. Hay. New York: Calvert, Vavasseur & Co., Inc.,1972.

process cracks the seed, exposing the oils to air and light, which cause oxidation. The oil is then extracted by squeezing the cooked seeds with screw presses, which generate heat again (approximately 185° to 203° F). These oils are sold as unrefined, but, as you can see, they have gone through at least two heat processes, which destroyed their nutritional value. Such heated oils are detrimental to your health because most of their fatty acids have been converted from the natural cis fatty acid form (present in unheated oil) to trans fatty acids, which are toxic and have been implicated as a causative factor in heart disease and cancer. (For more information on oils, *see* Chapter 11, "A Little Controversy.")

The avoidance of all heated oils is strongly recommended. (For genuinely cold-pressed oils, *see* "Flora and Barleans" in the Source Index.)

CRANBERRY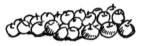

Always try to get organic cranberries where possible. Since the cranberry season is very short, I buy some extras and dehydrate them for occasional use in my recipes, during the rest of the year. Unfortunately, commercially dried cranberries usually have sugar, and sometimes oil, added to them.

CRUDITÉ

Crudité is a French term that refers to an appetizer made from a variety of raw vegetables that are cut into strips, sticks or bite-size pieces. A crudité is usually served with a dip or spread.

THE DEADLY WHITES

WHITE SUGAR	BAKING POWDER	WHITE OIL (processed-filtered-bleached)
WHITE FLOUR	ANIMAL FAT	
WHITE SALT	WHITE MEAT	PASTEURIZED DAIRY
WHITE BREAD	THE "OTHER" WHITE MEAT (pork)	WHITE DISTILLED VINEGAR
WHITE RICE		
CORNSTARCH	LARD	

The very first baby steps on the journey towards health are to eliminate ALL of the above. If you've been raised with these things, as I was, then you will have quite a time letting them go. If all this is new to you, you may have to take it one step at a time. Let one thing go. Substitute. Wait a while, and then let something else go. Substitute. Wait a while, etc. Or you could drop them all at once— it's up to you.

DIJON MUSTARD

Prepared Dijon mustard is formulated with grain vinegar and white wine vinegar. These vinegars are not beneficial to the body according to raw/live food guidelines (*see* listing for Apple Cider Vinegar in this section). The logical question then becomes: why do I use it? If I'm having a *Spinach Caesar Salad* for example, I will be eating a very large proportion of greens in relation to 1/2 tsp. of Dijon Mustard which is called for in the dressing. This salad serves two, so my ingestion of the mustard is 1/4 tsp. The touch of Dijon mustard flavor makes the salad very satisfying for me to eat. It may be a compromise that some "purists" are not willing to make and that's fine. They can just leave the ingredient out of the recipe. Tree of Life brand Dijon mustard uses organic wine vinegar (no grain vinegar) and the acetic acid percentage, as listed on their label, is 1.8%.

Others may object to the mustard seed in the Dijon mustard. I do not have any problem with this ingredient (*see* Chapter 11, under "Are Herbs and Spices Beneficial?")

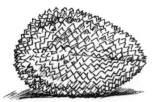

DURIAN

The durian fruit shows that Mother Nature has a sense of humor. It is most unusual in that it tastes like creamy custard, has a vivid yellow color and gives off the smell of dirty socks or stinky toes. If you can get over the smell, it's good eatin'.

GENETIC ENGINEERING OF FOOD

(See Chapter 9, "Frankenfoods: Biotechnology and Genetically Engineered Foods.")

GINGER

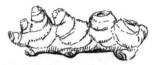

Ginger is a tropical herbaceous plant that yields a pungent, aromatic rhizome. It is used a lot in Oriental cooking.

If you need just a little ginger juice, squeeze cut-up ginger pieces through a garlic press. For more juice, you can use your juicer. I don't find it necessary to peel. Also, keep a small piece of ginger in your freezer—this makes it super easy to grate just a little bit into various dishes.

HIGH-RAW

High-Raw to me means a diet composed of 85-100% raw and living foods.

JERUSALEM ARTICHOKES

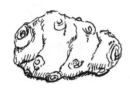

Jerusalem artichokes sometimes go by the name of sunchokes. This is a root vegetable in the sunflower family that is very easy to grow and looks somewhat like a knobby potato. If you put it in your garden once, it will come up year after year. When washing Jerusalem artichokes, be aware that soil can get trapped under the knobs. You can break the knobs off in order to clean out the soil.

JICAMA
(pronounced HEE-ka-mah)

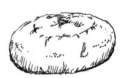

Jicama is a tuberous root vegetable in the legume family. It resembles a rock in appearance and tastes kind of like an apple, but not sweet. It has a refreshing flavor and is much used in Mexico. If you can't find it in your regular market, look for it in a Hispanic neighborhood produce store. Jicama needs to be peeled before using.

MISO
(pronounced MEE-soh)

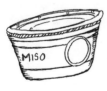

Miso is a pasty seasoning made by fermenting soybeans and sea salt (sometimes grains are also added) for at least 18 months, and up to 3 years. This is done by adding a culture to cooked soybeans. The end product, miso, is a storehouse of nutrients, such as protein, calcium, iron, B-vitamins including B-12, enzymes, and lactobacillus microorganisms. Miso also contains zybicolin, a substance first identified in 1972, which is an effective detoxifier and eliminator of radioactive elements[3] from the body.

---

[3]*Diet for the Atomic Age* by Sarah Shannon. Wayne, NJ: Avery Publishing, 1987.

Miso comes in different varieties and strengths, depending on the grains used and the fermentation time. In Japan, the making of miso is a centuries old tradition.

The important thing to remember, for the purpose of our recipes, is to only use organic, UNPASTEURIZED miso. This means that the miso, even though made with cooked soybeans in the first place, has not been recooked. (The culture that was added to the cooked beans, through the process of fermentation, processed the beans and created all that good stuff mentioned above. Not everyone agrees with this evaluation, however.)

The lighter, mellower misos, which have been fermented over a short term, have more lacto-bacillus activity than the darker, longer fermented misos.

See "Miso" in the Source Index.

MSG
(Monosodium Glutamate)

A white, crystalline, water-soluble powder used widely in the food industry to intensify the flavor of prepared foods. Glutamate is in a category of food additives, along with aspartate and hydrolyzed vegetable protein, known as excitotoxins. MSG is a powerful brain toxin which can produce neuron damage and death. "When neurons are exposed to these substances, they become very excited and fire their impulses very rapidly until they reach a state of extreme exhaustion. Several hours later these neurons suddenly die, as if the cells were excited to death."[4]

Chinese restaurants are notorious for using this additive. Some people get severe headaches from eating it. Other effects may include facial pressure, a burning sensation, nausea, and psychiatric reactions.

NAMA SHOYU

An organic, unpasteurized soy sauce, sold under the Ohsawa brand. It is generally available in health food stores. Even though this sauce is unpasteurized, initially the soy beans **are** cooked, before they are allowed to ferment. After the fermentation process, they are not cooked again, thus the claim that it is unpasterurized. In the fermentation process beneficial nutrients and enzymes are produced.

NUTRITIONAL YEAST FLAKES

This is not a raw product. I use it occasionally to impart a cheesy flavor to some dishes. Look for nutritional yeast flakes to which whey powder has not been added. We must also be vigilant in making sure that the manufacturers do not, in the future, use genetically modified organisms in its production.

OLIVES

The fruit of an evergreen tree grown chiefly in the Mediterranean and other warm regions. The fruit cannot be eaten as is, but must be cured in order to remove its bitterness. If you try to bite into a raw olive, as I did, you will quickly be dissuaded; it is terribly bitter. When some olives growing by the beach fell into the sand, it was accidentally discovered that soaking olives in sea water dispelled the bitterness.

---

[4]From *Excitotoxins—The Taste that Kills* by Russell L. Blaylock, M.D. Santa Fe, NM: Health Press, 1997.

Always purchase naturally processed olives; otherwise, they may have been treated with lye and other chemicals. Some distributors of naturally processed olives are Sunorganic Farm and Sun-Food (*see* Source Index).

HOW TO GET THE SALT OUT:

Soak olives in distilled water for a few hours to plump them up (which makes them easier to pit). Then put the olives through a cherry pitter. If you don't have a cherry pitter, pit them by hand. (The right cherry pitter saves a lot of time. I found mine in an antique store.) Remove the pits. Then once again, cover the olives with distilled water (distilled water draws minerals to it), and let sit at room temperature for 15 hours. Then drain and rinse them well. Yes, you will lose some of the flavor this way, but they are a lot healthier without all the salt.

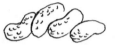

PEANUTS
(see "A Little Controversy", Chapter 11, page 79)

PECANS

Most pecans are steamed before they are taken out of the shell. The rationale given for the steaming is that the pecans will then come out of the shell in two neat halves, without splintering. For truly raw pecans, you have two options: either shell your own or buy from Sunorganic Farm (*see* Source Index). Sunorganic has found a supplier who shells the pecans without steaming.

PLANTAIN

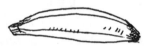

The plantain is a cousin to the banana, but is much larger. I have heard and read many times that it cannot be eaten raw, but this is not true. In order to eat plantain raw, you have to wait until it is completely ripe and most of the starch has turned to sugar. Usually this takes place when it is medium soft (NOT mushy soft) to the touch and the skin is halfway to or almost black. If you cannot find plantains in your supermarket, they can usually be located in an Hispanic neighborhood store.

PRUNES

A prune is a variety of plum that dries without spoiling.

People cook prunes to make them soft (stewed prunes), but this is totally unnecessary. All you have to do to soften up prunes is to soak them in water for a while, a few hours to overnight. If you want prunes for breakfast, just cover with some filtered water and leave at room temperature overnight. In the morning, you've got "unstewed prunes," soft enough for a baby. Well actually, **for a baby, I would blend them first and then strain them through a fine sieve or muslin cloth.**

Every time I eat soaked prunes, I am amazed at why anyone would choose a chemical laxative over something sweet and natural, which works sooo well. Yet, the evidence is there in every drugstore in the country.

SAD = STANDARD AMERICAN DIET

| MEAT, FISH, POULTRY HOT DOGS, HAMBURGERS | FOOD WITH ADDITIVES AND PRESERVATIVES ALL VINEGAR, (EXCEPT APPLE CIDER VINEGAR) | ALL CONVENIENCE FOODS ALL PROCESSED FOODS ALL PACKAGED, PREPARED FOODS |

COLD CUTS

BACON, SAUSAGE

FRENCH FRIES

WHITE "ENRICHED" BREAD

BREAD, IN GENERAL

FRIED FOODS

PASTEURIZED DAIRY FOODS

PASTEURIZED JUICES

SAUERKRAUT, THAT HAS
  BEEN PASTEURIZED

ALL PASTEURIZED FOODS

CHEMICALIZED PRODUCE

PESTICIDE, HERBICIDE LADEN
  PRODUCE

CANNED FOODS

MOST FROZEN FOODS

TV DINNERS

PROCESSED BREAKFAST
  CEREALS

PANCAKES

PANCAKE SYRUP

CORN SYRUP

JELLY AND JAM

SALTED CHIPS

IRRADIATED FOODS

MICROWAVED FOODS

PRE-COOKED FOODS

ALL FAST FOODS

MARGARINE

SODA POP

CANDY

CAKES

PIES

DONUTS

PASTRIES

ICE CREAM

PIZZA

PASTA

BARBECUE

EVERYTHING THAT IS REFINED

SALT
(White Refined Table Salt)

White table salt is a by-product of the processing of earth salt, after the valuable minerals have been extracted for sale to industry. The salt is subjected to a complicated process of refining, which includes heating the salt to over 2,000 degrees. The minerals are precipitated out of the salt, **going through numerous processes**, and then the salt is recrystallized. To make the salt free flowing, an anti-caking agent is added, which has the unfortunate side effect of turning the salt purple. Since no one is going to purchase purple salt, it is bleached, and then glucose, talcum, aluminum silicate and . . . a few other things are added. The end product is 97.5% sodium chloride with no trace mineral elements. **This salt is poison to the body**.

This is the salt used in most processed and prepared foods. This is the salt used in baked goods, and breads. This is the salt used in most restaurants and take-out places. And it is also used in canned and frozen foods.

SCALLIONS

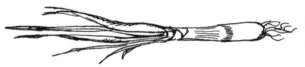

Scallions are also known as green onions. On the bottom of these scallions are white rootlets. Most often these are discarded, probably because soil gets trapped in there and it's hard to get it out. I like to use these parts. To get the soil out: With a sharp knife make two cuts (like a cross) down into the rootlets and a little into the white part of the scallion, then rinse thoroughly with water. The soil comes right out.

SEAWEEDS
(SEA VEGETABLES)

In China, Korea, Japan, Ireland, Scotland, Wales, Denmark, the coastal regions of Europe and Africa, Russia, Scandinavia and the South Pacific, sea vegetables are commonly used and appreciated. Other cultures, such as the Native Americans, the Aborigines of Australia, the Celts and the Vikings also valued these foods. In the United States, however, we turn up our nose at this most wonderful family of vegetables. Sea vegetables are a storehouse of vitamins, minerals, trace minerals, proteins, carbohydrates and other elements that, aside from feeding our body cells with first class materials, also assist it to expel radiation.[5] This is a most important function today, when there is so much nuclear fallout

---

[5] Ref: Tests conducted at McGill University.

all around us. The organic iodine found in many sea vegetables prevents the thyroid gland from taking up radioactive iodine.

Some sea vegetables (alaria, arame, kelp, hijiki, wakame, kombu) contain alginic acid, which binds with toxic metallic elements in the intestines, allowing them to be excreted. An abundance of alkalizing minerals in sea vegetables helps to purify the blood.

A taste for sea vegetables can be cultivated.

There are some precautions to take when purchasing sea vegetables. According to an informative booklet by Larch Hanson of the Maine Seaweed Company, it would be wise to find out how and where the sea vegetables you purchase are harvested. He states that aquacultured varieties are grown in calm waters, where there is more stagnation and pollution. Other things to be aware of and to avoid are:

- Seaweed grown on the waste of fish farming operations
- Seaweed that is harvested using boats with gasoline engines, or boats painted with lead-based or toxic bottom paints (copper)
- Seaweed harvested near harbors, factories or nuclear power plants
- Powdered seaweed, which is generally made from lower quality plants

Larch says you need "to find a harvester who has integrity, clear senses, and good intuition. This harvester should be working on outer islands, as much as possible, away from boat traffic."

Heat-treated seaweeds include nori sheets and blanched wakame from Japan. Up in Maine, Larch's seaweed harvest is sun/wind-dried, with no heat treatments. (*See* "Maine Seaweed" Company in the Source Index.)

SLIPPERY ELM POWDER

First used by the American Indians, Slippery Elm powder is derived from the inner bark of an American elm tree. The powder is cream colored, mucilaginous when wet, and extremely nutritious. It is one of the best foods to administer for people who are recovering from serious illness. Many miraculous properties have been attributed to this herb. *Heinerman's Encyclopedia of Healing Herbs & Spices* (by John Heinerman, Prentice Hall 1996) has an interesting account of one such healing. Look for Slippery Elm Powder in an herb shop.

STANDARDS OF IDENTITY

Basically, the "standards of identity" consist of food recipes developed by the Food and Drug Administration. The standards define what a given food product is, its name, and the ingredients that must (or may) be used in its manufacture. In the beginning, the standards were set up to protect the public from food manufacturers who watered down the milk with chalk, mixed coffee and other foods with sawdust, reformulated old and moldy cheeses into "processed" products and engaged in other unscrupulous practices. The standards set minimum amounts of some substances that certain foods may contain and maximum amounts of other substances. Where the standards went wrong was that by setting these percentages for a product, and also by designating what ingredients a "recipe" needed to contain, they inadvertently created a situation in which a manufacturer could make an inferior product which would conform to the standards while another manufacturer, producing a superior product, would not conform. The better quality product would then have to be labeled as artificial because it did not conform.

Ketchup made without sugar is a good example. To be allowed to call their product "ketchup," a manufacturer is obliged to include sugar. A company producing a natural ketchup without sugar is then precluded from calling its product "ketchup." Another example involves jams and preserves. The government set a range for the amounts of fruit and sugar (or other carbohydrate sweetening ingredients) to be included in these products. A company making a natural jam or preserves using all fruit, and honey as a sweetener (or without a sweetener at all), would not meet the standards and therefore could not call their product a jam or preserve. That is how the name "Conserve" came into being. There are no "standards of identity" for conserves.

Another disadvantage to the consumer of government-imposed standards is that a manufacturer does not have to list on its product label those ingredients that conform to the government's idea of what a recipe should include. Without full disclosure, the consumer has no idea what he is ingesting unless he obtains a copy of the standards to actually see what the food could potentially contain. And of course, the government recipes include non-food items as well, such as questionable additives and preservatives. Raw fooders don't have to worry about the standards because we do not buy packaged goods, only fresh ones.

TEFLEX™

Teflex™ is a flexible sheet, made of fiberglass, and coated with 6 layers of Dupont Teflon. Teflex,™ because of its non-stick surface, is used in dehydrators when making fruit leathers or drying any food that is liquefied. The Teflex™ sheet is placed on the mesh dehydrator tray and the liquid is poured onto it. When dehydrated, the food will easily peel off the sheet. The sheet is washable and can be reused again and again.

Teflon is a toxic substance when ingested. Most of us have seen cookware where the teflon surface has flaked off. Where did it go? Hopefully, not into the food. In speaking with the producers of Teflex™ and other non-stick, flexible sheets of this type, I tried to ascertain how the teflon could migrate into the food. They told me that when you see a damaged piece of teflon cookware, it was usually damaged because somebody used an abrasive on it, either to clean it, or to scrape the food away. In the scraping process, some of the teflon is loosened. I asked how we could avoid this with the flexible sheets. Where I could elicit a thoughtful response, the answer was to clean the flexible sheet with a soft sponge only. Do not use any abrasive to clean the Teflex™ sheet. I quickly realized that I had been using the abrasive side of my two-sided sponge to clean the sheets easily. I reordered new sheets and will treat the new ones as instructed.

Why use Teflex™ at all? The alternatives are not very workable. If you try to dehydrate liquids on parchment paper, wax paper, baking paper, or plastic paper (like Saran Wrap), your final product will not peel off easily. In fact, it will be very frustrating. For foods that hold together more, like cookies and crackers, parchment paper or baking paper can be used, or you can put the food directly onto the mesh dehydrator tray.

TOMATILLOS

Tomatillos are small green tomatoes with a papery husk around them. They are extremely easy to grow, come up like a weed, and they re-seed themselves each year. If you grow them yourself, you could let them ripen to the yellow stage, which is when I think they are the most delicious. At this ripe stage, the acid in them has mellowed out and they taste kind of cheesy. Unfortunately, I've never seen the yellow ones offered for sale in the markets.

VANILLA BEAN

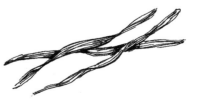

The vanilla bean is the fruit of certain varieties of tropical orchids. It originated in Mexico, but today is also cultivated in such exotic places as Tahiti, Madagascar and Bali. Vanilla is truly an intoxicating smell and taste experience.

VANILLA POWDER, as called for in some of the recipes, is simply ground vanilla bean: Cut 3 vanilla beans into small pieces, put them into a nut (or coffee) grinder, and grind as fine as possible. Store in a small glass jar in the refrigerator, and use as needed. It keeps for months. If it develops an off smell, then discard; but I've never had this happen. The alternative to making the vanilla powder would be to just cut a small piece of vanilla from the pod. Cut into small pieces and blend into the recipe. Depending on the quality of your equipment, it may or may not break down completely, and get blended.

If your vanilla bean is too moist and doesn't powder up in the nut mill, then leave the vanilla bean out at room temperature for a couple of days so that it dries a bit. Under no circumstances put the vanilla bean in a food dehydrator, because it will lose all its flavor.[6] You could even grind up this moist vanilla bean, but it will come out like the texture of ground tobacco, instead of as a powder. This has just as much flavor and works just as well in the recipes. Store in the refrigerator.

Commercial vanilla extract usually contains alcohol and may be extracted with solvents. Solvents have no place in a healthy diet.

VITAMIN B12

A properly functioning digestive tract produces all the B vitamins the body needs. For those who worry about getting enough Vitamin B12, include some of the following foods in your diet:

Sea Vegetables	Concord Grapes	Miso	Sauerkraut
Spirulina	Comfrey Leaves	Ginseng	
Seeded Bananas	Wheat Germ	Peanuts	
Sunflower Seeds	Mustard	Bee Pollen	

SOME PLANTS CONTAINING VITAMIN D

Do you remember being told as a child that no plants contained Vitamin D? And that this vitamin could only be obtained from the sun's rays touching and interacting with the natural oils on your skin? Or by drinking milk (which has been artificially "enriched" with synthetic vitamin D)? Well, surprise, surprise: here are some plants which do contain Vitamin D. Unfortunately, most of us do not generally consume plants from this list.

Fenugreek	Red raspberry	Papaya	Mullein
Chickweed	Rose hips	Agar-Agar	Nettles
Basil	Sarsaparilla	Sprouted seeds	Mushrooms
Alfalfa	Thyme	Wheatgrass juice	
Bee pollen	Watercress	Queen of the Meadow	
Eyebright	Irish Moss or Carrageen	Sunflower greens	

WASABI POWDER

Wasabi powder is made from a potent Japanese root. It is a very hot, mustard-flavored root that grows near water. Eden Foods offers a version that comes with horseradish and gardenia. You'll notice that sushi bars always serve this along with their raw fish. I think it's because wasabi probably kills any bacteria present in the fish.

---

[6] I think this is why you never see vanilla sold in a powder form like other spices. Actually, I have seen vanilla powder sold in some specialty stores, but then it is loaded with additives and I doubt it is a natural vanilla at all.

WHEATGRASS

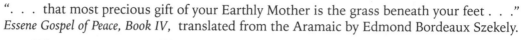

". . . that most precious gift of your Earthly Mother is the grass beneath your feet . . ." *Essene Gospel of Peace, Book IV*, translated from the Aramaic by Edmond Bordeaux Szekely.

Wheatgrass contains all known (and unknown) factors that are able to support life. It is rich in chlorophyll, vitamins (including B12), minerals (including trace minerals), amino acids (including the 8 essential ones), phytochemicals, antioxidants, 80+ enzymes, oxygen, fatty acids, and much, much more. The ingestion of wheatgrass juice has been reported to also have the following beneficial effects on the body: it reduces high blood pressure, helps eliminate heavy metals, reduces the effects of radiation, improves digestion, eliminates and/or counteracts toxins which have been ingested, purifies the liver, improves blood sugar problems, stimulates the growth of connective tissue cells and corrects the red blood cell count in anemia. (I saw this last effect in action when my mother's anemia was corrected in about 3 weeks.) All the live food institutes use wheatgrass juice in their programs and achieve amazing results.

For more information on wheatgrass, refer to *Wheatgrass—Nature's Finest Medicine*, a well-researched book on the subject by Steve Meyerowitz, Sproutman Publications, 1998, (www:Sproutman.com).

WILD RICE

Wild rice does not actually sprout, because it has been parched. I am searching for someone who has, or can conceive of, a different method of processing wild rice so that it need not be parched. I don't know, however, if this is even possible, or if soaked, sprouted unparched wild rice will soften up enough to eat.

To soften wild rice enough for eating, proceed **as if** you were sprouting it.

HOW TO PREPARE WILD RICE FOR EATING:

Soak 1 cup (or more) of wild rice for 36-48 hours in filtered water, changing the water twice. If you are in a hot and humid climate, you might have to change the water three times. At the end of the soaking period, drain and rinse the rice and spread out in a tapered bowl for sprouting. Rinse twice a day and let "sprout" for 2 to 6 days until "chewy." One cup dry rice equals 3 cups after "sprouting."

WILLARD WATER

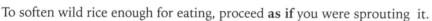

Willard Water was developed by Dr. John W. Willard, Professor Emeritus of the South Dakota School of Mines and Technology, who received his PhD in chemistry from Purdue University. Doc, as he was called, had been working on a product that would clean up sludge, grease and pitch. After many years of experimentation, refinement, trial and error, and most of all serendipity, he discovered a novel "catalyst altered water." CAW for short, is water with an altered molecular structure that behaves differently than normal water. It is a more activated form of water and this activation is due, in part, to micelle activity in the water. (A micelle is an electrically charged colloidal particle; a source of electrons and magnetism.) In addition the water also contains trace amounts of minerals extracted from lignite. Lignite is a soft coal which consists of carbonized vegetable matter from ancient plants. Through a proprietary process, the Doc was able to separate the toxic elements of the coal, leaving behind only the beneficial minerals. The resulting water (with a couple of other things added) is then referred to as a "concentrate.[7]"

This concentrate is mixed with either distilled water or with the purest water that you can find, at the ratio of one ounce (2 tablespoons) of concentrate to 1 gallon of water. It's this "mixed-up-gallon" that is the actual Willard Water you can employ for drinking and countless other uses. Both the

---

[7]The concentrate, however, is about 99% water. All the other ingredients combined make up only about 1% of the concentrate, which is then further diluted when you mix it for use.

concentrate and the Willard Water are stored in plastic containers, because of the water's ability to break things down which, Doc said, in theory, might mean it could/would break down the layers of film and glass involved in most glass products. Plastic is normally manufactured as a single sheet without layering, making that hypothetical possibility irrelevant.

Willard Water is an enigma to me. Normally, with a manufactured product, I run, don't walk, to the nearest exit. And this product contains minerals extracted from lignite[8] (coal). Even coal that is completely cleansed of toxic substances, as this is, seems like a turnoff.

But Willard Water is different, and I suppose, the phrase "there are exceptions to every rule" applies here. My rule has always been to follow Nature in every way that I can and yet, here is the exception. A manufactured product, yet an extremely beneficial one for practically anything that ails you (well almost). I've certainly had very good experiences with it. Even if you don't believe all the wonderful benefits that people have reported from its use, you can rest assured that it will do absolutely no harm. Willard Water has 21 US patents for a variety of uses in agriculture, animal husbandry, etc.

The following are some of the unusual characteristics of Willard Water that have been reported:

- It is a powerful antioxidant and free radical scavenger
- It breaks down waste materials and toxins in the body
- It boosts an organism's assimilation of nutrients
- It reduces swelling
- It reduces stress. Doc said, "It takes an organism under stress and helps it to return to its normal state."
- It works as a skin conditioner
- It increases bio-magnetism in a living organism by 50%
- Users have said it beneficially impacts the following conditions: back pain and other back problems, PMS, arthritis, burns and sunburn, bronchitis, stomach ulcers, digestive problems, dry and tearing eyes, constipation and diarrhea, asthma, high blood pressure, emphysema, low and high blood sugar, and the list goes on.

> **CAUTION–** **For those still taking medication.** It could change (reduce) the amount of medication you need. If changes occur in the underlying condition a medication is treating, the amount of medication needed may change. Consult your health care provider for information on what types of changes would indicate your dosages might need changing.

- Plants thrive on it. I've seen this both in my houseplants and in my garden. I once had two large houseplants growing in a **ONE AND A HALF INCH** layer of soil in the same container for years. I fed them Willard Water regularly, and they were both gorgeous and constantly putting out new leaves.
- Ranchers report fewer veterinary bills when using it for their animals.

If you decide to give Willard Water a try, **beware** of imitations or diluted products. *See* "Nutrition Coalition" in the Source Index for the genuine article.

---

[8]Tests conducted by reputable laboratories have shown that it is non-corrosive, non-toxic, non-carcinogenic, and non-mutagenic.

INDEX

SOURCE INDEX

I have endeavoured to provide accurate information from all of these sources. But remember, sometimes companies may experience changes in personnel, in ownership, policies or suppliers. The result may be that the products that you have counted on may no longer be available, or that other products which do not meet your standards are offered as substitutes. From time to time, therefore, it is wise to check out pertinent information for yourself. Also, in the case of dried fruits, those that are sun-dried are always my first choice. With dehydrator-dried fruit, you can never be sure of the temperature used in the process, unless of course, you dried the fruits yourself.

ACRES, U.S.A.

512.892.4400 - Fax: 512.892.4448
Website: www.acresusa.com

This newspaper, billed as "A Voice For Eco-Agriculture," is full of interesting information, not only for farmers, but for all of us. Published once a month, it covers topics dealing with food, health, technology, farming, sustainable agriculture, economics and politics. You won't find the standard view of things here, but you will be stimulated to think and gain a different perspective on vital issues of the day.

ANN WIGMORE NATURAL HEALTH INST.

Ruta 115, Km 20, Calle Moret, Bo Guayabo
Aguada, PR 00602
Mailing Address:
PO Box 429
Rincon, PR 00677
787.868.6307 - Fax: 787.868.2430
Website: www.annwigmore.org

At this institute you can learn the entire living foods program and lifestyle. It offers a comprehensive program in a very loving and supportive atmosphere where the teachings of the late Dr. Ann Wigmore are conscientiously followed. Classes on all aspects of health are offered, which begin at daybreak with yoga by the sea. Luscious tropical fruits, including coconuts like you've never seen, are also provided. The young coconut meat is soft like custard.

Dr. Ann's lifestyle and research have contributed to saving the lives of thousands of people who were abandoned, with no hope of recovery, by the conventional medical profession. The Institute is located right by the beach in Aguada, Puerto Rico. When you are ready to learn how to heal your mind, body and spirit . . . the Ann Wigmore Institute is an excellent choice. Call for more information and a brochure.

BARLEANS

4936 Lake Terrell Road
Ferndale, WA 98248
360.384.0485 - Orders: 800.445.3529

Barleans provides flaxseed oil and borage oil that is produced at temperatures which do not exceed 96° F.

CABBEC VEGETABLE SLICER available at:

www.zensuke.com/450024.html
605.341.7391

Carries the Cabbec Vegetable Slicer, which grates hard vegetables into spaghetti-like strips. Call to order by mail.

CHAMPION JUICER

Plastaket Manufacturing Company, Inc.
6220 East Hwy 12
Lodi, CA 95240
209.369.2154 - Fax: 209.369.7455

The Champion juicer is available in many health food stores. If you can't find it, contact the manufacturer for a distributor in your area.

CHER CARDEN

Health Educator
New York, NY
212.242.5127

Cher Carden is a multi-talented wellness consultant and living food instructor in New York City who offers assistance to health seekers through a variety of services. In her vegetarian living food classes you will prepare uncooked, tasty, easy meals that cleanse the body, enhance vitality and facilitate weight loss, while also learning how to maintain or reclaim vibrant health. She also offers colonics, ear conings, weight loss programs and individual counseling sessions for colon management.

CLOTHCRAFTERS, INC.

PO Box 1005
Sheboygan, WI 53081
920.457.7383

Provides the muslin bags used for making the seed and nut yogurts and milks in my recipes. These bags go by the name of "Salad Jelly Bags," because they are sold for storing salad vegetables and making jelly. Send for them by mail. They are also available at my website.

DAFNA MORDECAI

New York, NY
212.779.2395

Dafna Mordecai has 20-years experience in the Natural Hygiene way of life and in raw food preparation. She is a raw food coach and spiritual teacher focusing on a holistic approach.

DEER GARDEN REJUVENATIVE FOODS
PO Box 8464
Santa Cruz, CA 95061
800.805.7957 - 831.427.2196

Provides raw nut and seed butters and raw cultured vegetables which are available in the refrigerated section of some health food stores.

DORIS DJOLIT BEIGEL
Certified Colon Hydrotherapist
Natural Alternative
310 West 72nd St., #310
New York, NY, 10023
212.580.3333

Offering State-of-the-Art and Gravity Method Colon Hydrotherapy, detoxification programs, living food and raw food education, therapeutic massage, aromatherapy and foot reflexology.

DRIED SWEET CORN (*See* Organic Provisions)

ELYSA MARKOWITZ, TV Star of:
Elysa's Raw and Wild Food Show
17551 Mountain View Road, Ste. 47
Desert Hot Spring, CA 92240
760.251.7488

Elysa is an author/lecturer, with an exuberant personality, who travels around the country giving talks and raw food preparation workshops. One of her books, *Living with Green Power: A Gourmet Collection of Living Food Recipes*, has lovely color photographs of this fine tasting cuisine. Offering over 150 recipes to choose from, this book is a real treat. Elysa also makes available for purchase the videotapes of her TV shows.

EXCALIBUR DEHYDRATOR
EXCALIBUR PRODUCTS, A Division of KBI

6083 Power Inn Road
Sacramento, CA 95824
800.875.4254 - 916.381.4254

This company produces the Excalibur Food Dehydrator. The founder, Roger Orton, told me that to satisfy the needs of the growing raw/living foods community, he is developing a special dehydrator which will have the thermostat calibrated on the lower end for more accuracy. The temperature settings will range from 75° F to 120° F. It will also have a 26-hour timer. This special model, called the Living Food Dehydrator, will become available in the Autumn of 2000. I applaud Roger for recognizing and fulfilling the needs of the raw/live food community. (As of 2010 no special model has been produced. For their explanation on this, go to their website www.excaliburdehydrator.com)

FELICIA'S HEART LIGHT
Brooklyn, NY
718.469.7262

Felicia offers a raw, vegetarian, gourmet food catering service, providing sumptuous, mouth-watering live cuisine for the Tri-State area. She also conducts live food workshops and seminars for children and adults.

FLORA, INC.
PO Box 73
Lynden, WA 98264
800.446.2110 - Fax: 888.354.8138

Flora, Inc. sells organic, genuinely cold-pressed oils. They are sometimes found in the refrigerated section at health food stores. These oils are pressed at below "body temperature" (20–30° C), with no heat or chemical solvents ever applied. Flora oils are bottled with nitrogen (to prevent oxidation) in light-resistant, dark amber glass bottles. Organic flax, sunflower, olive, peanut, safflower and sesame oils are available. They also sell an oil blend called Udo's Choice, which is a combination of organic flax, sesame and sunflower seed oils, along with unrefined oils from the germ of rice, oats and wheat. Flora also offers walnut, almond, and pumpkin seed oils, which are not organically grown at this time. Send for their mail order catalog.

FOOD UNDER FOOT
Melissa & David Sokulski
Pittsburgh, PA
412.381.0116
www.FoodUnderFoot.com

Food Under Foot is a free educational website with detailed pictures, information, recipes and videos on using wild plants as food and medicine. Sign up to receive five free ebooks on common wild edible plants. The site was put together by licensed acupuncturists and herbalists Melissa Sokulski and David Sokulski. Based out of Pittsburg, PA, they also lead wild edibles walks and workshops. Check the website for information (www.FoodUnderFoot.com).

GOLD MINE NATURAL FOOD CO.
7805 Arjons Drive
San Diego, CA 92126
858.537.9830 - Fax 858.695.0811

Suppliers of Ohsawa brand organic, unpasteurized miso. They also carry a large variety of whole grains, beans, nuts, and other interesting stuff.

THE GRAIN & SALT SOCIETY
Four Celtic Dr.
Arden, NC 28704
800.867.7258 - Fax 828.654.0529

Providers of Celtic Sea Salt from Brittany. This salt is gray in color, because of all the trace minerals it contains.

HEALTHFORCE NUTRITIONALS
1835A South Centre City Pkwy., #411
Escondido, CA 92025-6504
Orders Only: 800.357.2717 (Visa, MC, DSC, Amex,
Checks or Money Orders accepted.)
Customer Service: 760.747.8822
Fax: 760.747.8922
Website: www.healthforce.com
Jameth Sheridan, N.D. & Kim Sheridan, N.D.

HealthForce offers the *Uncooking with Jameth & Kim*
recipe book as well as highly researched, select products that genuinely make a difference. This company
is run by my friends, Jameth and Kim, who really live
the raw/live foods lifestyle. They carry an excellent
selection of enzyme-active, whole foods-based vitamins and minerals, such as Vitamineral Green, (which
contains a wide range of organic green vegetation,
algae, grasses, etc.), Spirulina, natural Vitamin C in the
form of Acerola Cherry Powder, colon cleansers, digestive enzymes (essential if eating anything cooked),
etc. These supplements are non-toxic, truly bio-com-
patible, and based on live foods and Mother Nature.

HEIRLOOM SEEDS
287 East Finley Dr.
W. Finley, PA 15377
724.663.5356
Website: www.heirloomseeds.com

A source for heirloom, non-hybridized seeds for planting in your garden. They also have a selection of
organic seeds.

HIGH VIBE HEALTH & HEALING
138 East 3rd Street
New York, NY 10003
212.777.6645 - 888.554.6645
Website: www.highvibe.com

High Vibe regularly offers seminars, workshops and
raw food preparation classes. The owner, Dagger, goes
out of his way to stock many hard-to-find items for the
raw community in his store. Mail order catalog avail.

HIPPOCRATES HEALTH INSTITUTE
1443 Palmdale Court
West Palm Beach, FL 33411
561.471.8876
Website:www.hippocratesinst.com

A spa and alternative health education institute
where you can learn the entire live-foods program
in beautiful, conducive surroundings. They do Live
Blood Analysis while you are there, so you can
monitor the progress of your own blood picture.
This is fascinating. You are able to actually see on
a TV monitor how the bloodstream cleans up from
eating living foods and following the lifestyle, even
during a short stay. Send for a brochure.

KEFIR CULTURE available from:
Lifeway Foods, Inc.
6431 W. Oakton St.
Morton Grove, IL 60053
877.281.3874 - Fax 847.967.6558

Provides Kefir starter, an active culture for making Kefir.
Lifeway provided a letter for my files which states that
they use no genetically modified organisms in this
product.

LIVING LIGHT CULINARY ARTS INSTITUTE
301-B No. Main St.
Fort Bragg, CA 95437
800.816.2319 - 707.964.2420
Website: www.rawfoodchef.com

This institute provides certification courses in raw/live
food cuisine for individuals, chefs and teachers. Courses provided are suitable for novices as well as professionals and are taught by Cherie Soria, one of the
world's top raw food chefs.

LIVING TREE COMMUNITY FOODS
PO Box 10082
Berkeley, CA 94709
510.526.7106 - Fax: 510.526.9516
800.260.5534
Website: www.livingtreecommunity.com

Living Tree Community Foods is dedicated to providing quality, organic dried fruits, nuts, nut butters,
and gift packs. This company is justifiably proud of its
organic almonds and dried fruits, which are grown by
family farmers. Upon harvest, Living Tree almonds are
frozen as soon as possible to preserve freshness and
flavor and to destroy insect larvae. Conventionally
grown almonds, on the contrary, are fumigated with
methyl bromide, a toxic substance. Jesse Schwartz, the
owner, states that his company specializes in low-
heat dehydration of fruits. In addition, peaches, nectarines, figs and tomatoes are dried by the sun. Send
for their mail order catalog.

MAINE SEAWEED COMPANY
PO Box 57
Steuben, ME 04680
207.546.2875

This company provides a variety of high quality seaweeds (sea vegetables) which are sun/wind-dried. To
order some by mail, send for their flier and current
price list.

MISO (*See* Gold Mine Natural Food Co.)

MOTHERS FOR NATURAL LAW
Website:www.safe-food.org/welcome.html

This organization provides information on biotechnology and, with our assistance, is trying to get trans-
genic food products labeled, so that, at the very least,

we can identify them. As things stand now, we may be buying these products inadvertently. Genetically engineered produce is a serious threat to our health and the environment. Call this organization, get the facts and get involved.

MUSLIN BAGS (*See* Clothcrafters, Inc.)

MUSLIN HERB BAGS (*See* OrganzaBagg.com)

NATIVE SEEDS/SEARCH
3061 No. Campbell Ave.
Tucson, AZ 85719
520.622.5561 - Fax: 520.622.5591

This organization is dedicated to preserving ancient desert crops and heirloom farming practices. They offer both heirloom and wild seeds for your garden.

NESHAMINY VALLEY NATURAL FOODS (*See* Organic Provisions.)

NUTRITION COALITION
PO Box 3001
Fargo, ND 58108
US and Canada 800.447.4793 - 218.236.9783
Website: www.willardswater.com

For genuine Willard Water.

OHSAWA BRAND MISO (*See* Gold Mine Natural Food Company.)

OPTIMUM HEALTH INSTITUTE OF SAN DIEGO
6970 Central Ave.
Lemon Grove, CA 91945
800.993.4325 - 619.464.3346
Website:www.optimumhealth.org

The Optimum Health Institute offers a comprehensive program covering many aspects of health maintenance and recovery, including mental and emotional detoxification, live food preparation and spiritual matters. The entire program runs for 3-4 weeks, but you can attend for only one week also. Check-in is on Sunday and their prices are super-reasonable. Send for a brochure. A second Institute was recently opened in Austin, Texas.

ORGANIC PROVISIONS
PO Box 756
Richboro, PA 18954
Orders: 800.490.0044 – 215.674.2217
Website: www.orgfood.com

Mail order supplier of Neshaminy brand "dried sweet corn," used in *Hot Tamale Pie*, *Minestrone Soup* and other recipes.

ORGANZABAGG.COM
PO Box 19284
San Diego, CA 92159
619.861.6220 - Fax: 619.462.8155
Website: www.organzabagg.com

PERFECT FOODS INC.
New York
800.933.3288
Website: www.800wheatgrass.com

Delivers fresh, certified organic wheatgrass and sprouts to stores in New York, New Jersey and Connecticut and if you are near their delivery route they will deliver to you as well. They also will overnight their products nationwide.

PRICE-POTTENGER NUTRITION FOUNDATION
7890 Broadway
Lemon Grove, CA 91945
800.366.3748 - 619.462.7600
Website: price-pottenger.org

A non-profit organization that collects and disseminates information on a variety of health-related topics. It offers a catalog of books, reprints, and video and audio tapes; most notably the works of Dr. Weston Price (*Nutrition and Physical Degeneration*) and Dr. Francis M. Pottenger, Jr. (*Pottenger's Cats*).

RESTAURANTS SERVING RAW FOOD CUISINE:

105 DEGREES CAFÉ
5820 No. Classon Blvd., Ste. 1
Oklahoma City, OK 73118   405.842.1050

ARNOLD'S WAY VEGETARIAN RAW CAFÉ
319 West Main St., Store #4 Rear
Lansdale, PA 19446   215.361.0116

BEETS LIVING FOOD CAFE
1611 W. 5th St., Ste. 165
Austin, TX 78734   512.477.2338

BEVERLY HILLS JUICE CLUB
8382 Beverly Blvd.
Los Angeles, CA 94122   323.655.8300

CAFÉ GRATITUDE
2400 Harrison St. (@20th St.)
San Francisco, CA 94110   415.830.3014

CARAVAN OF DREAMS
405 East 6th St.
New York, NY 10009-6303   212.254.1613
(The menu is not raw, but Caravan does offer many and varied raw food options.)

THE CHACO CANYON CAFÉ
4757 12th Ave NE, on the corner of 12th and 50th
in the University District
Seattle, WA 98105   206.522.6966

ECOPOLITAN
2409 Lyndale Ave. South
Minneapolis, MN 55405   612.874.7336

ENZYME EXPRESS
1330 East Huffman Road
Anchorage, AK 99515   907.345.1330

GARDEN TASTE
1237 Camino Del Mar
Delmar, CA 92014   619.793.1500

GO RAW CAFÉ
2910 Lake East Dr.
Las Vegas, NV 89117   702.254.5382

GREZZO RESTAURANT (Grezzo, Italian for raw)
69 Prince St.
Boston, MA 02113   857.362.7288

KAREN'S RAW CAFÉ
1901 No. Halsted St.
Chicago, IL 60614   312.255.1590

LIFEFOOD GOURMET
1248 SW 22nd St.
Miami, FL 33145   305.856.6767

LIVE HEALTH CAFÉ
264 Dupont Street
Toronto, Ontario M5R 1V7   416.515.2002

NATURAL HIGH JUICE BAR & CAFÉ
At **Freshmart Aguadilla**
Plaza Victoria, Route #2, Km. 129.5
Rincon PR 00677   787.882.2656

ORGANIC GARDEN CAFÉ AND JUICE BAR
294 Cabot Street
Beverly, MA 01915   978.922.0004
Website: www.organicgardencafe.com.

PURE FOOD AND WINE
54 Irving Place (bet 17th & 18th Sts)
New York, NY 10003   212.477.1010

QUINTESSENCE
263 East 10th St.
New York, NY 10009   646.654.1823

SAF AKATLAR
Club Sporium (Mayadrom Arkası)
Cumhuriyet Cad. No: 4/8
TR 34626 Akatlar, Besiktas Istanbul
                    0212 2827946 / 7291

TREE OF LIFE CAFÉ
By reservation only – call
771 Harshaw Road
Patagonia, AZ 85624   866.394.2520

THE VEGETARIAN OASIS
431 West 13th St.
Escondido, CA 92025   760.740.9596

For a more complete list of raw restaurants, go to
www.RawFoodInfo.com and look in the Directories.

RHIO'S RAW ENERGY
New York, NY 10013
212.941.5857
Website: www.RawFoodInfo.com

Rhio is a proponent of the Raw/Live food lifestyle. She
offers classes and private consultations on the preparation of raw/live foods and information on the benefits of taking control of your own health and well
being. Her radio show *Hooked on Raw* can be heard
worldwide on www.NYTalkRadio.net and www.Raw-
FoodInfo.com. She also offers on her website a huge
selection of books, DVDs, kitchen equipment and
other products geared for the raw/live community.

Rhio is also available for lectures and presentations.
Contact: Rhio@RawFoodInfo.com

SALADACCO (*See* Rhio's Raw Energy)

SALADSHOOTER® SLICER/SHREDDER
National Presto Industries, Inc.
3925 N. Hastings Way
Eau Claire, WI 54703-3703
800.877.0441 - 715.839.2209

The SaladShooter® is a small, hand-held electrical
appliance, which very quickly slices or grates almost
all vegetables, nuts and seeds. Available at some
kitchen appliance stores. If you cannot locate it, call
the manufacturer for a distributor in your area.

SCHOOL OF SELF-RELIANCE
PO Box 41834
Eagle Rock, CA 90041
323.255.9502
Webpage: www.self-reliance.net

This school, under the direction of Christopher
Nyerges and assistants, teaches how to identify edible wild foods. Send for schedule of events throughout the year.

SEEDS OF CHANGE
PO Box 15700
Santa Fe, NM 87506-5700
800.957.3337 - 888.762.7333
Website: www.seedsofchange.com

Provides heirloom, certified organic, non-hybridized
seeds for planting in your garden.

SOIL REMINERALIZATION WITH ROCK DUST
Earth Health Regeneration
Don Weaver
PO Box 620478
Woodside, CA 94062-0478
650.851.3622
Email: earthdon@yahoo.com
Website: www.remineralize.org

THE SPICE HUNTER
PO Box 8110
San Luis Obispo, CA 93403-8110
Information request line 800.444.3061, Ext. 7000
805.597.8992 - Fax: 805.544.3824
Website: www.spicehunter.com

The Spice Hunter has organic herbs and spices available in their organic line. They do not purchase products grown from genetically altered seeds and their products are not irradiated. Ask for their mail order catalog.

SUNFOOD
1830 Gillespie Way, Ste. 101
El Cajon, CA 92920
800.205.2350 - 619.596.7979
Website: www.sunfood.com

This website is a source for many raw/living food books, juicers, dehydrators, the Saladacco, and other equipment useful for the raw food lifestyle.

SUNORGANIC FARM
411 So. Las Posas Rd.
San Marcos, CA 92078
888.269.9888 - Fax: 760.510.9996
Website: www.sunorganicfarm.com

An excellent mail order catalog that provides quality organic dried fruits, nuts, seeds, legumes, beans, grains, herbs, spices, gift baskets and more. The owners have gone out of their way for the raw/live food community. They understand the problems we face in trying to find low-heat processed products and actively search for the alternatives we need. For example, here you can find a viable, sproutable hulless oat. The fruits are unfumigated and unsulphured. Send for their catalog.

TREE OF LIFE REJUVENATION CENTER
PO Box 778
Patagonia, AZ 85624
866.394.2520
Website: www.treeoflife.nu

The Tree of Life Rejuvenation Center, founded and directed by Gabriel Cousens, M.D., is an innovative spiritual, live-food, holistic healing, eco-retreat. The center is committed to the integration of all healing life forces for complete body, mind and spiritual renewal. This residential retreat offers 100% gourmet, vegan, Kosher, organic live-food cuisine at their Tree of Life Café, which is also open to the public (by reservation). Many transformational programs, such as medically supervised individual fasting, and psycho-spiritual self-healing are offered throughout the year. The Tree of Life provides an excellent facility for inspiring and supporting the raw lifestyle.

URBAN ORGANIC
240 6th St.
Brooklyn, NY 11215
718.499.4321

Provides a service for home delivery of organic produce. They offer a choice of four different sized boxes, which they deliver once a week, right to your door, in the boroughs of New York City. The fruits and vegetables are of good to excellent taste and quality. If you refer someone who registers with them, they will send you a free box.

VITA-MIX
8615 Usher Rd.
Cleveland, OH 44138-2199
800.848.2649

See Kitchen Equipment for a description of the Vita-Mix. Call the 800 number for a distributor in your area.

WILD FOOD IDENTIFICATION See "Wildman" Steve Brill (New York area), School of Self-Reliance (Southern California area), and Food Under Foot (Pittsburgh, PA area).

"WILDMAN" STEVE BRILL
Westchester, NY
914.835.2153
Website: www.wildmanstevebrill.com

The "Wildman" provides *Wild Food and Ecology Tours* in New York City and surrounding areas throughout most of the year. This hands-on environmental program consists of field walks focusing on identifying and collecting common wild plants and mushrooms. The "Wildman" places special emphasis on key characteristics of these plants so all those present learn to recognize the various species. Look on his website for a schedule of activities.

WILLARD WATER (*See* Nutrition Coalition and Rhio's Raw Energy)

BIBLIOGRAPHY

Airola, Dr. Paavo, *How to Keep Slim, Healthy and Young with Juice Fasting*. Phoenix, AZ: Health Plus Publishers, 1971.

Anderson, Dr. Richard, N.D., N.M.D., *Cleanse & Purify Thyself*. 1988.

Arlin, Stephen, Fouad Dini and David Wolfe, *Nature's First Law: The Raw-Food Diet*. San Diego, CA: Maul Brothers Publishing, 1996.

Ausubel, Kenny, *Seeds of Change: The Living Treasure - The Passionate Story of the Growing Movement to Restore Biodiversity*. New York: HarperCollins, 1994.

Baroody, Dr. T. A., Jr., *Alkalize or Die*. Waynesville, NC: Eclectic Press, 1991.

Batmanghelidj, Dr. F., *Your Body's Many Cries for Water*. Falls Church, VA: Global Health Solutions, Inc., 1997.

Bircher-Benner, *The Prevention of Incurable Disease*. James Clarke & Co., 1981.

Bragg, Paul C., N.D., Ph.D., *The Miracle of Fasting*. Santa Barbara, CA: Health Science, 1966.

Braunstein, Mark M., *The Sprout Garden*. Summertown, TN: The Book Publishing Co., 1993

Brill, "Wildman" Steve, with Evelyn Dean, *Identifying and Harvesting Edible and Medicinal Plants in Wild (and Not So Wild) Places*. New York: Hearst Books, 1994.

Cichoke, Dr. Anthony J., *The Complete Book of Enzyme Therapy*. Garden City Park, NY: Avery Publishing Group, 1999.

Clark, Hulda Regehr, Ph.D., N.D., *The Cure for all Diseases*. San Diego, CA: ProMotion Publishing, 1995.

Clement, Brian R., with Theresa Foy DiGeronimo, *Living Foods for Optimum Health*. Rocklin, CA: Prima Publishing, 1996.

Cousens, Dr. Gabriel, *Conscious Eating*. Santa Rosa, CA: Vision Books International, 1992.

Dawn, Jesse Anson, *Never "Old"*. Hilo, Hawaii: World Changing Books, 1993.

De Vries, Arnold, *The Fountain of Youth*. Los Angeles, CA: Institute Press, 1946

Diamond, Harvey, *Your Heart Your Planet*. Santa Monica, CA: Hay House, 1990

Doyle, Jack, *Altered Harvest - Agriculture, Genetics and the Fate of the World's Food Supply*. New York: Viking Penguin, 1985.

Fowler, Cary & Pat Mooney, *Shattering: Food, Politics and the Loss of Genetic Diversity*. University of Arizona Press, 1990.

Fuller, DicQie, Ph.D., D.Sc., *The Healing Power of Enzymes*. New York, NY: Forbes, 1998.

Gerson, Max, M.D., *A Cancer Therapy, Results of Fifty Cases*. Barrytown, NY: Station Hill Press/Gerson Institute, 1958/1997.

Gray, Robert, *The Colon Health Handbook*. Emerald Publishing, 1990.

Hay, Louise L., *You Can Heal Your Life*. Santa Monica, CA: Hay House, 1982.

Howell, Dr. Edward, *Enzyme Nutrition*. Wayne, NJ: Avery Pub. Group, 1985.

Howell, Dr. Edward, *Food Enzymes for Health & Longevity*. Twin Lakes, WI: Lotus Press, 1994 (2nd edition).

Hunt, Charles J., III, *The Christ Diet*. La Jolla, CA: Heartquake Pub., 1992.

Hutchins, Imar, *Delights of the Garden*. New York: Main Street Books, Doubleday, 1994.

Jacobsen, Roy M., Aqua Vitae, *The Story of Dr. John W. Willard and His Breakthrough Discovery: Catalyst Altered Water*. Second Edition 1992.

Jensen, Dr. Bernard, *Tissue Cleansing through Bowel Management*. Escondido, CA: Pub. by author, 1981.

Jensen, Dr. Bernard, *Nature Has a Remedy*. Santa Cruz, CA: Unity Press, 1978.

Kirschner, Dr. H.E., *Nature's Healing Grasses*. Riverside, CA: H.C. White Publications, 1960.

Kirschner, Dr. H.E., *Live Food Juices*. Monrovia, CA: H.E. Kirschner Pub., 1957.

Kroeger, Rev. Hanna, *God Helps Those That Help Themselves*. Boulder, CO: 1984.

Kulvinskas, Viktoras, *Survival Into the 21st Century*. Fairfield, IA: 21st Century Publications, 1975.

Lee, Lita, Ph.D., *Radiation Protection Manual*. Redwood City, CA: Grassroots Network, 1990.

Loomis, Howard F., Jr., D.C., F.I.A.C.A., *Enzymes: The Key to Health, Volume 1*. Madison, WI: 21st Century Nutrition Publishing, 1999.

Lyman, Howard, *Mad Cowboy*. New York: Scribner, 1998.

Malkmus, Dr. George with Michael Dye, *God's Way to Ultimate Health*. Edison, TN: Hallelujah Acres Publishing, 1995.

Mander, Jerry, *In the Absence of the Sacred*. San Francisco, CA: Sierra Club Books, 1992.

Meyerowitz, Steve, *Sprout it*. Great Barrington, MA: The Sprout House, 1983.

Nolfi, Dr. Kristine, *My Experiences with Living Food—The Raw Food Treatment of Cancer and Other Diseases*. Denmark: Health Research (reprint).

Ott, Dr. John, *Health and Light*. Simon & Schuster, 1973.

Ponder, Catherine, *The Healing Secrets of the Ages*. Marina del Rey, CA: DeVorss & Co., 1967.

Pottenger, Dr. Francis M., Jr., *Pottenger's Cats*. La Mesa, CA: Price-Pottenger Nutrition Foundation, 1983.

Price, Weston A., *Nutrition & Physical Degeneration*. Santa Monica, CA: The Price-Pottenger Foundation, 1945/1972.

Priestley, R.J., *Effects of Heating on Foodstuffs*. Applied Science Pub., 1979.

Robbins, John, *Diet for a New America*. Walpole, NH: Stillpoint Publishing, 1987.

Santillo, Humbart, BS, MH, *Food Enzymes, The Missing Link to Radiant Health*. Prescott, AZ: Hohm Press, 1987.

Schaeffer, Severen L., *Instinctive Nutrition*. Berkeley, CA: Celestial Arts, 1987.

Schechter, Steven, N.D., *Fighting Radiation and Chemical Pollutants with Foods, Herbs and Vitamins*. Vitality, 1990.

Shannon, Sara, *Diet for the Atomic Age*. Wayne, NJ: Avery Pub. Group, 1987.

Shinn, Florence Scovel, *The Game of Life and How to Play It*. Marina del Rey, CA: De Vorss & Co, 1925.

Shiva, Vandana, *Biopiracy–The Plunder of Nature and Knowledge*. Boston, MA: South End Press, 1997.

Soria, Cherie, *Angel Food*. Santa Barbara, CA: Heartstar Productions, 1996.

Szekeley, Edmond Bordeaux, *The Essene Gospel of Peace*. International Biogenic Society, 1981.

Teitle, Martin, PhD., and Kimberly A. Wilson, *Genetically Engineered Food: Changing the Nature of Nature*. Rochester, VT: Park Street Press, 1999.

Tilden, J.H., M.D., *Toxemia Explained*. (1952) Photographic reprint, Mokelumne Hill, CA: Health Research.

Tobe, John H., *Hunza: Adventures in a Land of Paradise*. St. Catharines, Ont: The Provoker Press, 1960.

Tompkins, Peter & Christopher Bird, *Secrets of the Soil*. New York: Harper & Row, 1989.

Tompkins, Peter & Christopher Bird, *The Secret Life of Plants*. New York: Avon Books, 1973.

Walker, Dr. N.W., D. Sc., *Become Younger*. Phoenix, AZ: Norwalk Press, 1949.

Walker, Dr. N.W., D.Sc., *Fresh Vegetable and Fruit Juices*, (formerly titled *Raw Vegetable Juices*, 1st edition 1936). Phoenix, AZ: O'Sullivan Woodside & Co., revised 1978.

Wigmore, Ann, *Be Your Own Doctor*. Wayne, NJ: Avery Pub. Group, 1982.

Wigmore, Ann, *The Hippocrates Diet*. Wayne, NJ: Avery Pub. Group, 1984.

Williams, Roger J., *Biochemical Individuality*. University of Texas Press, 1979.

RAW LIFESTYLE SUPPORT

Check out Rhio's website:
www.rawfoodinfo.com
for additional support and
abundant health resources

- Order *What's Not Cookin' in Rhio's Kitchen* DVDs
- Order more *Hooked on Raw* books
- Check out other raw/live food books
- Lectures on CD by raw lifestyle experts
- Food prep DVDs
- Food-based supplements
- Kitchen supplies and equipment
- Unique products and gifts and more

Many of the products in the Source Index are available on our website

Email us at: **orders@rawfoodinfo.com**
Call us at 212.941.5857
Fax us at 212.274.0978

Listen to Rhio's radio show *Hooked on Raw* on
www.NYTalkRadio.net and www.RawFoodInfo.com

RHIO'S RAW ENERGY
New York, NY
Email Rhio: Rhotline@rawfoodinfo.com
Website: www.rawfoodinfo.com

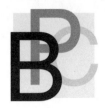

BOOK PUBLISHING COMPANY

since 1974—books that educate, inspire, and empower

To find your favorite vegetarian and soyfood products online, visit:
www.healthy-eating.com

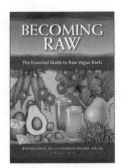

Becoming Raw
Brenda Davis, RD, and
Vesanto Melina, MS, RD,
with Rynn Berry
978-1-57067-238-5 $24.95

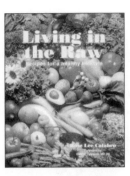

Living in the Raw
Rose Lee Calabro
978-1-57067-176-0 $19.95

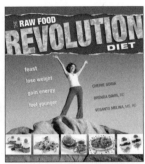

The Raw Revolution Diet
Cherie Soria,
Brenda Davis, RD, and
Vesanto Melina, MS, RD
978-1-57067-185-2 $21.95

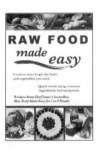

Raw Food Made Easy: DVD
Jennifer Cornbleet
978-1-57067-302-3 $19.95

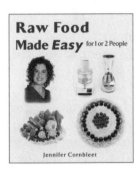

Raw Food Made Easy
Jennifer Cornbleet
978-1-57067-175-3 $17.95

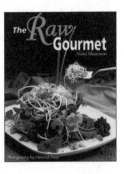

The Raw Gourmet
Nomi Shannon
978-0-92047-048-0 $24.95

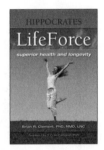

Hippocrates LifeForce
Brian R. Clement, Ph.D,
NMD, LNC
978-1-57067-249-1 $14.95

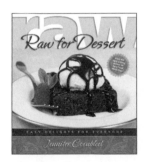

Raw for Dessert
Jennifer Cornbleet
978-1-57067-236-1 $14.95

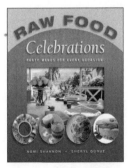

Raw Food Celebrations
Nomi Shannon and
Sheryl Duruz
978-1-57067-228-6 $19.95

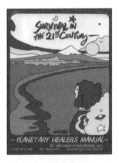

Survival in the 21st Century
Victoras H. Kulvinskas, MS
978-1-57067-247-7 $29.95

Purchase these health titles and cookbooks from your local bookstore or
natural food store, or you can buy them directly from:

Book Publishing Company • P.O. Box 99 • Summertown, TN 38483
1-800-695-2241

Please include $3.95 per book for shipping and handling.

I am truly impressed with *Hooked on Raw* by the raw-foods rising star, Rhio. Here we have a well-researched and documented work that is fun, informative and yummy. Although our points of view may differ on some issues, I applaud Rhio's talent, imagination and dedication to the raw-foods movement. Bravo!!

> **Mark Solomon, Ph.D., Pres.,**
> **Vibrant Health**
> **Centers Worldwide**

Rhio is a shining example of what each and every one of us are capable of. Enjoy this writing and become well.

> **Brian Clement,**
> **Hippocrates Health Institute**

I can enthusiastically recommend *Hooked on Raw* to my patients and students as a further step towards getting in touch with nature, and towards experiencing vibrant good health and well-being. I have been in long-time agreement with, and have used many of the concepts that Rhio advocates; e.g. vegetarianism, the teachings of Natural Hygiene, and the idea that all diseases stem from autointoxication. I also embrace the book's anti-aging philosophy. The few areas where I don't totally concur hardly matter; since reading Rhio's book, in fact, I'm even reconsidering some of those. Her Source Index is invaluable too, and I can't wait to try some of the mouth-watering recipes. This book is an impressive labor of love!

> **Phyllis-Terri Gold, Ph.D., NCC.**
> **Board Certified Clinical Mental Health**
> **Counselor and Psychologist.**
> **Founder/Director of**
> **Mindworks Center for The Self**